Social Indicators Research Series

Volume 86

This series provides a public forum for authored and edited volumes on social indicators research. It is a companion series to the journal Social Indicators Research. The book series deals with problems associated with the quality of life from a broad perspective. It welcomes research on a wide range of substantive areas, including health, crime, housing, education, family life, leisure activities, transportation, mobility, economics, work, religion and environmental issues. The topics represented in this series cover and involve a variety of segmentations, such as social groups, spatial and temporal coordinates, population composition, and life domains. The series presents empirical, philosophical and methodological studies that cover the entire spectrum of society and are devoted to giving evidence through indicators. It considers indicators in their different typologies, and gives special attention to indicators that are able to meet the need of understanding social realities and phenomena that are increasingly more complex, interrelated, interacted and dynamic. In addition, it presents studies aimed at defining new approaches in constructing indicators. An international review board for this series ensures the high quality of the series as a whole.

Available at 25% discount for International Society for Quality-of-Life Studies (ISQOLS). For membership details please contact: ISQOLS; e-mail: office@isqols.org Editors: Ed Diener, University of Illinois, Champaign, USA; Wolfgang Glatzer, J.W. Goethe University, Frankfurt am Main, Germany; Torbjorn Moum, University of Oslo, Norway; Ruut Veenhoven, Erasmus University, Rotterdam, The Netherlands.

R. Allan Freeze

The Metrics of Happiness

The Art and Science of Measuring Personal Happiness and Societal Wellbeing

Springer

R. Allan Freeze
Surrey, BC, Canada

ISSN 1387-6570 ISSN 2215-0099 (electronic)
Social Indicators Research Series
ISBN 978-3-031-10912-6 ISBN 978-3-031-10913-3 (eBook)
https://doi.org/10.1007/978-3-031-10913-3

This Springer imprint is published by the registered company Springer Nature Switzerland AG
The registered company address is: Gewerbestrasse 11, 6330 Cham, Switzerland

Acknowledgements

I would like to thank my friend and colleague Tony Hodge for his long-standing support for this project, his review of some of the material, and our many stimulating discussions.

I was also lucky to be put in contact with Alex Michalos at a critical stage in the development of this book. His review of the entire manuscript was invaluable. I especially appreciate the help and support he was willing to offer to someone from outside the community of recognized happiness experts.

I want to thank Shinjini Chatterjee and Daniel Jagadisan at Springer Nature for shepherding me through the publication process.

I have probably bored my wife, family, and friends to death with my plethora of tales and anecdotes from the world of happiness research, and I want to thank them for their tolerance for what must have seemed at times my obsessive interest in this somewhat esoteric field.

Contents

List of Tables

Part I
The Multi-faceted World of Happiness and Wellbeing

Chapter 1
An Introduction to the Concepts and Ideas

Measuring the Unmeasurable

Sometime, not too long ago, you have almost surely picked up your local newspaper and encountered a headline about happiness or wellbeing. Not *the* headline on page one, but a smaller item on a later page, perhaps in the op-ed section. The headline, and the article beneath it, may have told you that Denmark, or New Zealand, or some other country you don't live in, has just been determined to be the very best country in the world. Or, if you live in the United States or Canada, that they rank in the top ten, but not at the very top. You may have learned where your city ranks on a list of the "most livable cities" in the world. Or that the "gross national happiness" of the world has gone up or down. Or that your quality-of-life has been assessed and found wanting. Or that the United Nations has just issued its latest World Happiness Report, and that it did so on March 20, which has now been proclaimed as the International Day of Happiness.

Haven't you ever wondered how they come up with these lists? How do they go about defining, and measuring, and comparing happiness, or wellbeing, or livability, or quality-of-life?

And who are "they" actually?

And what about those happiness questionnaires that pop up from time to time in your weekend supplement, or on that web page when you're checking out the latest news of the Kardashians? "Taking all things together," asks some anonymous questioner, "how would you say things are going these days?" You are given five choices and asked to choose one. Are you: Very Happy? Happy? Neither Happy nor Unhappy? Unhappy? Or Very Unhappy?

What did you answer?

Happy?

Most people do.

So if you chose "Happy," what exactly did you take into account? You probably thought about your financial situation. Maybe, your level of marital contentment?

R. A. Freeze, *The Metrics of Happiness*, Social Indicators Research Series 86,
https://doi.org/10.1007/978-3-031-10913-3_1

How about your kids? Do they make you more happy or less happy? What about the current success (or lack thereof) of your favorite college football team? Or the state of live theater in your town? Or whether there is a good supply of butterscotch ripple ice cream in your fridge?

If you checked the "Happy" box on that questionnaire, and not the "Very Happy" box, what would it take to move you up a notch from "Happy" to "Very happy?"

There are tangles here. Surely there is more than one kind of happiness. Surely there are a host of things that contribute to our happiness, some that come from within our own hearts, and some that reflect the external influences of the world around us. And how does our rating of our own personal happiness feed into assessments of the communal wellbeing of our towns and cities? Who decides what is important and what isn't? How in the world might we go about trying to measure all this?

This book is an attempt to address these types of questions; a joint quest if you will, between author and reader to uncover what is important in the tangled history and current resurgence of the happiness movement. It is, at root, a book about measurement. It is about the now-decades-long striving, sometimes quixotic, sometimes more-or-less successful, to pin numbers onto the illusive chimera of personal human happiness and communal wellbeing.

In the eyes of some, it is about trying to measure the unmeasurable.

What About the Dow-Jones and the GDP?

Of course, in the eyes of many, the wellbeing of every nation is already being measured. One can pick up any newspaper in the country and find the latest values of the Dow-Jones Industrial Average, and with lesser regularity, but easily discovered nevertheless, the current estimate of this year's Gross Domestic Product. Some see these economic indicators as a suitable proxy for happiness and wellbeing. But as we shall see, many others do not.

One of the strongest demurrals came from Robert F. Kennedy in a speech at the University of Kansas in 1968 [1]. His take on the Gross Domestic Product: "It does not allow for the health of our children, the quality of their education, or the joy of their play. It does not include the beauty of our poetry or the strength of our marriages, the intelligence of our public debates or the integrity of our public officials. It measures neither our wit nor our courage, neither our wisdom nor our learning, neither our compassion nor our devotion to our country. It measures everything in short, except that which makes life worthwhile."

In recent years, there has been an ever-growing philosophy of social governance which holds that public policy ought to lead to an improvement in the levels of happiness, wellbeing, and life satisfaction of the citizenry, and that the accomplishment of such policy prescriptions requires consideration of a much wider suite of concerns than just the wealth and economic prosperity of the favored few. As the economist Andrew Clark puts it: "Surely the ultimate aim of human endeavour must be to produce flourishing communities of people who are profoundly satisfied with their lives. It cannot be simply the creation of wealth." [2].

More to the point, this philosophy requires some way to *quantify* the success or failure of public policy, not just in terms of Gross Domestic Product or the Dow Jones Average, but in terms of the happiness that is engendered in individual citizens, and the wellbeing that is engendered in the population as a whole.

The Four Fountainheads

This philosophy has given rise to a whole new enterprise in the halls of academe (and in the self-help aisles of your local Barnes and Noble), one that emphasizes the development and assessment of happiness and wellbeing. It has grown helter-skelter across a wide spectrum of disciplines, both hard science and soft, but it owes its genesis to four paradigm-shifting transformations that have taken place in the way that scholars probe the human condition, all of which have pushed society closer to a more universal and meaningful perception of human happiness and wellbeing.

First of all, in psychology, the leaders of the *positive psychology movement* have changed the way we look at mental health, away from an obsessive interest in the identification and treatment of abnormal behavior, and toward a more preventive approach that emphasizes the development and nurturing of positive life skills that lead to personal fulfillment.

Secondly, we can turn to the domain of economics, where the *social indicators movement* has fostered a move away from sole dependence on economic indicators like the Dow-Jones and the GDP to measure our state of wellbeing, and toward a more inclusive assessment of the quality of life, one that includes consideration of social, spiritual, and health-based considerations, as well as giving value to the safety and security that is enabled by good governance.

Thirdly, in the latest incarnation of the environmental awakening that swept over the world in the second half of the twentieth century, the *sustainability movement* has made us all realize the negative impacts that decrease our happiness and wellbeing due to environmental contamination, resource depletion, and climate change, and the positive impacts that arise from a healthy and sustainable ecosystem.

And lastly, in the so-called hard sciences, there has been a move toward *happiness studies in the biological and medical sciences*, particularly in the areas of endocrinology, the neurosciences, and genetics. Studies in these areas have clarified the role of hormones, the promise of brain imaging technology, and the explanatory power of genetic coding, all of which. Have important implications for the understanding and measurement of human happiness and wellbeing.

In the next four chapters that make up Part I of this book, each of these movements will be taken in turn, examining their historical development, identifying the leaders of the new paradigms in each of the separate disciplines, and assessing the role that each sub-discipline has to play in the evolving multidisciplinary world of happiness and wellbeing research.

Detailed descriptions of the actual measurement tools will be saved until Part II, and the implications for social action and governance until Part III.

In the remainder of this introductory chapter, the goal will be to set the table, defining and differentiating between happiness and wellbeing, introducing the basic building blocks of indicators and indexes, drawing the distinctions between subjective and objective measures, and identifying a hierarchy of possible scales of study. In all these cases, the treatment in this chapter will be introductory. There will be much more to say about all these issues in later chapters.

The Human Desire for Quantification

Human beings have been measuring things since time immemorial. Our earliest ancestors must have utilized some rough prototypical ideas of measurement in order to carry out the tasks in their daily lives: in the barter of goods, the construction of dwellings, or the scheduling and planning of migratory travels. As civilization progressed, the needs of trade and commerce required the development of common units of measurement, defined by science, enshrined in trade agreements, and eventually legitimized in the laws of individual countries and in the treaties between them.

The first consistent *system* of measure probably dates to the third century BC in Mesopotamia and Egypt [3]. It is known for sure that a unit of length was developed by that time. The *cubit* was defined as the length of one's forearm from one's elbow to the tip of one's middle finger, and despite the obvious vagaries of such a definition, this unit was widely used in the design and construction of the pyramids. Weights and volumes are also mentioned in the Bible, in the context of providing fair measure. The Magna Carta of 1215 specifies that the quart shall be the official measure used in the sale of wine throughout the British realm.

If temperature is taken as a representative proxy, we learn that Galileo Galilei invented the first device for measuring it in 1592, and that Anders Celsius was the first to suggest a scale of 0 to 100 degrees between the freezing point and the boiling point of water (although his scale was inverted, with 0 for boiling and 100 for freezing, and it was left to later scientists to reverse the scale to the one we use today). The point is that in the hard sciences, in medicine, and in engineering, there are myriad well-defined properties and parameters that are measured routinely with ever-more-accurate measurement instruments, using widely-accepted units of measurement. Physicists measure the mass, volume and density of solids. Chemists measure the concentrations and solubility of chemicals in water. Engineers measure the stresses and strains in engineering structures. Meteorologists measure the temperature and pressure of the atmosphere. And so on.

The question is: Can one conceive of a comparable system of measures, with well-defined units of measurement, and reliable instruments of measurement, that can be applied in the social sciences? Specifically, can one hope to quantify personal happiness and/or communal wellbeing in a meaningful way?

There is no doubt that this has been the hope of social scientists for a long time. As early as 1881, the economist Francis Edgeworth dreamed of the future development of a *hedonimeter* that would measure human happiness directly [4]. In 1940, the sociologist Hornell Hart promoted his *euphorimeter*, which was not actually a direct measure, but one based on interviews and questionnaires [5]. A similar approach has led to the *eurobarometer*, which is currently used to track wellbeing in the European Union.

Certainly, in economics, which can be viewed as the hardest of all the soft sciences, there is much quantification of measurable entities, from stock market prices, to worker wages, to government deficits (all of which are measured in units of currency such as the dollar). There are many other parameters like interest rates, unemployment rates, and rates of inflation, which are not measured in units of currency, but which have numerical values that are open to mathematical and statistical analysis. The subfield of economics that handles this quantitative analysis is well-enough established to have its own name, *econometrics*, its own journals and societies, and its own specialized college courses [6].

The comparable subfield in psychology is called *psychometrics*, and it, too, is now a highly-developed discipline [7]. It is defined as the objective measure of an individual's skills, knowledge, abilities, attitudes, personality traits, and educational achievements. It includes the quantitative assessment of happiness and wellbeing as part of its mandate.

The question of whether psychological traits such as happiness can be sufficiently quantified to qualify as measurements was answered in the affirmative in 1946 by the Harvard psychologist Stanley Smith Stevens. He argued that "any number that can be assigned to objects or events according to some rule constitutes a measurement." [8] Under this definition, numerical scores that are derived from psychological assessments such as IQ tests, or tests that measure ability in, say, mathematics, or self-reported scores from any type of happiness questionnaire that uses a numerical scale, all qualify as measurements that can be analyzed mathematically and interpreted quantitatively. Such tests and surveys constitute the *measurement instruments* for psychometric evaluation.

Perhaps the most-well-known quantitative approach to psychological assessment is the Minnesota Multiphasic Personality Inventory (MMPI), first developed at the University of Minnesota in 1943, updated most recently in 2008, and still in wide use [9]. It is a standardized psychometric test of adult personality. The questionnaire at the heart of the MMPI requires the test candidate to answer 338 true-or-false statements, which are then assessed with the aid of 10 clinical scales, 4 validity scales, and 32 additional supplementary scales. The final result is a set of numbers, one for each clinical scale, that lie in the range 30 to 120. A set of "codetypes" aids the psychologist in interpreting these numbers. The MMPI is used primarily in the diagnosis of mental illness and the development of treatment plans, but it has also found application in non-medical applications such as in job screening, personnel selection, and as a forensic tool in legal cases.

So, suppose you decide to sign on for one of the many available happiness surveys. Most of them will feature a questionnaire with many questions, maybe even many pages of questions, but some of them use only one question. If there is only one question, it may look something like the one that was introduced earlier: "Taking all things together, how would you say things are going these days? Would you say you are: Very Happy, Happy, Neither Happy nor Unhappy, Unhappy, or Very Unhappy?" Suppose you check the second box. You are Happy. If the test designer has assigned the numerical values 5, 4, 3, 2 and 1 to the five choices, you have just recorded a 4. You have given the tester a numerical estimate of your happiness. You have given him or her a measurement. And if there was a prologue to the questionnaire that required you to identify your age, gender, marital status, level of educational attainment, line of work, and other personal info (kept scrupulously anonymous, of course), he or she will be able to add your numerical score into the database that has been built from the results of others who have filled in the questionnaire, and it will now be possible to carry out statistical analyses on the data to correlate personal happiness with some of the possible contributing factors. Moreover, the database as a whole will provide the tester with much information that is pertinent to the assessment of happiness on a communal scale. And if there are trends to that assessment over time, it may be possible to relate them to possible external causes, including changes in public policy.

In short, we have taken the initial steps towards measuring the unmeasurable. The parameter under investigation is happiness. The units of measurement are derived from the numerical scales used to interpret qualitative expressions of personal emotion. The instruments of measurement are the questionnaires that produce the numbers and the statistical databanks that store the data. Admittedly, these soft-science "measurements" (and the "instruments" that measure them) are not quite the same as in the hard sciences, but they do satisfy Stanley Smith's requirement that they are numerical, and that they can be interpreted "according to some rule." All this is not to say that designing a meaningful questionnaire is easy or trivial; there are issues of bias, and scaling, and representativeness, and more. At this point, it is just the concept of this type of "measurement" that has our attention; a full and thorough discussion of the potential pitfalls is saved for Chap. 6.

It is probably appropriate to end this section with a pause for thought. While measurement is a powerful and essential ingredient in assessing wellbeing, it is certainly not the only way to do it. Despite our emphasis on measurement and our search for quantification, let us not lose sight of the value of more qualitative approaches to the assessment of happiness and wellbeing. There is a long history of *hermeneutic* ideas in the social sciences; the art of understanding and communication through story, contemplation, and allegory; and the recognition of the role of experience and world-view in interpreting human social behavior. We have begun to see how happiness can be expressed as a number, but clearly it is much more than a number.

Happiness and Wellbeing Defined and Differentiated

Thus far, the terms *happiness* and *wellbeing* have been presented as if they were synonyms of one another. However, there must be some uneasiness in every reader's mind that this is not quite so, that the two terms are related, but that they do not mean exactly the same thing. In fact, there are two distinctions that are often drawn to differentiate happiness from wellbeing.

The first distinction relates to their meanings when applied to a single individual. Most psychologists see *happiness* as a short-lived feeling of contentment, a positive emotion to be sure, but one that comes and goes with one's mood. The synonyms for happiness that are listed in the various versions of Roget's Thesaurus appear to support this concept of happiness. They include such words as bliss, delight, elation, glee, and joy, all of which seem to refer to the enjoyment of momentary high spirits. You may be happy as a lark, happy as a clam, or happy as a king. Happiness may make you sing, purr, smile, laugh, walk on air, or be on cloud nine, but presumably not forever.

The *wellbeing* of an individual, on the other hand, is seen as a term of wider scope, based on a more contemplative evaluation of life satisfaction, a cognitive rather than an emotional assessment of one's physical, intellectual, and social state of mind. Roget's synonyms include such words as contentment and good fortune, and recognize wellbeing as somehow related to safety, security and success. The wellbeing of an individual is a state or condition of existence characterized by ongoing good health, happiness, and prosperity. In this view, happiness is "a necessary but not sufficient condition for high levels of wellbeing." [10].

The second distinction uses *happiness* as a term to be ascribed mainly to individuals, while *wellbeing* is reserved mainly for a communal or societal scale. The conceptual equivalents of wellbeing under this distinction include such terms as public welfare, quality of life, and livability, all of which tend to reflect a societal focus. Wellbeing at this scale implies the existence of a civil society. Much of this book reflects this second distinction, referring as it often does to "personal happiness" and "communal wellbeing." However it is not possible to be slavish. The concept of "gross national happiness," for example, highlights happiness, but is clearly meant to be applied at a societal scale. The terms are too closely related, and too widely-used in a variety of senses, in both academic research and popular self-help literature, to try to enforce any clear-cut rules.

Another issue that arises in this regard is that of culture and language. Are the concepts of happiness and wellbeing universal? Is the happiness and wellbeing experienced in rich developed countries similar in kind to that experienced in poorer less-developed countries? Do citizens of individualist societies honor the same characteristics of wellbeing as those in collectivist societies? What about religious traditions? Is the concept of happiness for Buddhists or Muslims more or less the same as it is for Christians? As it turns out, much of the wellbeing literature that is quoted in this book is produced by happiness researchers who are based in the so-called WEIRD countries (Western, Educated, Industrialized, Rich, and

Democratic), especially those nations of northern Europe and North America with a long history of economic success and democratic freedoms. Perhaps not surprisingly, the country rankings that their studies produce tend to favor these same countries. Skeptics see an opportunity for bias. Suffice it to say for now that there are many diverse concepts of happiness and wellbeing in the many cultures and languages of the world, and there will be more to say about their possible impacts on studies of happiness and wellbeing in later chapters.

Hedonic and Eudaimonic Happiness

There are many types of happiness, but most of them can fit into a twofold classification which happiness researchers call *hedonic* and *eudaimonic* [11].

Hedonic happiness focuses on sensual gratification, the attainment of pleasure, and the avoidance of pain. The ideas date to the Greek philosopher Epicurus (341-271 BCE). We are all familiar with the Epicurean mandate to "eat, drink, and be merry," but in fact Epicurus' tracts were more nuanced than that, emphasizing the value of "healthy souls." He recommended a peaceful life, as well as a merry one [12]. Nevertheless, the concept is a selfish one at root, with so much stake laid on personal pleasure. In modern dress, the search for hedonic happiness can lead to an undue focus on material wealth, and the shallow pleasures that accompany the consumer society. It can also lead one onto the so-called "hedonic treadmill," whereby satisfaction never arrives; the more you have, the more you want. Many of the articles in a volume of research papers sponsored by the American Psychological Association found that those who lived their lives governed by materialistic drives tended to exhibit lower self-esteem, greater narcissism, less empathy, and more conflicted relationships [13].

Sigmund Freud's *pleasure principle* is basically a restatement of hedonic theory, but one where the central tenets are instinctual rather than the result of rational thought [14]. He defined the pleasure principle as an innate seeking of pleasure and avoidance of pain in order to satisfy one's biological and psychological needs, wants, and urges. When the needs of the pleasure principle are not met, anxiety and tension arise. In general, Freud seemed more interested in *arresting unhappiness* than in *promoting happiness*, and under his leadership, the field of psychotherapy settled into to a reactive approach to mental health issues, rather than a preventive one that might have focussed more on the pursuit of happiness and wellbeing.

To some degree, Freud was building on the evolutionary theories of Charles Darwin, which also featured an involuntary selection of hedonic biological attributes. Clearly the arrival of pleasure and the delay of pain are attributes that will be favored in species that are most successful in their adaptation to their environment. With the later developments of genetic theory now in hand, there is a better understanding of how our "selfish genes" play a role in this game of survival of the happiest [15].

The hedonic tradition is also usually credited as the forerunner of utilitarianism, the philosophical movement founded by Jeremy Bentham in the late 1700's, which holds that individuals will generally make decisions that are in their own rational self-interest [16]. They do so by maximizing their *utility*, where utility is defined as the aggregate pleasure derived by the decision-maker from any action. Utilitarian economists tend to believe that almost every decision made by a rational human being can be translated into the form of a "purchase," whether of goods or services, and that economic measures therefore provide a suitable proxy for happiness and wellbeing. To an economist of this stripe, "*having* is everything. There is no room in this world view for *being or doing*." [17].

Bentham argued that utilitarian decision-making would lead to "the greatest good for the greatest number." As originally presented, utilitarianism paid little attention to the impact of one's decisions on others, or to the so-called *externalities* in the form of aesthetic or environmental outcomes for which it is difficult to assign a specific value of utility. John Stuart Mill tried to raise utilitarian ideas onto a higher plane by giving greater value to pleasures of the intellect than to those of mere sensation, but the emphasis on self remains. Adam Smith, who is generally acknowledged as the founder of modern economics, used rational self-interest as the basis for his formulations of a free market economy.

The tenets of utilitarianism are carried to ultimate economic fruition in the ideas of Bayesian decision-making, where every outcome of every decision has a utility, usually measured in units of currency such as dollars. The Bayes approach does take explicit consideration of the externalities, but it does so by employing *utility functions* that use subjective weighting schemes to convert non-monetary outcomes into dollars (even up to and including the value of life, which may arise in the making of life-and-death decisions, such as those that occur in military strategy, or in risk-laden technical decisions like the development of nuclear power). In this line of thinking, everything has its price, and a straightforward summing of the resulting utilities leads to the preferred decision from a suite of possible alternatives. It is implicit in all these economic systems with hedonic or utilitarian roots that the maximization of utility also maximizes personal happiness.

The concept of *eudaimonic happiness* introduces a moral dimension into the discussion. The term *eudaimonia* is a Greek word that can be parsed into its two parts: *eu*, meaning "good," and *daemon*, meaning "spirit." Aristotle (384–322 BCE), who may have coined the word, viewed eudaimonia as a "virtuous life, well-lived." He wrote of "flourishing," and emphasized the pursuit of excellence, and kindness to others. He was the first of the Greek philosophers to see happiness, not just as the result of fate or good luck, but as an attainable pursuit over which we have some control. In his view, failure to attain happiness is at least partially our own fault [18].

In its modern usage, psychologists see the eudaimonic approach to life as one that breeds happiness from a wider and less-selfish suite of activities than just those that deliver the narrow pleasures of hedonism. Eudaimonic happiness arises from having a purpose in life, from maximizing personal growth, and from using ones strengths in helping and developing positive relations with others. It values the feelings of belongingness, and the pleasures brought by making contributions to society. It is a philosophy of self-realization and self-acceptance, but one where these traits grow at least in part from contributing to the greater good. Joar Vitterso, the editor of the *Handbook of Eudaimonic Well-Being* argues that eudaimonic happiness is "the most important idea in the world" and defines it as "the good composed of all goods." [19].

The appropriateness of the two-fold classification of happiness into hedonic and eudaimonic spheres has been widely discussed and debated in the happiness literature. Aristotle apparently favored a threefold breakdown featuring "goods of the mind" (like moral virtue and wisdom), "goods of the body" (like health, beauty, and strength), and "external goods" (like wealth, friends, and good government) [20]. Another paper identified 12 distinct conceptions of happiness held by the ancients [21]. Vitterso presents a table of 41 different descriptions of happiness from the literature. Most of the alternative classifications fall in the two-fold to four-fold range. They are often based on a differentiation of various "states of mind."

At the other end of the spectrum, perhaps even the two-fold subdivision is one too many. In most of these alternative conceptualizations, pleasure is seen at best as a "handmaiden" of eudaimonia but never the central component. Hedonic happiness implies good feelings, and the satisfaction of basic psychological needs, while eudaimonic happiness implies something more. In this context, eudaimonic happiness is the more encompassing term and hedonic happiness is just a subset of it.

In this book, despite these somewhat esoteric controversies, the basic two-fold classification is retained, and the techniques that are presented for the measurement of happiness and well being will reflect both hedonic and eudaimonic contributing factors. However, it will be accepted that the eudaimonic term is the more encompassing, and for this reason it has been highlighted in the title of Part II. The term *eudaimetrics* is coined there, in parallel to such terms as *econometrics* and *psychometrics,* as the art and science of measuring happiness and wellbeing.

A Little History

The Greek philosophers were not the first to think about happiness. It is likely that ancient peoples had some recognition of their own moods; certainly they would have been familiar with both pleasure and pain. However, they probably ascribed the comings and goings of the good times to fate and luck and the fickle will of their Gods. It is unlikely that they saw their own personal happiness as something over which they had any control.

The first real attempts at self-analysis may have come from the Buddha in the fifth Century BC [22]. Buddhist doctrine charts an eightfold path to inner peace that recommends meditation as a route to mental equanimity and a deeper form of happiness. Some twenty-one centuries later, these ideas still have resonance. Tenzin Gyatso, the 14th Dalai Lama, spends his life traveling the world spreading his Buddhist-based message of "educating the heart" and practising the "art of happiness." [23].

Buddhism is not the only religion to address the question of wellbeing. Almost all religions recognize the need to engender happiness in the minds of their followers, if only to keep their flocks faithful to the teachings of their prophets. However, most of them try to do so by promising peace and harmony if, and only if, their adherents observe the tenets of their church's particular dogma. Early Christian thought held that true happiness could only be found in a knowledge of God. The Roman Catholic scholar, Thomas Aquinas, in the thirteenth Century, concluded that perfect happiness, in the form of pure and everlasting bliss, was possible only in the afterlife. In his view, in this life we are limited to an imperfect happiness which he called *felicitas* [24].

Most historians trace the beginnings of happiness as we know it, as an attainable goal in the earthly realm, to the arrival of the Renaissance in 15th and sixteenth Century Europe [25]. The blossoming of art and literature during this period brought with it a more humanist and secular view of man's place in the firmament, with less emphasis on the afterlife. The Protestant Reformation, at least in its dour Calvinist trappings, may have been a bit of a setback, but during the Enlightenment of the eighteenth Century, with its emphasis on reason, tolerance, and liberty, it once again became legitimate to seek personal happiness. And of course it was around this same time that the pursuit of happiness became enshrined as a basic right in the newly-minted Constitution of the United States.

The Kingdom of Bhutan

No history of happiness can ignore the landlocked Asian country of Bhutan. It was in this Himalayan mountain kingdom, in 1972, that the then-king, Jigme Singye Wangchuk, declared that his government's policies would no longer be based on Gross National Product, but rather on a more inclusive measure of Gross National Happiness. According to the king, the four pillars of GNH are the promotion of equitable and sustainable socio-economic development, the preservation and promotion of cultural values, conservation of the natural environment, and the establishment of good governance. In 1999, a Centre for Bhutan Studies and GNH Research was established. It now publishes its own English-language academic journal, and has sponsored four international conferences, the most recent of which took place in 2013. The appearance of a best-selling book on Bhutan in 2004 generated media coverage for the GNH revolution in Time and the New York Times [26].

Sadly, despite all these good intentions, it was not until 2008 that Bhutan began the difficult transition from absolute monarchy to full-fledged democracy, holding its first free elections in that year. More discouraging yet, Bhutan remains one of the poorest countries in the world, and appears on the radar of Amnesty International for serious human rights violations with respect to its Nepalese minority.

Even with the questionable success in its home country, the idea of Gross National Happiness remains strongly on the radar screen of the happiness movement. In 2005, an American economic think tank, the International Institute of Management, with headquarters in Las Vegas, was the first to develop a GNH Index, based on the original concepts from Bhutan. In doing so, they beat the Bhutanese at their own game, who did not come out with their homegrown version until 2010. Both these indices were designed to replace the GDP as a more-inclusive measure of national wellbeing. In their reports both groups make a plea for the consideration of "softer values," including environmental and social "intangibles," in the assessment of national success.

There are literally hundreds of programs and projects around the world that take their lead from the original ideas of GNH. If you type "Gross National Happiness" into your Google browser, it will produce over five million hits. A more complete coverage of the GNH indexes, along with their many competitors, is presented in Chap. 9.

The Hierarchy of Scales of Study

In earlier sections of this chapter, a clear differentiation has been presented between personal happiness and communal wellbeing. However, it is certainly more complicated than that. At the communal level, there are many possible scales of study, and it is possible to arrange them in a hierarchal order, with each level in the hierarchy representing an ever-larger pool of subjects available for measurement and statistical study. From the *individual*, one can move to the *family* as the unit of study, and from the family to *groups*, like service clubs or sports teams. The next level of study would be in the *workplace,* or in educational institutions, or in the military. At the further end of the societal spectrum are *communities*, *cities*, *states*, and *nations*, and ultimately, the *world* as a whole.

Studies of happiness and wellbeing have been carried out at all these scales. Some of the measurement techniques and methods of statistical or mathematical analysis are common to all the scales, but many are not. By the same token, some of the factors that contribute to happiness and wellbeing are also common to all the scales, while others are not. In the simplest light, when studies are carried out at the level of individual happiness, the contributing factors are often more hedonic and self-centered. When studies are directed to wellbeing on a communal scale, they are likely to be more eudaimonic, more centered on the common good.

In Part II of this book, the various available measurement tools are organized in terms of this hierarchy of scale. There are separate chapters on personal happiness, satisfaction in the workplace, the livability of cities, and the wellbeing of nations.

Perhaps the thing that most separates these scales one from another is the fact that each of them has roots in a different academic discipline, and the histories of the development of ideas and methodologies for each of them reflect the traditions of the root disciplines. At the individual level, the assessment of happiness lies in the domain of psychology, and most Departments of Psychology at academic institutions now host programs in happiness studies. Questions of workplace satisfaction and how best to achieve it have historically been addressed in Faculties of Commerce, and in programs in Business Administration or Industrial Relations. The enhancement of the quality of life in schools and colleges, for both students and instructors, has been the concern of Faculties of Education. The livability of cities has been the domain of programs in Urban and Community Planning, some of which are housed in Schools of Architecture. The move toward more all-inclusive assessments of the quality of life at the scale of states and nations has taken place primarily in Departments of Economics and/or Political Science, almost all of which now host programs in the new economics of wellbeing.

Clearly, there are huge differences in the histories and traditions of psychology, commerce, education, architecture, and economics. The paradigm shift that has seen more psychologists embrace the positive psychology movement has taken place in a milieu that was created by the history of development of the field, by the influences of Freud and Jung, and the relatively late emergence of quantitative rather than qualitative methodologies. Programs in commerce and business administration, at least the ones in Europe and North America, have almost all developed within a capitalist, free-market framework and its utilitarian traditions. Most early studies were generally carried out from the employer's perspective rather than the employee's. The history of education reflects its roots in religious doctrine and an early emphasis on discipline and rote learning. Concern with student happiness has arisen only as a by-product of the various theories of teaching and learning, such as those of Jean Piaget and Maria Montessori, which lean on a background in childhood developmental psychology. Urban planning dates back to the efforts of Baron Georges-Eugene Haussmann and the architect Le Corbusier in nineteenth-century Europe, whose city plans were designed to create showpieces of national pride. Current academic programs in urban studies lie at the intersection of architecture and engineering, and deal primarily with the functional questions of infrastructure, and the efficiency of civic governance. The economics and politics of wellbeing have arisen as a kind of antidote to the prevailing utilitarian doctrines in these various fields, influenced in part by the liberal sentiments of John Maynard Keynes and Thorsten Veblen.

Human Wellbeing and Ecosystem Wellbeing

In general, the emphasis in this book is on the happiness and wellbeing of humans, but the need for a harmonious relationship between human wellbeing and ecosystem wellbeing is recognized and supported. In fact, the importance of environmental sustainability is sufficiently highly regarded that it is acknowledged as one of the fountainheads of the human happiness movement (Chap. 4). More significantly, environmental health is seen as a direct contributor to human wellbeing, and environmental degradation as a serious negative influence. Concern over such issues as climate change, water contamination, air quality degradation, resource depletion, and loss of species diversity, weigh heavily on both personal happiness (as described more fully in Chap. 6) and on communal wellbeing (as elaborated in Chaps. 8–10).

Subjective and Objective Measures

There is another distinction that needs to be made sooner rather than later. Happiness researchers distinguish between subjective and objective measures. *Subjective measures* are based on privately observable phenomena as seen from the perspective of a particular person. *Objective measures* are based on publicly observable phenomena as seen from the perspective of any independent, unbiased, and well-informed person [27]. Subjective measures depend on the judgement of the observer, while objective measures depend on external evidence that is independent of the observer. In communal happiness studies, subjective data come from personal assessments of the hopes, fears, desires, and levels of life satisfaction of a cohort of citizens. They are usually gleaned from answers to questions posed on happiness questionnaires. Objective data are based on measures of external factors that directly impact quality of life such as housing availability, secondary school graduation rates, or income distributions. They are generally taken from publically-available databases like census results, health outcomes, crime statistics, or government economic information.

In general, subjective measures are more widely used in assessments of individual happiness, while objective measures tend to find greater application in assessments of communal wellbeing. Once again, however, the separation is not clear-cut. The results of individual subjective happiness surveys, when viewed as a communal database, certainly have a place in studies of societal wellbeing. Conversely, an objective measure, say the distance of a respondent's home to the nearest park, may have a role to play in assessing a particular respondent's personal happiness.

There is also the question of whether one wants to take a single snapshot in time, or track trends over time. Both subjective and objective measures, either separately or together, may be used, on the one hand, to compare levels of happiness and wellbeing in different groups or jurisdictions at a particular moment in time, or alternatively, to track the levels of happiness and wellbeing in a single group or jurisdiction through time. The first approach is used in the annual country-by-country rankings one regularly sees reported in newspapers and TV clips. The second approach produces the time trends that are the stuff of every federal election, with one side telling us how much better off we are than we were a decade ago, and the other telling us that we are all going to hell in a hand-basket.

In their book *Soft Systems Methodology in Action* Checkland and Scholes note that "while subjectivity is never a problem for those whose inclinations are towards arts and humanities, it can be difficult for numerate scientists and engineers whose training has not always prepared them well for the drama, tragedy and farce of the social process." [28] In a book such as this one that searches for "numerate" findings, care must be taken not to ignore the "drama, tragedy and farce of the social process."

Indicators and Indexes

There are going to be many references in this book to indicators and indexes of happiness and wellbeing. The reader will encounter economic indicators, social indicators, and environmental indicators. You will be introduced to the Social Progress Index, the Crime Severity Index, the Environmental Performance Index, the Global Peace Index, and many others. It is appropriate that one understand what is implied by each of these two terms at the outset.

An *indicator* is a numerical or statistical measure of a single variable that changes its value over time, and that is thought to reveal some underlying aspect of social reality, in our case, the happiness and wellbeing of individuals and/or communities. An indicator must be easily identified and clearly defined. There must be an unimpeachable, non-partisan, non-ideological source of data for the indicator, usually in the form of publicly-available databases hosted by national governments or international agencies. Among the thousands of indicators of wellbeing that might be gleaned from such sources could be such diverse items as life expectancy at birth, seasonally-adjusted unemployment rates, urban air quality, levels of internet connectivity, or high school math literacy.

An *index* is a higher-level concept that usually involves the integration of several indicators into a single measure of greater breadth than that represented by the individual indicators. As a simple example, consider the two-indicator index known as the *Misery Index*, which is a kind of index of unhappiness. It is defined as the seasonally-adjusted unemployment rate plus the annual inflation rate (both in percent). It claims to reflect how an average citizen is doing economically. From the perspective of communal wellbeing, low is good, high is bad. Despite its ironic name, it is actually a respected measure of financial health (or lack thereof) developed by Arthur Okun, a Yale economist who was a member of the Council of Economic Advisors to both the Kennedy and Johnson administrations [29]. The values of the two component indicators, the unemployment rate and the inflation rate, are both easily found in widely-available databases at any point in time for any or all of the countries in the world. In 2013, a comparison of the Misery Index for 89 countries in the word showed values running from 5.4 to 79.4, with Japan at the top and Venezuela at the bottom. In the USA the MI value in January 2017 was 6.8.

Almost all the indexes that come into play in the world of wellbeing integrate a much larger suite of indicators than the two included in the Misery Index. The State of Caring Index, for example, put out by the United Way of America, uses 36 indicators. The Worldwide Press Freedom Index uses seven criteria, with several indicators defined for each of them. The Global Opportunity Index tracks five major areas, using 54 distinct indicators. In all these cases, the ability to come up with a single numerical score for the index itself involves some kind of subjective weighting of the various basic indicators. The indicators used in the State of Caring Index, for example, include measures that reflect charitable donations, volunteer activities, and engagement in civic activities. The designers of the index have to decide how to integrate and weight these various contributions to civic health, differing as they do in function and impact, and, more importantly, in the units of measurement that might be used to chart them, say dollars for the first indicator, hours donated to the cause for the second, and some kind of subjective scoring for the third [30].

All of the indexes noted thus far are *single-dimensional*, that is, they reflect conditions in just one aspect of happiness and wellbeing. The Misery Index is an economic index. It says nothing about the social or environmental components of human happiness. The State of Caring Index charts volunteerism, and only volunteerism. The Press Freedom Index is similarly unidimensional. Economics, volunteerism, and press freedom are often identified as each having a role to play in communal wellbeing, but taken alone they are certainly not the whole story.

There has always been a yearning for a single score that might be developed for any given jurisdiction, be it a workplace, a city, or a country, that tells the whole story, a numerical value that can be used to rank these jurisdictions one against another, or to track conditions in a single jurisdiction over time. For this, the eudaimetric world has turned to *multi-dimensional* indexes. These are composite indexes, or "indexes of the indexes" if you will, that integrate not just many indicators but many unidimensional indexes as well. In principle, one could imagine a composite index that includes the Misery Index, the State of Caring Index, and the Press Freedom Index, all as subcomponents of an overall Happiness and Wellbeing Index. In fact, many such attempts are already on the books. In Chap. 7, the various dimensions that have been proposed to describe the multi-dimensional world of happiness are laid out, and Chap. 9 catalogs many of the most successful ventures, including the Human Development Index, the Quality of Life Index, the Happy Planet Index, and many more.

Self-Help, Inc.

There are two distinct wings to the happiness movement, one based in the hallowed halls of academia, and the other scrambling for the big bucks in the down-and-dirty competitive world of self-help. The paradigm-shifting breakthroughs in human psychology, economic theory, sustainability, and medical science are all first reported by academically-based happiness researchers in the specialized journals of their diverse disciplines. However, the man-on-the-street does not monitor the *Journal of Positive Psychology* or the *International Journal of Wellbeing*, and if he did, he would probably drown in the sea of jargon and lack of background knowledge. The message needs to be taken to the masses.

And so it has. Modern times have seen the birth and growth of the happiness doctrine as a money-making industry that has featured an explosion of self-help in the form of books, videos and seminars. Cyberspace is awash in motivational speakers, personal coaches, and new-age philosophers. Take a stroll down the self-help aisle at your nearest Barnes and Noble. Peruse the latest New York Times bestseller list. Or just punch in "happiness" on your smartphone and take a spin through the lead offerings at Amazon.com. What you see there will leave you in little doubt as to the universal longing for happiness, and the omnipresence of authors who promise to deliver it. Titles that offer joy, bliss, contentment, and success fill the bookshelves and Kindles of the nation.

It is not a completely new thing. One of the earliest happiness-centered self-help books was penned in 1930 by the celebrated philosopher, Bertrand Russell, who provided a rationalist prescription for living a happy life [31]. He was followed by such noteworthy purveyors of optimism as Dale Carnegie, who taught us how to make friends and influence people, and Norman Vincent Peale, who emphasized the power of positive thinking.

However, the sheer volume of output is a new thing. Many of the authors of these do-it-yourself, feel-good books that now crowd the non-fiction best-seller lists are the very same academic researchers whose research findings have fueled the happiness movement. It takes experimental studies and learned articles in the best academic journals to get tenure, but it is the popular press that leads to fame and fortune. Table 1.1 introduces us to a suite of academic authors who have parlayed their special knowledge about happiness into best-selling self-help books designed for the man on the street.

Right away, we are introduced to the names of Martin Seligman, Ed Diener, and Mihaly Czikszentmihalyi, all of whom will figure prominently in Chap. 2. So too will the academic contributions of Sonja Lyubomirsky, David Myers, and Emma Seppala. With respect to David Myers, it is worth noting that his book "The Pursuit of Happiness" is by far the oldest on Table 1.1, dating back to 1993. It bears the honor of being the first trade paperback to bring the new science of positive psychology to the masses.

Four of the other listed authors have connections with Harvard University. Shawn Achor was a lecturer there before leaving academia to form the business motivational firm, GoodThink, Inc. Tal Ben-Shahar is noted for teaching the most popular course ever offered at Harvard, a positive psychology class that annually attracts over 1000 students. Daniel Gilbert is the most renowned of the foursome. His book "Stumbling on Happiness" has been translated into 30 languages, and was honored as the best popular science book of 2007. It promises "all that science has to tell us about the uniquely human ability to envision the future, and how likely we are to enjoy it when we get there," Gilbert's ideas have also been highlighted in the PBS series, "This Emotional Life."

Several of the academic authors on Table 1.1 come from fields other than psychology. Richard Layard, who sits as Baron Layard in the British House of Lords, is a labor economist and the Program Director of the Centre for Economic Performance at the London School of Economics. Richard Thaler is a behavioral economist at the University of Chicago's Booth School of Business. Cass Sunstein is a professor at Harvard Law, and also served as the Head of the Office of Information and Regulatory Affairs in the Obama administration. He is an amazingly-prolific author, having written over 20 books that run the gamut from "The Politics of Libertarian Paternalism" to "The World According to Star Wars." In addition to

Table 1.1 Academic authors of popular self-help happiness books

Author	Academic affiliation	Published self-help happiness books
Martin Seligman	University of Pennsylvania	• *Authentic Happiness: Using the New Positive Psychology to Realize Your Potential for Lasting Fulfillment*, Free Press, 2002. • *Flourish: A Visionary New Understanding of Happiness and Well-Being*, Free Press, 2011.
Ed Diener and Robert Biswas-Diener	University of Illinois, Portland State Univ.	• *Happiness: Unlocking the Mysteries of Psychological Wealth*, Wiley-Interscience, 2008
Mihaly Czikszentmihalyi	Claremont Graduate University	• Czikszentmihalyi, Mihaly, *Finding Flow: The Psychology of Engagement with Everyday Life*, Basic Books, 1998.
Daniel Gilbert	Harvard University	• *Stumbling on Happiness*, Vintage, 2007.
Sonja Lyubomirsky	University of California, Riverside	• *The How of Happiness: A New Approach to Getting the Life You Want*, Penguin, 2008. • *The Myths of Happiness: What Should Make You Happy But Doesn't, What Shouldn't Make You Happy But Does*, Penguin, 2014.
Richard Layard	London School of Economics	• *Happiness Lessons from a New Science*, Penguin, 2005.
Richard Thaler and Cass Sunstein	University of Chicago, Harvard University	• *Nudge: Improving Decisions about Health, Wealth and Happiness*, Yale University Press, 2008.
David Myers	Hope College	• *The Pursuit of Happiness: Discovering the Pathway to Fulfillment, Well-Being, and Enduring Personal Joy*, William Morrow, 1993.
Tal Ben-Shahar	Harvard University	• *Happier: Learn the Secrets to Daily Joy and Lasting Fulfillment*, McGraw Hill, 2007. • *Being Happy: You Don't Have to Be Perfect to Lead a Richer, Happier Life*, McGraw Hill, 2010.
Shawn Achor	Harvard University	• *Before Happiness: The Five Hidden Keys to Achieving Success, Spreading Happiness, and Sustaining Positive Change*, Crown Books, 2013. • *The Happiness Advantage: The Seven Principles of Positive Psychology that Fuel Success and Performance at Work*, Crown Business, 2010.
Emma Seppala	Stanford University	• *The Happiness Track: How to Apply the Science of Happiness to Accelerate Your Success*, HarperOne, 2017.

the book highlighted on Table 1.1 that Sunstein coauthored with Richard Thaler, he is also the author of a 2010 treatise on "Law and Happiness."

While academic authors have been prevalent in the self-help happiness explosion, they are certainly not alone. There are literally thousands of writers, journalists, practicing psychologists, motivational speakers, New Age philosophers, and just plain hockey moms, who have found a niche in the movement. Sometimes it has been in the form of published books, sometimes under the klieg lights out on the

Table 1.2 A selection of happiness gurus

Deepak Chopra	• Author of *The Ultimate Happiness Prescription: Seven Keys to Joy and Enlightenment*, Harmony Books, 2009. • Founder of the Chopra Center for Well-Being, Carlsbad, CA.	[www.deepakchopra.com]
Gretchen Rubin	• Author of *The Happiness Project*, Harper Collins, 2012. • Host of weekly podcast "Happier with Gretchen Rubin."	[www.gretchenrubin.com]
Neil Pasricha	• Author of *The Book of Awesome*, Penguin, 2010. • Author of *The Happiness Equation: Want Nothing, Do Anything, Have Everything*, Putnams, 2016. • Founder of the Institute for Global Happiness.	[www.1000awesomethings.com] [www.globalhappiness.org]
Debbie Gisonni	• Author of *The Goddess of Happiness: A Down-to-Earth Guide for Heavenly Balance and Bliss*, New World Library, 2010. • CEO, Stillheart Institute	[www.goddessofhappiness.com]
Dan Baker	• Author of *What Happy People Know*, St. Martins Griffin, 2004. • Director of the Life Enhancement Program, Canyon Ranch, Tucson, AZ.	[www.canyonranch.com]
Chade Meng Tan	• Author of *Joy on Demand: The Art of Discovering the Happiness Within*, HarperOne, 2016. • Developer of the Search Inside Yourself motivational program. • Google's "Jolly Good Fellow."	[www.ChadeMeng.com]
Billy Stream	• Author of *The Hoho Dojo: Lighten Up and Love Life Laughing*, Random House, 2008. • Director of the Association for Applied and Therapeutic Humor.	[www.billystrean.com]
Steve Wilson	• Founder of the World Laughter Tour. • Founder of the Laughter Arts and Sciences Foundation.	[www.worldlaughtertour.com]
Ken Walker	• The Happiness Guy	[www.thehappinessguy.com]

speaking circuit, sometimes on internet websites. Interesting backgrounds and a talent for self-promotion abound. Table 1.2 highlights a few of the best-known of these happiness gurus.

The top name on the list is probably known to us all. Deepak Chopra is a widely-followed speaker, a TV celebrity, and the author of many books on health and happiness. He is an advocate of transcendental meditation, a populariser of many New Age practices, and a zealous supporter of alternative medicine. On the latter front, he has espoused a placebo-based approach called "quantum healing," which has been pilloried by the medical establishment as pseudoscientific quackery. On the happiness front he has published several books, and hosts several websites, each of which promises to reveal the keys to joy, happiness, and worldly success. The number of keys to happiness in Chopra's offerings is usually highlighted in the come-on; originally it was five or six, then in the book highlighted on Table 1.2, it became seven, and more-recently he has promised as many as ten. Among the keys: Start Now; Think Well; Get Clear; Expect Less; Do Good; and Be Present.

Gretchen Rubin is the author of the #1 bestseller, "The Happiness Project," and all its many spinoffs. The New York Times Book Review calls her the "queen of the self-help memoir." She is a lawyer by training, and once served as a clerk to Supreme Court Justice Sandra Day O'Connor. She has also been a columnist for *Good Housekeeping* magazine.

Neil Pasricha is a Canadian advocate of the so-called "positivity" movement. His series of books that started with "The Book of Awesome" in 2010 have all been bestsellers. The Vancouver Sun described one of them in a review as "a snappy Jerry Seinfeld monologue by way of Maria von Trapp."

Debbie Gisonni and Dan Baker both come to their happiness prescriptions from a New Age perspective. Gisonni is a "holistic lifestyle advisor," and Baker is director of the "life enhancement program" at a Tucson health resort. Gisonni and Ken Walker, call themselves, respectively, "The Happiness Goddess" and "The Happiness Guy." Billy Strean and Steve Wilson both promote the value of laughter in finding happiness. Who would have known that there are *two* organizations dedicated to the promotion of this idea: the Association for Applied and Therapeutic Humor, and the Laughter Arts and Sciences Foundation? Strean's website promises "Exhilarated Performance." The motto of Wilson's World Laughter Tour is "Think globally; Laugh locally." He calls himself "The Cheerman of the Bored." [32].

Chade Meng Tan, the author of "Joy on Demand," began his career at Google, Inc. as a software engineer, but as the years went by, he morphed into a spiritual motivator for the company. He developed a mindfulness-based course called "Search Inside Yourself" that eventually turned into his first self-help book. His official title at Google was "Jolly Good Fellow" (which nobody can deny). His meditation catchphrase: "Joy is when you're in deep sit."

Most of these books do not discuss the *measurement* of happiness per se. Their value to us lies in the advice they provide to attain happiness, oodles and oodles of it. Their many suggestions can be used to define the tableau of questions that might be asked of respondents in a self-reported subjective happiness survey, or the types of information that would be useful in an objective happiness assessment based on publically-available databases.

The positive psychology movement has often been touted as bridging the gap between the ivory tower and Main Street. If so, some of its most illustrious lights have jumped onto Main Street with both feet. One of Martin Seligman's websites offers access to a set of "happiness building exercises" for $9.95 per month. Martin Gilbert has appeared on a series of Prudential Life TV ads that have him proffering financial advice for a secure future. If you would like to meet some of these folks close-up, many of them are interviewed in the documentary film "Happy" directed by Academy Award nominee, Roco Belic.

Put on a Happy Face

Corporate America has not missed out on the cult of happiness. Disney's motto is "Make People Happy." McDonalds sells "Happy Meals." Coke ran an ad campaign that urged us to "Open Happiness." Pepsi countered with "Happiness is a Choice." Even that ubiquitous, yellow, "Happy Face" that we all sport on buttons and caps is not a freebie. It was designed in 1963 by an advertising executive named Harvey Bell, and in its first decade on the scene, it generated annual licensing revenues of over $50 million.

Tin Pan Alley has fully embraced happiness over the years. On the website of Billboard Magazine one can find a list of the 20 happiest songs of all time, which includes Barbra Streisand's "Happy Days Are Here Again," Judy Garland's "Get Happy," and Blood, Sweat and Tears' "You've Made Me So Very Happy." The Number One happiest song? Bobby McFerrin's "Don't Worry, Be Happy." The sentimental favorite: Jimmy Durante rasping through the lyrics of "Make someone happy. Make just one someone happy. And you will be happy, too."

To close out this chapter, one might want to ponder the quotes in Table 1.3 [33]. They are presented more for their wit and charm than for any role they play in our primary objectives. Yet, one cannot help but notice that the issues they raise are some of the very ones that have been subjected to the measurement approaches of happiness researchers, as will be reported in later chapters. Looking at the quotes in Table 1.3, one has every right to wonder, as Charles Darwin did, whether having children brings happiness or misery. And what about the claims of Martin Luther King and the Dalai Lama that true happiness requires kindness to others? Is this true or just wishful thinking? Or Franklin Roosevelt's emphasis on creative effort and achievement? Will any or all of these down-home homilies stand up to the objective measurements of happiness researchers. And finally, there is perhaps the most fundamental and long-debated question of all: What is the role of money in all this? Can you buy happiness or not?

Outline of the Book

The book is presented in three Parts. Part I introduces the reader to the *Multi-faceted World of Happiness and Wellbeing*. The four chapters that follow this one summarize the four scientific revolutions highlighted at the beginning of this chapter. Chapter 2 describes the impact of the *positive psychology movement* on the *social* foundations of wellbeing. Chapter 3 addresses the changes that have been wrought by the *social indicators movement* on the *economic* foundations of wellbeing. Chapter 4 highlights the influence of the *sustainability movement* on the *environmental* foundations of wellbeing. And Chap. 5 describes the happiness studies that have been carried out in the *biological and medical sciences*.

Table 1.3 Some miscellaneous quotes on happiness

Buddha	"If one speaks or acts with a pure thought, happiness follows one, like a shadow that never leaves."
Aristotle	"Happiness is an activity of the soul, expressing virtue."
Omar Khayyam	"Be happy for this moment. This moment is your life."
Emmanuel Kant	"Happiness is not an ideal of reason, but of imagination."
Mahatma Gandhi	"Happiness is when what you think, what you say, and what you do are in harmony."
Dalai Lama	"If you want others to be happy, practice compassion. If you want to be happy yourself, practice compassion."
Marcel Proust	"Let us be grateful to the people who make us happy; they are the charming gardeners who make our life bloom."
Albert Schweitzer	"Happiness is nothing more than good health and bad memory."
Albert Einstein	"A table, a chair, a bowl of fruit, and a violin; what else does a man need to be happy?"
Charles Darwin	"Children are one's greatest happiness, but often, and often still, a greater misery."
Sigmund Freud	"The goal towards which the pleasure principle impels us—of becoming happy—is not attainable; yet we may not—nay, cannot—give up the efforts to come nearer to realization of it by some means or other."
Franklin Roosevelt	"Happiness is not in the mere possession of money; it lies in the joy of achievement, in the thrill of creative effort."
John Barrymore	"Happiness often sneaks in through a door you didn't know you left open."
Martin Luther King	"The surest way to be happy is to seek happiness for others."
Charles Schulz	"Happiness is a wet puppy."
Guru Meher Baba	"Don't worry. Be happy."
Howard Hughes	"Money can't buy happiness."
Gertrude Stein	"Whoever said that money can't buy happiness, just didn't know where to go shopping."
Oscar Wilde	"Some cause happiness wherever they go, others whenever they go."
George Burns	"Happiness is having a large, loving, caring, close-knit family—in another city."
Henny Youngman	"What's the use of happiness? It can't buy you money."

Part II is entitled *Eudaimetrics.* It encompasses the six chapters that present the nuts and bolts of the measurement of happiness and wellbeing, both at the personal and communal levels, and at a variety of scales of study. Chapter 6 summarizes the methods of measurement and analysis used for subjective studies of *personal happiness*. Chapter 7 provides a template for the later chapters by defining the *dimensions of communal wellbeing*. Chapter 8 clarifies the role played by single-dimensional indexes as the *building blocks of communal wellbeing*. Chapter 9 provides descriptions of the most holistic of all the quantitative assessments, those that use multi-dimensional indexes to assess the *wellbeing of nations* as a whole. Chapter 10 addresses the *livability of* cities. Chapter 11 covers the measurement techniques used in the assessment of *workplace satisfaction*.

Part III is the *Nexus*. Its single Chap. 12 returns to the *raison d'être* for this whole exercise: the value of measurements of happiness and wellbeing in policy prescriptions, and their impact on the *politics of happiness*.

References

1. As quoted in: Antolini, F., The evolution of national accounting and new statistical information: Happiness and GDP, Can we measure it, *Social Indicators Research*, 129(3), 1075-1092, 2016.
2. Clark, A.E. et al, *The Origins of Happiness: The Source of Well-Being Over the Life Course*, Princeton University Press, 2018.
3. Kisch, Bruno, *Scales and Weights: A Historical Outline*, Yale University Press, 1965; Alder, Ken, *The Measure of All Things*, Little Brown, 2002.
4. Edgeworth, F.Y., *Mathematical Psychics: An Essay on the Application of Mathematics to the Moral Sciences*, Paul Rudd, 1881.
5. Hart, Hornell, *Chart for Happiness*, Macmillan, 1940.
6. Heckman, James J. and Edward Learner, *Handbook of Econometrics*, Elsevier, 2007.
7. Porter, T.M., *Trust in Numbers: The Pursuit of Objectivity in Science and Public Life*, Princeton University Press, 1995; Michell, J., *Measurement in Psychology*, Cambridge University Press, 1999; Boorsboom, D., *Measuring the Mind*, Cambridge University Press, 2005.
8. Stevens, Stanley S., On the theory of scales of measurement, *Science*, 103, 677-680, 1946. See also: Griffin, James, *Well-Being: Its Meaning, Measurement and Moral Importance*, Oxford Clarendon Press, 1986. For a modern take on the measurability issue, see: Veenhoven, R., Greater happiness for a greater number: Is that possible or desirable? *Journal of Happiness Studies*, 11, 605-629, 2010; and Angner, Erik, Is it possible to measure happiness? The argument from measurability, *European Journal for Philosophy of Science*, 3(2), 221-240, 2013.
9. Buchanan, R.D., The development of the Minnesota Multiphasic Personality Inventory, *Jour. History Behavioral Sciences*, 30(2), 148-161, 1994; Tellegen, A. And Y.S. Ben-Porath, *MMPI-2-RF (Minnesota Multiphasic Personality Inventory-2 Restructured Form): Technical Manual*, University of Minnesota Press, 2008.
10. Raibley, J.R., Happiness is not well-being, *Journal of Happiness Studies*, 13(6), 1105-1129, 2012.
11. Waterman, A.S., Two conceptions of happiness: Contrasts of personal expressiveness (eudaimonia) and hedonic enjoyment, *Journal of Personality and Social Psychology*, 64, 678-691, 1993; Ryan, R.M. and E.L.Deci, On happiness and human potentials: A review of research on hedonic and eudaimonic well-being, *Annual Reviews in Psychology*, 52, 141-166, 2001; Huta, V. and A.S. Waterman, Eudaimonia and its distinction from hedonia: developing a classification and terminology for understanding conceptual and operational definitions, *Journal of Happiness Studies*, 15(6), 1425-1456, 2014.
12. Bergsma, A., G. Poot and A.C. Liefbroer, Happiness in the garden of Epicurus, *Journal of Happiness Studies*, 9(3), 397-423, 2008. See also: Michalos, A,C., *Ancient Views on the Quality of Life*, Springer Nature, 2015.
13. Kasser, T. And A.D. Kanner, eds, *Psychology and Consumer Culture: The Struggle for a Good Life in a Materialistic World*, American Psychological Association, 2004.

14. Gay, Peter, Freud: *A Life for Our Times*, Anchor Books, 1988.
15. Dawkins, Richard, *The Selfish Gene*, Oxford University Press, 1976.
16. Goodin, R.E., *Utilitarianism as a Public Philosophy*, Cambridge University Press, 1995; Rosen, F., *Classical Utilitarianism from Hume to Mill*, Routledge, 2003.
17. Cobb, Clifford W., *Measurement Tools and the Quality of Life*, Redefining Progress, 2000.
18. Haybron, D.H., Happiness, in the *Stanford Encyclopedia of Philosophy*, E.N. Zalta, ed., 1995. [plato.stanford.edu]
19. Vitterso, J., The most important idea in the world: An introduction, in *Handbook of Eudaimonic Well-Being*, J. Vitterso, ed., 1-12, Springer Nature, 2016.
20. Michalos, A.C. and K.C. Land, Replies to our commentators, *Social Indicators Research*, 135(3), 1057-1078, 2018.
21. Michalos, A.C. and S.R. Robinson, The good life: Eighth century to third century BCE, in *Handbook of Social Indicators and Quality of Life Research*, A.C. Michalos and M.J. Sirgy, eds., 23-61, Springer, 2012.
22. For coverage of the history of happiness, see the following: Kingwell, Mark, *In Pursuit of Happiness: Better Living from Plato to Prozac*, Crown, 1998; McMahon, Darrin M., *Happiness: A History*, Atlantic Monthly Press, 2006; White, N.P., *A Brief History of Happiness*, Blackwell, 2006; Bok, D., *Exploring Happiness: From Aristotle to Brain Science*, Yale University Press, 2010; Estes, R.J. and M.J. Sirgy, eds., *The Pursuit of Human Well-Being: The Untold Global History*, Springer, 2017.
23. Gyatso, Tenzin, Dalai Lama, *The Art of Happiness: A Handbook for Living*, Tenth Anniversary Edition, Riverhead Books, 2009; Ricard, M., The Dalai Lama: Happiness from within, *International Journal of Well-Being*, 1(2), 274-290, 2011.
24. Setton, Mark K., *History of happiness*, [www.Pursuit-of-Happiness.org].
25. Zevnik, Luca, The origin of happiness in Renaissance and Reformation, in *Critical Perspectives in Happiness Research*, Luca Zevnik, ed., Springer, 2014.
26. Carpenter, Russ and Blythe, *The Blessings of Bhutan*, University Hawaii Press, 2004. See also: Biswas-Diener, R., E. Diener and N. Lyubchik, Wellbeing in Bhutan, *International Journal of Wellbeing*, 5(2), 1-13, 2015.
27. Michalos, A.C. and P.M. Hatch, Good societies, financial inequality and secrecy, and a good life: from Aristotle to Piketty, *Applied Research in Quality of Life*, 15(4), 1005-1054, 2020.
28. Checkland, P. and J. Scholes, *Soft Systems Methodology in Action*, Chichester: Wiley, 1990.
29. [www.miseryindex.us]
30. [www.unitedwayof america.org], [www.rsf.org], [www.freetheworld.com]
31. Russell, Bertrand, *The Conquest of Happiness*, Liveright, 2013. (Reprint of original publication of 1930.)
32. See also: Prilleltensky, Isaac, *The Laughing Guide to Well-Being: Using Humor and Science to Become Happier and Healthier*, Rowman and Littlefield Publishers, 2016.
33. Edberg, Henry, *101 Inspiring Happiness Quotes*, The Positivity Blog [www.positivityblog.com]. Also [www.quotegarden.com], [www.wisdomquotes.com], and [www.brainyquote.com].

Chapter 2
The Positive Psychology Movement

Half-Baked Psychology

The seminal moment in the modern era of the positive psychology movement is usually credited to Martin Seligman's inauguration speech as incoming President of the American Psychological Association at their annual meeting in 1998. Seligman, a professor in the Department of Psychology at the University of Pennsylvania, was by that time already a household name in the world of psychological research, having published many papers in his chosen field of "learned optimism." In his speech, he railed against the focus of many of his peers on mental illness and abnormal behaviors. "Psychology is half-baked," he argued. "We have baked the part about mental illness (but) the other side is unbaked, the side of strength, the side of what we're good at." [1] In a later article, he elaborated: "The exclusive focus on *pathology* that has dominated so much of our discipline, results in a model of the human being lacking the *positive features* that make life worth living." [2].

The charge was certainly valid. A study of the psychological literature in 1995 found that there were 17 times more articles on mental disorders than on positive aspects of human psychology [3]. However, any implication that consideration of the sources of happiness and wellbeing had not been addressed at all in the psychological world would have been misleading. There is a rich, albeit minority, tradition of work on these topics by researchers in two sub-genres of psychological research. Some of this research falls under the rubric of *humanistic psychology*, and some under the mantle of *subjective wellbeing*. Both these areas were well established by 1998 and deserve a full measure of respect as precursors of the current positive psychology movement [4]. Both grew in some measure as an antidote to the widely-used bible of psychological therapy, the American Psychiatric Association's "Diagnostic and Statistical Manual of Mental Disorders" (DSM). In the following subsections, we will follow this historical route, from the DSM, through the humanistic psychology movement and subjective wellbeing, to the modern emphasis on positive psychology.

R. A. Freeze, *The Metrics of Happiness*, Social Indicators Research Series 86,
https://doi.org/10.1007/978-3-031-10913-3_2

The DSM

The first authoritative attempt to gather information on mental health in the United States was the recording of the incidence of "idiocy and insanity" in the federal census of 1840. No attempt was made at that time to identify or differentiate between the different forms that the idiocy or the insanity might take. However, during the latter 1800s and the early 1900s, there was growing interest among psychologists, psychiatrists, and psychoanalysts in the occurrence of the various types of mental illness, and concern over the lack of an accepted system of classification. This desire for structure and standardization led the newly-formed American Psychiatric Association in 1921 to arrange for the inclusion of mental disorders in the American Medical Association's Standard Classified Nomenclature of Diseases [5]. By 1952 the APA had decided to go it alone with the first publication of their own "Diagnostic and Statistical Manual of Mental Disorders." It defined 60 types of mental illness, clearly differentiating between life-altering *psychoses* like schizophrenia and paranoia, and more-treatable *neuroses* like anxiety and depression. In the years since, the DSM has undergone several revisions, the most recent being the fifth edition, DSM-5, in 2013 [6]. DSM-5 enjoys widespread application by clinicians, researchers, the legal profession, the health insurance industry, pharmaceutical and medical organizations, regulatory bodies, and government policy makers. Sales of the DSM provide income of around $5 million per year to the American Psychiatric Association, perhaps as much as $100 million over the life of the publication to date.

The DSM has not been free from controversy. The question of what constitutes abnormal behavior has always been contentious, and charges of cultural bias have been common. As late as 1968 the DSM still listed homosexuality as a mental disorder. At the time of publication of the DSM-5, the psychiatrist Allen Frances, writing in the New York Times, claimed that the new category of Behavioral Addiction "makes a mental disorder of everything we like to do," while a diagnosis of Anxiety Disorder could easily be made for a patient who is suffering nothing more than "everyday worries." [7].

Humanistic Psychology

Clearly, the DSM is not about happy people, and there were many psychologists, even in the earliest days, who found the DSM's emphasis on "mental disorders" unduly pessimistic. The complaint also applied to the psychoanalytic theories of Sigmund Freud, which were much in vogue in those days. As early as the mid-1950s, a new subfield had begun to emerge under the name of *humanistic psychology*. Its practitioners focused on human strengths rather than neuroses and pathologies. They emphasized the development and expression of one's own capabilities and creativity. An Association for Humanistic Psychology was founded in

Table 2.1 A brief summary of Maslow's hierarchy of needs (Adapted from the source materials listed in Reference [8])

Self-actualization	Morality/creativity/spontaneity/problem-solving/lack of prejudice
Esteem	Self-esteem/confidence/achievement/respect for others
Love and belonging	Friendship/family/sexual intimacy
Security	Body/employment/resources/morality/family/health/property
Physiological	Air/food/water/sleep

1961, and the Society for Humanistic Psychology was established as Section 32 of the American Psychological Association shortly thereafter.

Abraham Maslow of Brandeis University was one of the leaders of the humanistic psychology movement in the 1950s. He felt strongly that too much of the current thinking in psychology at that time reduced humans to almost machine-like status, treating people as automatons responding instinctively to external stimuli. He preferred to think of his fellow humans as having free will, and able to make choices that affect their wellbeing. With regard to the "mental-disorder" approach of Freudian psychology and the then-recently-published DSM, he offered the following: "The study of crippled, stunted, immature, and unhealthy specimens can yield only a cripple psychology and a cripple philosophy." Politically incorrect it may have been (by modern standards), but the message was pretty clear. In 1954, Maslow put all these ideas into his *magnum opus* "Motivation and Personality." [8] The title of one of the book's appendices contains the term: "A Positive Approach to Psychology." In the eyes of many historians of the social sciences, this usage can be construed as the beginning of the positive psychology movement.

In fact, Maslow's book contains a paragraph that is eerily similar to Seligman's arguments forty-four years later in his presidential address. Maslow writes: "The science of psychology has been far more successful on the negative than on the positive side; it has revealed much about man's shortcomings, his illnesses, his sins, but little about his potentialities, his virtues, his achievable aspirations, or his full psychological height. It is as if psychology had voluntarily restricted itself to only half its rightful jurisdiction, and that the darker, meaner half." [9].

Maslow's most lasting contribution to the field was his *hierarchy of needs* which is presented in brief form in Table 2.1. It is supposed to be read from the bottom up, with the most basic physiological needs as the pedestal on which the higher needs of security, love, esteem, and self-actualization are built. The detailed human needs that are listed under each of these main headings bear a great resemblance to the factors that will be identified later as the main correlates of happiness and wellbeing.

The early humanistic psychologists were not quick to pick up on the traditional quantitative research methodologies derived from the physical sciences. They preferred qualitative approaches that they felt were more appropriate to the social sciences. This disdain for quantitative analysis on the part of the humanists is perhaps the main reason that Seligman and his colleagues in the new positive psychology movement are not willing to give greater credit to the humanistic psychology movement as a valid bridgehead to their own. The positive psychology movement is unabashedly quantitative, and researchers base their findings on what they see as objective measurement programs, not on intuitively-based theories.

Subjective Wellbeing

The other precursor of the positive psychology movement is the concept of *subjective wellbeing* [10]. The guru of SWB was Ed Diener, longtime professor of psychology at the University of Illinois, who passed away in 2021. Diener wrote and spoke widely on wellbeing and happiness for many years in both academic and public forums. His work was featured on two different occasions in Time magazine. His outspoken public support for the new positive face of psychology led to his being anointed with the affectionate title of "Doctor Happiness."

Assessments of subjective wellbeing are usually based on self-reported answers to questionnaires. By definition, emphasis is placed on the personal subjective assessment of life satisfaction by individuals, rather than a reliance on objective demographic measures of communal wellbeing. SWB assessors are more interested in internal expectations, experiences, values, and social environment, less so in external demographic and societal influences. Having said this, one can only note that promoters of SWB do not deny the value of objective indicators, and many of them have worked closely with those in other branches of the positive psychology movement, blurring whatever weak boundaries may exist, united in their goal to develop a more positive, preventive approach to psychological health.

In 1999, Diener was the lead author on a review paper titled "Subjective well-being: Three decades of progress," which implies that this sub-field of psychology has roots that go back to at least 1969 [11]. In fact, in this paper Diener and his coauthors send the roots back even further by quoting widely from a 1967 paper by University of Alabama psychologist Warner Wilson, who reviewed the progress to that date of what he called *avowed happiness*, a concept much akin to subjective wellbeing [12]. In his review, Wilson concluded that the happiest soul in a random sample of respectable citizens would be a "young, healthy, well-educated, well-paid, extroverted, optimistic, worry-free, religious, married person with high self-esteem, strong job morale, and modest expectations." This person might be a he or a she, and could exhibit a wide range of intelligence. Part of the purpose of the Diener article was to examine each of these implied indicators of happiness, and bring the picture up to date in light of the many quantitative studies that had been carried out between the two reviews.

Strengths and Virtues

As the new millennium dawned, the positive psychology movement blossomed under the leadership of Seligman and Diener. They saw it as encompassing the scientific study of the strengths and virtues that enable individuals and communities to thrive. Seligman joined forces with Christopher Peterson, a psychologist from the University of Michigan, to carry out a 3-year project involving 55 distinguished social scientists to review, assemble, and classify the identifiable positive traits in human beings that lead to individual happiness and a civil society. They tried to examine human goodness across cultures, nations and beliefs. The result was the publication in 2004 of "Character Strengths and Virtues: A Handbook and Classification." [13] The CSV, as it is known, was designed as the antidote and complement to the DSM, giving psychologists and therapists a handbook of strengths to counter the DSM's handbook of weaknesses.

The CSV identifies six broad areas of "virtue" and 24 "character strengths." Table 2.2 provides a summary of them. The authors further identify those strengths listed under Wisdom and Knowledge as *cognitive strengths*, those under Courage as *emotional strengths*, those under Humanity and Justice as *social strengths*, those under Moderation and Temperance as *protective strengths*, and those under Transcendence as *spiritual strengths*. At the individual level, it is held that those who discover and exploit their unique mix of character strengths, their honesty, vitality, love, forgiveness, and the rest, ought to find personal happiness. At the community level, it is held that civic institutions that foster such strengths as leadership, teamwork, love of learning, and moderation, will lead to a more civil society and a greater sense of communal wellbeing.

The growth in the field of positive psychology has been accompanied by a profusion of specialized university programs, well-funded research projects, and both private and academic think tanks. Table 2.3 lists a few of the most visible ones, the titles of which give some idea of the breadth of the movement. However the list is far from complete. It seems that every university worth its salt, and every psychological organization on the planet, now has its own positive psychology shop. This profusion of programs has led to greater specialization in the various aspects of positive psychology. Table 2.4 lists a few of the best-known researchers and their special interests [14]. Seligman's cry for change has been heeded.

There has also been an explosion in the number of specialized academic journals in recent years where the researchers at all these think tanks can place articles that report the findings of their studies. The grandfather of the quality-of-life/well-being/happiness journals is *Social Indicators Research* which first appeared in 1974. The *Journal of Happiness Studies* began publication in 2000, the *Journal of Positive Psychology* in 2006, *Applied Research in Quality of Life* in 2006, *Applied Psychology: Health and Well-Being* in 2009, the *Psychology of Well-Being: Theory, Research, and Practice* in 2011, the *International Journal of Wellbeing* in 2011, and the *International Journal of Happiness and Development* in 2012. All of these outlets encourage contributions on the measurement of happiness. In the founding

Table 2.2 A summary of Peterson and Seligman's character strengths and virtues (Adapted from the source materials listed in [13])

Virtues	Wisdom and knowledge	Courage	Humanity	Transcen-Dence	Justice	Moderation and temperance
	Creativity	Bravery	Love	Appreciation of Beauty and Excellence	Teamwork	Forgiveness and Mercy
	Curiosity	Persistence	Kindness	Gratitude	Fairness	Humility and Modesty
Strengths	Open-mindedness	Honesty and Integrity	Social Intelligence	Hope	Leadership	Prudence
	Love of learning	Vitality and Zest		Humor and Playfulness		Self-Regulation and Self Control
	Perspective			Spirituality and Sense of Purpose		

Table 2.3 A sampling of academic research centers and private institutes that focus on positive psychology

	Name	Location
Academic Research Centers	Positive Psychology Center	University of Pennsylvania
	Hedonic Psychology Laboratory	Harvard University
	Center for Investigating Healthy Minds	University of Wisconsin
	Greater Good Science Center	University of California Berkeley
	Positive Emotions and Psychophysiology Laboratory	University of North Carolina
	Center for Compassion and Altruism Research and Education	Stanford University
	Laboratory for the Study of Meaning and Quality of Life	Colorado State University
	Quality of Life Research Center	Claremont Graduate University, CA
	Center for Trauma, Resilience and Growth	University of Nottingham, UK
	Happiness Laboratory	Carleton University, Canada
	Well-Being Institute	Cambridge University, UK
	Center for Mindfulness in Medicine, Health Care and Society	University of Massachusetts
	Institute of Communitarian Policy Studies	George Washington University
	Center for Advancement of Well-Being	George Mason University
	Behavioral Science Centre	University of Stirling, UK
	Laboratory for the Study of Meaning and Quality of Life	Colorado State University
	Australian Centre on Quality of Life	Deakin University, Melbourne
Private Institutes	Values in Action Institute	Cincinnati, Ohio
	International Network of Personal Meaning—Meaningful Living Project	Toronto, Canada
	Centre for Applied Positive Psychology	United Kingdom
	Centre for Confidence and Well-being	Glasgow, Scotland
	Positive Psychology Program	The Hague, The Netherlands
	Chopra Center for Wellbeing	Carlsbad, CA
	International Happiness Observatory	Montpelier, France
	Mayo Clinic Mind Body Institute	Rochester, MN
	Happiness Research Institute	Copenhagen, Denmark

Table 2.4 Examples of specialization in the positive psychology movement

Researcher	Institution	Specialization
Roy Baumeister	Florida State University	Will-power and self-control
Mahzarin Banaji	Harvard University	Unconscious bias
Fred Bryant	Loyola University	Savoring
Victor Chan	Dalai Lama Centre for Peace and Education	Compassion
Angela Duckworth	University of Pennsylvania	Grit and perseverance
Elizabeth Dunn	University of British Columbia	Giving, altruism, affective forecasting
Robert Emmons	University of California, Davis	Gratitude
Walter Mischel	Columbia University	Delayed gratification
Timothy Pychyl	Carleton University	Procrastination
Kennon Sheldon	University of Missouri	Goal-setting
C.R. Snyder	University of Kansas	Hope
Everett Worthington	Virginia Commonwealth University	Forgiveness
John Zelinski	Carleton University	Nature-related happiness
Alex Michalos	University of Northern British Columbia	Personality, education, living conditions
John Helliwell	Canadian Institute for Advanced Research	Trust
Carol Ryff	University of Wisconsin	Eudaimonic happiness
Daniel Batson	University of Tennessee	Altruism, religion
Jonathan Haidt	University of Virginia	Morality, awe
Felicia Huppert	Cambridge University	Wellbeing over life's course
Christopher Boyce	University of Stirling	Personality
Gordon Brown	University of Warwick	Economic factors
Mark Holder	University of British Columbia, Okanagan	Happiness in children
Derek Isacowitz	Northeastern University	Age-related happiness
Michael Marmot	University College London	Status
Sonja Lyubomirsky	University California Riverside	Gratitude and affirmation
Tal Ben Shahar	Harvard University	Self-esteem and leadership
David Myers	Hope College	Faith
Amital Etzioni	George Washington University	Civil society
Emma Seppala	Stanford University	Compassion and resilience
Frederic Luskin	Stanford University	Forgiveness
Nancy Fagley	Rutgers University	Appreciation
Jean Decety	University of Chicago	Empathy
Kristin Neff	University of Texas	Self-compassion
Todd Kashdan	George Mason University	Mindfulness

editorial in the first issue of the Journal of Happiness Studies the editors, Ed Diener, Alex Michalos, and Ruut Veenhoven, announced their desire "to learn more about the ways we can assess how people feel about life and what are the best measures for that purpose." [15].

One result of this profusion of journals has been a huge increase in the number of published papers in the field. Ruut Veenhoven, a Dutch sociologist at Erasmus University in Rotterdam, is the founder of the World Database of Happiness, an "archive of research findings on the subject of enjoyment of life." His bibliographic files show an increase in published academic articles on happiness from less than 10 per year prior to 1965 to more than 200 per year in 2010 [16].

The positive psychology movement is not just an American phenomenon. It has become an international fascination. The International Wellbeing Group based at the Australian Centre on Quality of Life at Deakin University in Melbourne has over 100 institutional members from over 40 countries. The Fifth World Congress on Positive Psychology was held in Montreal in 2017. The United Nations has been active. In 2011 they issued a resolution that "happiness is a fundamental human goal and aspiration." In 2012, the UN began issuing its World Happiness Report. In 2013, the UN General Assembly decreed that March 20th would henceforth be celebrated every year as the International Day of Happiness.

And so the positive psychology movement marches on. Mihaly Czikszentmihalyi, another of the pioneer researchers in the movement continues to develop his concept of a *state of flow*, first enunciated as early as 1990, which holds that the best moments in a person's life occur when he or she is immersed in an activity that requires creative engagement and which leads to an accomplishment that is difficult and worthwhile [17]. Martin Seligman has followed up on his original 2002 bestseller on *authentic happiness* with a new book that hails *flourishing* as a "visionary new understanding of happiness and well-being." [18] In it, he introduces his "Pillars of PERMA," an acronym for what he sees as the five basic building blocks of wellbeing. The P stands for Positive Emotions, the E for Engagement, the R for Relationships, the M for Meaning (as in a purposeful existence), and the A for Achievement (a sense of accomplishment and success). One of the many self-help websites that offers the visitor a chance to test his or her happiness does so with the question: "Are you Permalicious?" [19].

Mindfulness

There is another movement in psychological circles that can be seen as closely related to the positive psychology movement, and which has at least peripheral importance in the assessment of happiness and wellbeing. The concept of *mindfulness* is rooted in Buddhist teachings and the rites of meditation. The American godfather of mindfulness is Jon Kabat-Zinn, an emeritus professor of medicine at the University of Massachusetts. Starting in the early 1970s, Kabat-Zinn began carrying out research designed to integrate the Buddhist traditions with North

American medical science. His work led to the development of a therapeutical approach known as Mindfulness-Based Stress Reduction, which has proven helpful in the alleviation of stress, anxiety, and chronic pain. The American Psychological Association has endorsed MBSR as a "hopeful strategy" for combating depression and pain.

Jonathan Haidt, a professor of ethical leadership at New York University's Stern School of Business, is another author who has mined the Buddhist tradition. His book, "The Happiness Hypothesis: Finding Modern Truth in Ancient Wisdom," promises to find the nuggets of wisdom from both Eastern and Western religious and philosophical traditions, "from Buddha to Plato to Freud to Dr. Phil." [20].

On Table 2.4, the final entry is that of Todd Kashdon, a psychology professor at George Mason University. Of the literally hundreds of researchers in the mindfulness game, his name has been selected because he was the lead editor of a book that brings the mindfulness movement and the positive psychology movement most closely together. It is titled "Mindfulness, Acceptance, and Positive Psychology: The Seven Foundations of Well-Being." [21] The seven foundations are Functional Beliefs, Mindfulness and Awareness, Perspective, Values, Experiential Acceptance, Behavioral Control, and Cognitive Skill.

Rick Hanson is the founder of the Wellspring Institute for Neuroscience and Contemplative Wisdom, and a Fellow at the Greater Good Science Center at the University of California at Berkeley, one of the academic think tanks highlighted in Table 2.3. His research and popular writings try to bring together ideas from the Eastern traditions of meditation with the Western breakthroughs in the neurosciences [22]. Like Kashdon and his coworkers, he has produced a set of "foundations of well-being," but he has gone them five better, coming up with 12 foundations rather than seven. They include Self-caring, Mindfulness, Learning, Vitality, Gratitude, Confidence, Calm, Motivation, Intimacy, Courage, Aspiration, and Service. Of particular interest here is the appearance of mindfulness as one of the 12 foundations.

Since the turn of the new millennium, mindfulness has been much in the news. There are lots of sources of information, from an "The Complete Idiot's Guide to Mindfulness," [23] to academic treatises that review the history and development of the ideas [24]. If you doubt the mainstream acceptance of this Buddhist-rooted approach to wellbeing, it is worth noting that Time Magazine, that beacon of Middle America, published a special issue on Mindfulness in 2016 [25].

Hygge and Ikagai

The Danish concept of *hygge* has much in common with mindfulness, and it too has reached the North American mainstream in recent years through two best-selling self-help books: *The Book of Hygge: The Danish Art of Contentment, Comfort and Connection*, by Louisa Thomsen Brits, and *The Little Book of Hygge: The Danish Way to Live Well*, by Meik Wiking [26]. Both books champion a simple lifestyle with lots of good food and drink, a careful reckoning of one's work/life balance, the amiable acceptance of disagreement, and an anti-elitist approach to social relationships in which everyone is treated with dignity, equality and trust.

Hygge is not the only happiness doctrine rooted in the cultural lore of a specific country. The Japanese celebrate *ikagai* which can be loosely defined as the "joy and a sense of wellbeing that comes from a life worth living." One Japanese study found that a lifestyle based on ikagai lowered the risk of cardiovascular heart disease and increased life expectancy [27].

Convergence

Perusal of the several sub-sections in this chapter reflects a coming together of the many strands in the positive psychology movement. As we follow the path from Maslow, to Seligman, to Kashdan, to Hanson; as we move along from humanistic psychology, to subjective wellbeing, to strengths and virtues, to mindfulness; we see the same concepts and ideas packaged and repackaged. We encounter the same headings and catchphrases. The need for self-esteem and connection run through all the ideologies. So too do concepts like compassion, perseverance, vitality, gratitude, hope, forgiveness, and courage. These very words form the chapter headings in the Oxford Handbook of Positive Psychology, published in 2005 [28]. As we move forward we will have to learn more about the measurement of the emotions and attitudes identified by all these various investigators, and the role they play in the assessment of human happiness.

References

1. The biographical information and historical quotes in this section come in part from the references that follow; from Wikipedia articles; and from the websites: [www.pursuit-of-happiness.org] and [https://positivepsychologyprogram.com].
2. Seligman, Martin E.P. and M. Czikszentmihalyi, Positive psychology: An introduction, *American Psychologist*, 55(1),5-14, 2000.
3. Myers, D.G. and E. Diener, Who is happy, *Psychological Science*, 6, 10-19, 1995.
4. Froh, J.J., The history of positive psychology, truth be told, *The Psychologist*, 16(3), 18-20, 2004; Angner, Erik, The evolution of eupathics: The historical roots of subjective measures of wellbeing, *International Journal of Wellbeing*, 1(1), 4-41, 2011.
5. Benjafield, J.G., *A History of Psychology*, Third Edition, Oxford University Press, 2010.
6. American Psychiatric Association, *Diagnostic and Statistical Manual of Mental Disorders*, DSM-5, 2013
7. Frances, Allen, Diagnosing the DSM, *New York Times*, May 11, 2012.
8. Maslow, Abraham, *Motivation and Personality*, Harper, 1954. See also [en.wikipedia.org/wiki/maslow]
9. Maslow, 1954, op. cit., as quoted in Froh, 2004, op. cit.
10. Larson, R.J. and M. Eid, eds, *The Science of Subjective Well-Being*, Guildford Press, 2008
11. Diener, E., E.M. Suh, R.E. Lucas, and H.E Smith, Subjective well-being: Three decades of progress, *Psychological Bulletin*, 125, 276-302, 1999.

12. Wilson, Warner, Correlates of avowed happiness, *Psychological Bulletin*, 67, 294-306, 1967.
13. Peterson, C. And M.E.P. Seligman, *Character Strengths and Virtues: A Handbook and Classification*, Oxford University Press, 2004. See also: [www.positivepsychology.com/classification-character-strengths-virtues]
14. A list of 175 active researchers in positive psychology can be found at [https://positivepsychologyprogram.com]
15. Veenhoven, R., E. Diener and A. Michalos, Editorial, *Journal of Happiness Studies*, 1(1), 5-8, 2000.
16. [http://worlddatabaseofhappiness.eur.nl]
17. Czikszentmihalyi, Mihaly, *Flow: The Psychology of Optimal Experience*, Harper and Row, 1990; Czikszentmihalyi, Mihaly, *Finding Flow: The Psychology of Engagement with Everyday Life*, Basic Books, 1998.
18. Seligman, Martin E.P., *Authentic Happiness: Using the New Positive Psychology to Realize Your Potential for Lasting Fulfillment*, Free Press, 2002; Seligman, Martin E.P., *Flourish: A Visionary New Understanding of Happiness and Well-Being*, Free Press, 2011.
19. [www.gostrengths.com]
20. Haidt, Jonathan, *The Happiness Hypothesis: Finding Modern Truth in Ancient Wisdom*, Basic Books, 2006.
21. Kashdan, Todd and Joseph Ciarrochi, eds., *Mindfulness, Acceptance, and Positive Psychology: The Seven Foundations of Well-Being*, New Harbinger Publ., 2013.
22. Hanson, Rick, *Hardwiring Happiness: The New Brain Science of Contentment, Calm and Confidence*, Harmony, 2013. [www.thefoundationsofwellbeing.com]
23. Ihnan, Anne and Carolyn Flynn, *The Complete Idiot's Guide to Mindfulness*, Penguin, 2008.
24. Black, David S., Hot topics: A forty-year publishing history of mindfulness, *Mindfulness Research Monthly*, 1(5), 2010.
25. Time Magazine, Special Edition, *Mindfulness*, March 21, 2016
26. Brits, L.M., *The Book of Hygge: The Danish Art of Contentment, Comfort and Connection*, Ebury Publ., 2016; Wiking, M., *The Little Book of Hygge: The Danish Way to Live Well*, Penguin, 2016
27. Sone, T., Sense of life worth living (ikagai) and mortality in Japan: Ohsaki study, *Psychosomatic Medicine*, 70(6), 709-715, 2008.
28. Snyder, C.R. and S.J. Lopez, eds., *Handbook of Positive Psychology*, Oxford University Press, 2005.

Chapter 3
The Social Indicators Movement

The Dow-Jones and the GDP

Throughout much of modern American history, the only widely-publicized measures of progress have been economic ones. We live and die with the *Dow Jones Industrial Average* (DJIA), which reflects the performance of the stock market, and the *Gross Domestic Product* (GDP), which tracks nation-wide manufacturing output. It is not really clear why these two somewhat esoteric measures of financial health should have become the proxies for our overall wellbeing, but they have. Perhaps Calvin Coolidge had it right when he said that "the business of America is business."

The DJIA has been with us almost since the founding of the country. The New York Stock Exchange dates back to 1792 and it moved into its current Wall Street headquarters in 1865. The Wall Street Journal began publication in 1896 with Charles Dow as its editor, and in that same year Dow developed and published the first version of the DJIA. The current version is published in almost every newspaper in the nation every day, and is applied on almost every smartphone. It is based on the stock market performance of a surprisingly small sample of only 30 companies, widely-held and influential companies to be sure, but still only 30 of them. In 1957, the financial services firm, Standard and Poor's, began producing their *S&P 500 Index*, boosting the number of companies included in a widely-published market analysis from 30 to 500. In 1966, the NYSE began reporting its own *NYSE Composite Index* based on all common stocks traded on the exchange [1].

To find the genesis of the GDP, we must go back to the 1930s, when the shock of the Great Depression generated a vocal movement to develop some meaningful national economic indicators that would provide advance warning of tough times ahead, and point the way to policy prescriptions to avoid the economic downturns. The dream was a single measure on a national scale that would rise in good times and fall in bad, "a statistic to end all statistics," a measure that would provide "a window on our economic soul." [2] The job of developing such a measure was turned over to

R. A. Freeze, *The Metrics of Happiness*, Social Indicators Research Series 86,
https://doi.org/10.1007/978-3-031-10913-3_3

the National Bureau of Economic Research in the Department of Commerce. At the NBER, the task was put under the leadership of a young economist named Simon Kuznets, who had immigrated with his family to the USA from Belorussia at the age of 21 in 1927, and had moved rapidly up the ladder at the NBER. In 1934, he was asked to report on his progress to the US Congress. In his report, titled simply *National Income*, he described his work on a set of country-wide accounts (that later became the National Income and Product Accounts, or NIPAs), and mused about the development of a new statistic, originally presented as the Gross National Product (GNP), and much later (in 1991) refined as the Gross Domestic Product (GDP). In 1971, he was awarded the Nobel Prize in Economics. In 1999, the Department of Commerce recognized Kuznets's work as the "achievement of the century" in the Department.

Both the GNP and the GDP reflect the total net market value of all goods and services produced by the nation during a given period (that is, the gross value minus the costs of materials and services used to produce the final products). Their calculation involves the summation of all consumer spending, investment, government spending, and net exports (exports minus imports). The two measures differ in that the GNP is calculated for all enterprises owned by any citizen of the country, no matter where the goods are produced, whereas the GDP is calculated for all enterprises within the country's borders, regardless of the citizenship of its owners.

There is a third version, known as Gross National Income (GNI), which is defined as the GDP plus all income paid into the country from other countries for such things as interest and dividends minus all similar payments paid out to other countries (which makes it similar, but not quite identical to the GNP).

The United States and Canada use the GDP as their favored statistic. The European Union and the World Bank use the GNI. Despite their differences, the two measures seem to track each other very closely. For example, in early 2017, the US GDP per capita was $46,436, and the GNI per capita was $46,730. The comparable numbers in Canada were $37,946 and $37,590 [3].

The GDP is adjusted for inflation so that comparisons can be made year to year. What such comparisons usually show is a long-term growth in economic activity. It is held by economic purists that such growth is a robust measure of a country's wellbeing. The Harvard economist, Benjamin Friedman, in his book *The Moral Consequences of Economic Growth* states that economic growth is essential to "greater opportunity, tolerance to diversity, social mobility, commitment to fairness, and dedication to democracy." He claims that during times of economic expansion, nations tend to liberalize their social policies, leading to expanded benefits for the needy and higher living standards for all [4]. Economic think tanks, especially those with a conservative bent, tend to pick up on these ideas, arguing for lower corporate taxes and greater foreign investment to spur economic growth, and providing strong support for the continued use of the GDP as a valid measuring stick of national wellbeing.

Of course, many in the economic community recognize that the GDP is not a perfect measure, even by economic standards. Economists with a more holistic worldview have been taking potshots at the GDP almost since its inception. For example, it doesn't take into account the plethora of non-market activities that take place in a vibrant community, things like household work, volunteerism, and other unpaid contributions to the economy. The GDP also fails to record the non-monetary transactions that take place through bartering and in the second-hand and recycling trade. In some countries, black-market dealings and trade in the so-called shadow economy can represent a significant component of the economy. It is also not clear that present methods of calculation correctly capture contributions to the economy from the recent boom in the personal services trade, dot-com technology, and internet commerce. Critics also claim that the value of health care is underrepresented, as are the positive pleasures of leisure time.

Household work in particular represents a considerable slice of the economy, and the fact that it is not included in the GDP represents a significant flaw in its calculation. The loudest and most effective voice in this regard has been that of Marilyn Waring, a professor of public policy at the Auckland University of Technology in New Zealand. In her book *If Women Counted* she reflects on the need for a new feminist economics, and calls for a redefinition of the GDP to properly take women's work into account. How in the world, she argues, can we have an accounting system that "counts oil spills and wars as contributors to economic growth, while child rearing and housekeeping are deemed valueless." [5].

Most egregiously, the GDP fails to take into account what economists call the externalities, those consequences of commercial activity that affect other parties without being reflected in the cost of goods or services provided. Most often, these externalities impose a cost on parties who did not choose to incur that cost, and had no input into the decision that led to it. Among the most-widely identified externalities that are not represented in GDP calculations are the social costs associated with environmental pollution, climate change, resource depletion, and the imposition of unwanted societal risk.

The GDP counts anything that generates economic activity as positive. When natural disasters strike, the money spent on rescue and rebuilding contributes to the GDP, but the human cost of trauma and displacement is not. Money spent on medical, social, and legal services boosts the GDP without consideration of the counterbalancing human costs to families that need such services. The negative financial impacts on society of crime, illness, drug and alcohol addiction, and family breakdown are not included in GDP calculations.

Perfect or not, the GDP has become a standard measure of national economic health. Like the Dow-Jones, it is widely reported in the popular press. Moreover, it is widely used internationally. At the United Nations Monetary and Financial Conference held at Bretton Woods, New Hampshire, in 1944, a group of 730 delegates from 44 Allied nations established two economic institutions that have stood the test of time: the International Monetary Fund (IMF) and the World Bank (originally called the International Bank for Reconstruction and Development). It was agreed that in these international institutions, the GDP would be the standard measure for assessing and comparing the economies of each member country. As noted above, the World Bank and most European countries now favor the GNI rather than the

GDP, but given the almost exact equivalence of these two measures for most countries, the point remains the same.

In the United States, the GDP is currently reported by the Bureau of Economic Analysis (BEA), a branch of the Department of Commerce. The quarterly calculation of the GDP is based on the data encapsulated in the NIPA accounts, first put together by Kuznets, and expanded in scope over the years. The latest NIPA reports feature almost 300 double-entry tables of economic inputs and outputs, grouped under seven summary accounts: the *domestic incomes product* account, *the private enterprise income* account, the *personal income and outlay* account, the *government receipts and expenditures* account, the *foreign transactions current* account, the *domestic capital* account, and the *foreign transactions capital* account. It is held that these accounts taken together represent the most consistent and comprehensive picture available of the U.S. economy [6].

When it comes to comparison of GDP across countries, one can turn to either of two respected sources. The International Comparison Program (ICP) is administered by the World Bank under the auspices of the United Nations Statistical Commission [7]. The Penn World Tables (PWT) are a compendium of worldwide national accounts originally developed at the University of Pennsylvania, but now maintained jointly by the University of California at Davis and the University of Groningen in Sweden [8]. Both the ICP and the PWT came to an early realization that comparison of national GDPs on the basis of market exchange rates does not provide an accurate picture of the relative sizes of the various national economies. Instead, they both now use the Purchasing Power Parity (PPP) approach to convert national accounts into a common currency. The PPP between two countries, A and B, measures the number of units of country A's currency required to purchase a basket of goods and services in country A, as compared to the number of units of country B's currency required to purchase a similar basket of goods and services in country B. The ratio so determined is used as the conversion factor to be applied to the comparative data for the two countries.

There are many other widely-used economic indicators that are not related to stock market performance or the GDP, many of them published on a regular basis by the federal bureaucracy. The government routinely reports on the *rate of inflation*, the *balance of trade*, the current *budget deficit*, and the *national debt*. Labor statistics like the *seasonally-adjusted unemployment rate* and the current *minimum wage* are reported regularly. There are indicators of importance to consumers such as the *consumer price index* and *consumer confidence* indices. The business community is interested in the latest numbers on the *interest rates* set by banks on commercial loans, the schedule of *corporate tax rates*, and bellwether stats like monthly *vehicle sales* and *housing starts*. In addition, there are literally thousands of economic indicators published on websites, in newsletters put out by the financial investment community, and kept proprietarily by special interests. The World Bank publishes data on 1519 World Development Indicators, many of which are economic or quasi-economic in nature (e.g. patent applications, employment statistics, tax policies). The Wall Street Journal has published an investment guide that suggests there are at least 50 economic indicators that "really matter" to an investor [9].

There are also quite a few that don't matter. The *Hemline Theory*, for example, holds that the length of women's skirts moves in the same direction as the stock market. The *Super Bowl Theory* predicts a bull market in years when the NFC team beats the AFC team in the January football showdown. And the politically-incorrect *Vixen Index* has something to do with the number of attractive waitresses in your hometown.

There are a couple of others that sound like they might also fit into this list of tongue-in-cheek indicators, but which actually have some merit. The *Big Mac Index*, first quoted by The Economist magazine in Britain in 1986, uses the price of a Macdonald's hamburger in various cities of the world to identify whether the exchange rate of that country's currency is over- or under-valued. The *Rapture Index* integrates 45 indicators of activities that are thought to be harbingers of the coming of the apocalypse (plagues, terrorist attacks, drug wars, etc.). More importantly, perhaps, it charts the response of evangelical Christian believers to this perceived threat. Surprisingly, this "Dow-Jones Average of the end-times" seems to be a somewhat reliable indicator of economic perceptions in the Americas [10].

Gini Coefficients and One-Percenters

If the GDP is a reasonable indicator of a nation's economic health, shouldn't the *GDP per capita* be a reasonable indicator of each individual's wellbeing, or at least his or her *economic* wellbeing? Well, sort of. Certainly, those of us who live in high-GDP nations like the US or Canada are probably building on a more secure economic base than those who live in low-GDP nations like Nigeria or Moldova. There is, without doubt, a country-by-country relationship between GDP per capita and the percent of those who are "satisfied with life as a whole," with Moldova near the bottom and Canada near the top. But within the framework of a single country, GDP per capita is not a very useful measure of individual wellbeing. The problem is the inequality in wealth that is found within every country. The GDP reflects only a country's total wealth, not the distribution of that wealth among its citizens. The economic indicators that have been highlighted in the previous sub-section really only reflect the wellbeing of the wealthy. Higher GDP or a higher Dow-Jones Average undoubtedly bode well for business owners and upscale investors whose economic interests lie in the market or the import/export trade, but they probably have almost no influence on the wellbeing of the man-on-the-street whose happiness has little to do with stock markets or the GDP.

On a global scale, statistics on the inequality of wealth are truly shocking. Approximately 80% of worldwide wealth is held by just 20% of the population, almost all of it in the developed countries. The 500 richest billionaires in the world have a collective wealth that is greater than the combined wealth of the three billion people in the poorest half of humanity.

The inequality in standard of living can also be viewed from the point of view of annual income rather than total wealth. The standard measure of income inequality is a statistical parameter known as a *Gini coefficient* named after the Italian statistician, Corrado Gini, who first defined the term away back in 1912. It is used to calculate the degree of dispersion in the frequency distribution of household incomes in a country. A Gini coefficient of 1 would imply maximum inequality (with all of a countries' income concentrated in one household); a Gini coefficient of 0 represents maximum equality (with every household having exactly the same income). Clearly, neither of these endpoints is likely to arise. The Gini coefficient for most countries lies in the range 0.25 to 0.70. Canada and most western European countries are in the range 0.25–0.35 (indicating a relatively equitable balance between rich and poor). Most countries in Africa and South America are in the range 0.55 to 0.65 (indicating a much larger and more inequitable gap). The United States comes in at 0.40 to 0.45, which places it in the bottom 30% of countries in the world, and among the least equitable of the western democracies.

In the US, between 1973 and 2005, the wealthiest 10% of the population snared over 30% of the total income. At the very top, between 2000 and the present, the so-called one-percenters have garnered more than 20% of the total income. In 2012 the average annual income of the 400 highest earners in the country was almost $350 million each. The average ratio of CEO salaries to worker salaries was 335 to 1. On the flip side, the poorest 50% of the population took home less than 10% of the total income. The current poverty level set by the federal government for a single person is roughly $12,000 per year, and for a family of two adults and two children, it is $24,000 per year. Under these guidelines, almost 15% of Americans live in poverty. And the situation is worsening over time; in the period 1950–2000 the gap between rich and poor in the USA has widened by almost 40% [11].

On a global basis, the picture is even more shocking. Half of the world's population (three billion people) have incomes less than US$10 per day.

Despite these inequities, one can still ask whether a *rise* in the GDP might actually lead to significant improvement in the personal happiness of individual citizens, regardless of their position on the totem pole. Is a rising GDP in any sense a proxy for a rising level of happiness in the populace? These are questions that have rankled economists for many years. Even Simon Kuznets in his 1934 speech to Congress felt impelled to warn the legislators that he didn't think that the welfare of the nation could be inferred from the GDP. By 1959, leading economists, like Stanford's Moses Abramovitz were being quoted as "highly skeptical" of the use of the GDP as a measure of society's overall wellbeing. In his book *The Progress Paradox*, Greg Easterbrook, a writer of popular books on social issues, reports that between 1950 and the present, the inflation-corrected annual GDP per capita has risen from less than $15,000 to more than $50,000, yet the average level of personally-reported happiness in the populace has remained remarkably steady, with 60% of us "happy" and 6–7% of us "very unhappy." [12] Moreover, during this same time frame, while GDP per capita rose, there were many signs of deteriorating community health. In 2004, Ed Diener and Martin Seligman, two psychologists who figured prominently in the previous chapter, made a widely-quoted foray into the economic literature entitled "Beyond Money: Toward an Economy of Well-Being." [13]. In that article, they pointed out that rates of clinical depression and anxiety in the U.S. have increased many fold in recent years. Trust in governmental institutions has fallen dramatically. Neighborhood cohesion has softened. Long-standing homilies like "helping one's neighbor" and "turning the other cheek" seem to have been replaced by the "me generation" with its emphasis on personal financial growth and material wealth.

On reflection, it seems pretty clear that national economic health, as reflected in the GDP, is just one facet of wellbeing, and attempting to use it as the sole indicator, or perhaps even the primary one, is inappropriate. In fact, the lack of correlation between increased income and increased happiness is sufficiently well-established that it has a name. It is called the *Easterlin paradox*, named after the UCLA economist, R.A. Easterlin, who first proposed it many years ago, and who has continued to develop the thesis over his career [14]. He recognized that in poorer countries, at the bottom end of the social hierarchy, there may still be a meaningful correlation, but in wealthier countries like the USA and Canada, and even in the poorer ones, once a minimum threshold has been reached that allows for adequate food and shelter, the paradox comes into play.

The diminishing returns of happiness that accompany increasing per capita income in the USA are well-documented [15]. It seems apparent that income *per se* does not drive happiness. If it did, then one might be able to make the argument that economic indicators are a suitable proxy for wellbeing, and that public policy need only direct its attention to increasing incomes. The fact that the correlation between wealth and happiness is so weak indicates the need for a broader suite of social indicators to capture all the necessary aspects of wellbeing. In a 2019 article, Alex Michalos and Maurine Hatch discount the impact of wealth and income on overall quality of life, and emphasize the importance of wants, needs, expectations, hopes, and experiences. They see quality of life as being controlled largely by the circumstances in which we live and what we make of them, with the latter strongly influenced by our perceptions, attitudes, beliefs, choices, actions, and all their attendant consequences [16]. Martin Seligman and Mihaly Czikszentmhalyi, in their seminal article outlining the tenets of the positive psychology movement, may have said it best. "The United States can continue to increase its material wealth while ignoring the human needs of its people and those of the rest of the planet. Such a course is likely to lead to increasing selfishness, to alienation between the more and less fortunate, and eventually to chaos and despair." [17].

Or as overconsumption activists David Batker and John De Graaf put it in the title of their book: "What's the Economy for Anyway? It's Time to Stop Chasing Growth and Start Pursuing Happiness." [18].

A Little History

Of course, these ideas did not just spring from a vacuum. The leading edge of the modern social indicators movement can be traced back to the 1960s, and there were even glimmers as far back as the 1930s. A little history is in order.

The 1960s were a time of social ferment in the United States. The assassinations of John F. Kennedy, Robert Kennedy, and Martin Luther King shocked the nation. The civil rights movement took its case into the south. Vietnam War protests escalated. And it was in this era of heightened awareness that strong voices were first heard decrying the fact that economic considerations were still being given what was felt to be undue priority in policy making. Edward Mishan, a British economist at the London School of Economics, published his book on *The Costs of Economic Growth* to academic acclaim in 1967 [19] and soon thereafter, the public learned of this perspective from The Club of Rome, an international think tank based at MIT, in their widely-read book on *The Limits to Growth*, which was billed as a report on the "predicaments of mankind." [20] In the 1964 presidential elections, Lyndon Johnson found common cause with the electorate in his promises of a "Great Society."

The question of what type of social indicators might be added to the existing economic indicators to create a more holistic measure of wellbeing depended to some degree on just what the concerns of the populace were that needed government attention. Fortunately, there were two studies published in the mid-60s that addressed exactly these issues. The first was a book published in 1965 by the Princeton psychologist, Hadley Cantril, titled *The Pattern of Human Concerns* [21]. Cantril was an early convert to the use of public-opinion polls of the type pioneered by George Gallup and Elmo Roper. It was his aim to appropriate these techniques for use in social psychology research. In his "Human Concerns" book, he used the burgeoning availability of polling results to identify strong correlations between individual wellbeing and widespread concerns about, yes, income, but also about education, health care, employment, and governance.

The second study came from an unexpected source. In the early 60s, the National Space and Aeronautics Administration set up a project to investigate the impact that the American space program might have on US society. The project director was Raymond A. Bauer of the Harvard Business School, and in 1966 he reported his results in a treatise that was simply titled *Social Indicators*. In it he argued that NASA's concerns were just the tip of the iceberg with respect to citizen concerns over governmental actions. He recommended that governments ought to be collecting social data, carrying out statistical analyses, and publishing the results in reports that could be easily-accessed and widely-used by policy decision-makers [22].

Interestingly, there had been precursors of these ideas as far back as the turn of the century. In the early 1900s the Russell Sage Foundation funded studies of housing and working conditions across the USA, and their reports used measures that look remarkably similar to some of the social indicators of today. The Russell Sage Foundation is still in operation out of its New York Headquarters, describing itself as "the principle American foundation devoted exclusively to research in the social sciences." The leaders of the foundation host a visiting scholars program and their own academic periodical, the RSF Journal.

In 1929, at the dawn of the Great Depression, President Herbert Hoover appointed a Research Committee on Social Trends, with William F. Ogburn, a University of Chicago sociologist, as Director. In 1933 Ogburn presented the findings of the committee in a report entitled *Recent Social Trends in the United States* [23]. It, too, provided an early blueprint for measuring social wellbeing, but for whatever reasons, the committee did not survive the 1936 election and their one and only report did not galvanize the social indicators movement at that time. Perhaps they laid the seeds, but if so, germination apparently required the more fertile soil of the 60s.

By the late 1960s, the idea that non-economic indicators might be needed to fully describe the wellbeing of the nation was beginning to percolate into economic thinking, thanks in large part to the work of two researchers at the Institute for Social Research at the University of Michigan, Frank M. Andrews and Stephen B. Withey. Their 1976 book, *Social Indicators of Well-Being*, was a major contribution to the assessment of the quality of life in America [24]. They argued for the use of social indicators to identify social problems that require action, and to prioritize government programs and public policies. They saw the need for both subjective "direct measures" of wellbeing, and "indirect" objective measures available in public databases.

Interest in social indicators also spread from its US roots into the international community. At the United Nations, the Department of Economic and Social Affairs had been putting out a report on the "world social situation" since 1952. Building on this groundwork, the UN set up a Research Institute for Social Development which published a report on *The Measurement of Levels of Living and Welfare* in 1970 [25]. All of these works had influence, but they did not lead to a full-fledged paradigm shift in the economic world. The GDP was still king, even though more and more economists saw that the crown did not fit very well.

Commodities and Capabilities

In the early 1980s, the brilliant Indian-born economist and future Nobel Prize winner, Amartya Sen, began his work on what has come to be known as the human development approach to wellbeing. He argued firstly that the GDP was flawed as a measure of wellbeing because it was based on production rather than consumption. While it might be a pertinent measure for industrial producers, it had little relevance to man-on-the-street consumers. For the latter, living standards are much more highly correlated with factors on the consumption side of the equation than on levels of industrial production.

Secondly, and related to the first point, he contended that measures of wellbeing ought to emphasise "capabilities" rather than "commodities." He argued that what really matters to people is their capability to live the life they value. To do so, they need to live a long and full life, have opportunities to develop their skills, and be able to participate in the economic and political life of their community. In this view, one's quality of life is determined more by "being" and "doing," than by "having." "Being" requires good health, strong social connections, and the development of self-esteem. "Doing" requires the freedom to engage in community affairs and work in a stimulating workplace. In Sen's eyes, poverty is nothing more than capability deprivation [26].

Martha Nussbaum, a professor of law and ethics at the University of Chicago, has outlined a list of ten core capabilities [27]. There is no question that her list includes many items that are not included in the calculation of economic measures of wellbeing; things like imagination, love, and freedom of expression. To some degree, her core capabilities can be seen as an updating of Maslow's "hierarchy of needs" presented back in Chapter Two.

In 2005, Paul Anand, an economist at Oxford University's Health Economics Research Centre in the UK, reported the results of a study designed to investigate whether capabilities can be measured, and if so, whether such measures would be useful in assessments of wellbeing. He and his coauthors conclude that the capabilities framework is a good fit for assessing quality of life and human wellbeing [28]. They estimate that a "dashboard" of 40 to 50 basic social indicators would be required to bring such an endeavour to fruition.

One of the issues that has arisen in the capabilities movement is whether it is feasible and/or desirable to try to integrate the various core capabilities into a single composite measure that might compete with the GDP, or whether it would be more defensible to leave the results as a dashboard of indicators. More defensible or not, most researchers in the field recognize the strong demands on the part of the public and the media for a single measure. Amartya Sen is part of this latter group, and it is for this reason that he played such a central role in helping the United Nations develop its Human Development Index. This index has become the most visible post-GDP composite index, and we will learn much more about it later in this book. Sen has described his creation as "an index as vulgar as the GDP, but more relevant to our lives."

Like so many of these paradigm-shifting advances, the *capabilities movement* has also developed its own internal cosmos. The Human Development and Capabilities Association was founded in 2005, and now publishes its own specialized journal, the Journal of Human Development and Capabilities.

A Revolution in Economics

Economics is a conservative enterprise. Change is resisted. Paradigm shifts come only under intense internal or external pressures. Yet, since the turn of the new millennium, a revolution has occurred in the staid world of economics [29]. Happiness has come to the "dismal science." Research on wellbeing, until recently the exclusive province of the positive psychology movement, has been spilling over into the research studies of economists. It simply became impossible for economists to ignore the findings of psychological research or to fail to incorporate these findings into their economic models. There is an ever-increasing cadre of economists and social scientists of many stripes, honing in on social indicators as a needed antidote to the sole reliance on traditional economic indicators. In academia, the new

Table 3.1 A sampling of academic research centers and private institutes that focus on the economics of wellbeing

	Name	Location
Academic Research Centers	Gund Institute for Ecological Economics	University of Vermont
	Well-Being Institute	Cambridge University, UK
	Centre for Economic Performance, Wellbeing Programme	London School of Economics, UK
	Institute for Social Research	University of Michigan
	Levy Economics Institute, Measure of Well-Being Program	Bard College, NY
	Happiness Economics Research Organization	Erasmus University, Netherlands
Private Institutes	Canadian Institute for Advanced Research, Program for Social Interactions, Identity, and Well-Being	Toronto, Canada
	Redefining Progress	San Francisco, CA and Washington, DC
	New Economics Foundation	London, UK
	Legatum Institute, Commission on Wellbeing and Policy	London, UK
	Organization for Economic Cooperation and Development (OECD), Better Life Initiative	Paris, France
	International Institute of Management	Las Vegas, NV
	Russell Sage Foundation Program in Behavioral Economics	New York, NY
	Alliance pour une Economie Responsible, Plurielle et Solidaire	France
	Happiness Alliance	Seattle, WA

economics has caught on big time. Most economics departments on campus now feature research teams that work on "happiness studies." Table 3.1 lists a few of the research centers and private institutes that focus on the economics of wellbeing. In 1974, a specialty journal on *Social Indicators Research* began publication. The editors describe it as "an international and interdisciplinary journal of quality-of-life measurement." There is also an International Society for Quality-of-Life Studies that puts out a quarterly newsletter called the Social Indicators Network News (SINET).

The primary message from the psychologists is that economic utility is not a good model for the assessment of wellbeing. In their view, the concept of utility needs to be imbued with more psychological insight. They have shown that people are not that good at predicting their future utility. In other words, they are not that good at predicting what will make them happy. They tend to overestimate the value of wealth and status, and underestimate the value of relationships with friends and family, the importance of workplace satisfaction, the desire for safety and security, and the benefits of good physical and mental health. In 2002, the psychologist Daniel Kahneman of Princeton University became the first non-economist to win the Nobel Prize in Economics, and he did so for his work that questioned many of the concepts inherent in classical utility theory.

Even indicators that appear at first glance to be economic in nature have costs and benefits that are not purely economic. Unemployment statistics, for example, are often viewed solely from the perspective of the business world, but such a viewpoint fails to capture the full social costs of unemployment in terms of the humiliation of the out-of-work breadwinner and the family chaos that results. Inflation rates have economic significance, but they also have social costs in the form of lost economic security for workers and their families. On the benefit side, there is value that does not appear on economic spreadsheets, in having purpose in life, in having opportunities for personal growth, and in gaining recognition and increased status from work well done. In the past, these types of social externalities were seldom taken into account in economic models.

The basic concept of an indicator variable was introduced back in Chapter One and examples of *economic* indicators appear in our news sources every day. So how do *social* indicators differ and what exactly do they look like? The dictionary definition identifies a social indicator as a numerical measure that describes the wellbeing of individuals or communities. A social indicator is seen as having three main uses: (1) to monitor changes over time in a broad range of social phenomena that extend beyond traditional economic matters and include indicators of wellbeing and quality of life, (2) to contribute to public enlightenment through social reporting both to the general public and policy makers, (3) to provide information for monitoring and evaluating public policy, searching for the common good, and deciding on how to reach it [30]. According to Judith Innes, an urban planning professor from Berkeley who has published widely on social indicators: "the measures must be pertinent to questions of concern; the concepts underlying the measures must be clear and agreed upon; the measure must relate to the concept which it is assumed to, and do so in a well-understood way; the methods to produce the measure must provide reliable results, measuring what they purport to without hidden or unexpected bias; and the measure must be understandable and understood in its concept and limitations." [31] Diener and Seligman, in their "Beyond Money" article, add the further proviso that social indicators ought to reflect both the big-picture facets of wellbeing such as life satisfaction, having purpose in life, engagement, and positive and negative emotions, and the more down-to-earth measures of wellbeing like work, health, family, community, and leisure [32].

Key National Indicators

The problem with all this should be obvious. There are just so many facets to the non-economic components of wellbeing that it is difficult to see how this material can be presented to the public in a way that competes with the simplicity of the

Dow-Jones or the GDP. It is highly unlikely that the media is going to publish regular easy-to-decipher statistics on all the relevant issues: the percentage of happy marriages, the level of trust in government institutions, the membership numbers in voluntary and charitable organizations, and so on.

Clearly, what is required is a single index that somehow integrates all these diverse threads into an easy-to-digest format. The United Nations Human Development Index mentioned above purports to do this, but as we will see in later chapters, its focus is very narrow, and in no way can it claim to cover the waterfront of non-economic social indicators.

There have been many public calls for the US government to get in the game. In 2000, Ed Deiner, who we met earlier in coverage of the positive psychology movement, was perhaps the first to call for a single-value national wellbeing index that would provide the necessary impact [33]. In 2004, Nobel prizewinner Daniel Kahneman jumped into the fray with a call for "national wellbeing accounts." [34] Then, as recently as 2012, two economists working at the John F. Kennedy School of Government at Harvard, Ben Beachy and Justin Zorn, prepared a report at the request of US Congressman Hansen Clarke, entitled "Twenty-First Century GDP: National Indicators for a New Era," that put it all very plainly. "The congress," they wrote, "should prescribe the broad parameters of new, carefully-designed supplemental national indicators. It should launch a bipartisan commission of experts to address unresolved methodological issues." [35] They placed this recommendation in the context of a proposed piece of legislation, never acted upon, which they called the "Twenty-First Century GDP Act."

It is not as if the US government has never done anything along these lines. Back in the early 1970s, the Office of Management and Budget started a program, later taken over by the Bureau of the Census, that eventually published three volumes in 1973, 1977 and 1980, all titled *Social Indicators: Selected Data on Social Conditions and Trends in the United States*. As early as 2003, the Government Accountability Office (GAO), the National Academy of Sciences (NAS), and the Congress began working together to create a non-profit, non-partisan agency that would "help all Americans assess the nation's progress for themselves, at all levels, with the best quality measures and data on the most important issues facing the nation." Then in 2007, the State of the USA Program was founded, with the charge to create a Key National Indicator System (KNIS). In 2010, Congress actually created a Commission on Key National Indicators, with the NAS in the lead role. The State of the USA Program and the KNIS Commission are funded, not by the government itself, but by prominent national foundations and private donors [36]. Studies are ongoing, but the dream of a full-bore government-sponsored wellbeing index to buttress the GDP remains elusive.

While the US government has been slow to act, other countries, Canada, Britain, Switzerland, and Australia among them, have developed national wellbeing indices. Bhutan is no longer alone.

There are also several indices sponsored by international agencies that are in various stages of development and use, among them the aforementioned United Nations Human Development Index, and the Better Life Index of the Organization of Economic Co-operation and Development (OECD). Then too there are the many indices developed by private institutions in the USA and elsewhere that would appear to at least partially meet the needs of a national index of wellbeing: The Gallup-Healthways Well-Being Index, The Happy Planet Index, the Genuine Progress Indicator, and many more. A full analysis of the strengths and weaknesses of such indices will be covered in the detailed treatment of nationwide wellbeing in Chapter Nine.

The Sarkozy Commission

In 2009, then-president Nicolas Sarkozy of France made a highly-publicized call for the nations of the world to develop alternatives to the GDP. He established a Commission on the Measurement of Economic Performance and Social Progress, chaired by Joseph Stiglitz of Columbia University, with a membership of 21 of the leading social scientists in the world, including Nobel Prize winners, Amartya Sen, Kenneth Arrow and Daniel Kahneman. The report that they produced had loud repercussions in the press around the world [37].

In their report, they likened those who are currently in charge of guiding the economies of the world to "pilots trying to steer a course without a reliable compass." They argued that reliance on GDP-like economic indicators fails to capture many phenomena that have an increasing impact on the wellbeing of citizens. Furthermore, they noted that such reliance does not reflect the newly-available access to data on many other fronts that has accompanied the development of the "information society." Their report called for a global "statistical system which goes beyond commercial activity to measure personal well-being," one that incorporates these recent advances in metrics.

Among the structural changes they identify in the evolution of modern economics is the growing share of the service sector: medical services, educational services, financial services, communication technologies, research activities, recreational support, and public housing, all of which contribute to higher living standards and are increasingly valued by citizens.

More specifically, in discussing the 2008 economic meltdown, they argue that had there been more awareness of the limitations of then-current metrics, there might have been less euphoria over the economic performance in the years prior to the crisis, and more recognition of the unsustainable levels of indebtedness that were growing in the personal lives of the citizenry.

In a critique of the Sarkozy Commission Report, Alex Michalos commended the authors for their clear recommendations to shift the emphasis in national accounting procedures from measuring economic production to measuring the well-being of the citizenry, but he chided them for their failure to link the requirements of an acceptable measure of well-being to those of an acceptable measure of sustainability. He was also disappointed that the Commission did not address the lack of coordination between academic researchers and government statistical offices, or make recommendations that would improve the situation [38].

Social Capital

There is another movement based primarily in economic circles that deserves our attention. It concerns the concept of *capital*. Most of us would define this term in the traditional way, as Webster does, as "the value of a stock of accumulated goods, especially at a specified time, and in contrast to income received during a specified period." [39] In other words, it is our *income* that allows us to save money, and to buy and stockpile goods, but the money and goods themselves represent our capital, or in more common parlance, our *wealth*. The question arises whether there are more components to wealth than just money and goods? It seems that there are, because another common definition of capital holds that it is wealth in the form of money *or other assets* owned by a person or organization. It is these other assets that interest us here.

In fact, the modern social indicators movement identifies at least five different types of capital [40]. *Manufactured capital* (material goods and fixed assets) and *financial capital* (in the form of shares, bonds and money) represent the two traditional types of capital. The newer boys on the block are *natural capital*, which reflects the value to society of a healthy environment and the renewable and non-renewable resources contained therein; *human capital*, which recognizes the value of peoples' knowledge, skills, motivation, and health; and *social capital*, which values the institutions that help develop and maintain human capital in the family, the workplace, and the community.

It is the last of these that has especially caught the attention of the social indicators movement, largely under the influence of Robert Putnam, a professor of public policy at Harvard University, whose book, *Bowling Alone: The Collapse and Revival of American Community*, published in 2000, was an influential best-seller [41]. Putnam defined social capital as "a form of economic and cultural capital in which social networks are central; transactions are marked by reciprocity, trust and cooperation; and market agents produce goods and services not mainly for themselves but for a common good." The accumulation of social capital is marked by a set of mental dispositions and attitudes that favor cooperative behavior within society, and which can lead to an improvement of living conditions for the whole community. The primary premise is that social networks have value, and that social capital is built up through participation in networks of friends, neighborhood activities, church and school involvement, membership in clubs and organizations, and civic engagement. The ideas have much in common with a parallel movement that promotes a *civil society*. Clearly, the concepts of social capital and a civil society have much to do with individual and societal happiness and wellbeing.

The greatest weakness in the concept of social capital is probably the absence of consensus on how to measure it. Critics recognize the concept as a "remarkably productive idea" but find it too soft and fuzzy, and used in so many multicultural contexts that it defies meaningful measurement [42]. Putnam himself recommended a 14-item social capital index based on public polling of peoples' levels of networking, civic engagement, organizational activities, and attitudes toward trust and reciprocity in the marketplace. Under Putnam's leadership, a "Saguaro Seminar" of the John F. Kennedy School of Government at Harvard engaged the Roper Center for Public Opinion Research to carry out two Social Capital Community Benchmark Surveys in 2000 and 2006 to gauge the level of social capital in America. Comparison of the two sets of results revealed a decline in membership in service clubs, declining church attendance, and an overall decline in social capital [43].

Emphasis in the social indicators literature has always been on the positive contributions of social capital, but dissidents have recognized many potential negative aspects, sufficiently so that a 2010 special issue of the journal *American Behavioral Scientist* was dedicated entirely to the examination of this "dark side." The consensus is that networking probably always produces positive value for the individual, but not necessarily for society as a whole. Consider for example "families" of criminal activity, or groups that promote political cleavages or religious intolerance. Among the possible downsides of many so-called old-boy networks are the exclusion of outsiders, and the maintenance of long-standing inequalities [44].

The accepted bottom line seems to be that the concept of social capital is an intriguing integration of sociology and economics. There are several non-profit organizations that try to spread the word (Social Capital Foundation, Social Capital, Inc., among others). The World Bank has issued "a multidisciplinary toolbox for practitioners." [45] The Organization for Economic Co-Operation and Development sponsored an international conference on the subject [46]. These various groups all argue that social capital is not just about warm and cuddly feelings but also about tangible benefits (and perhaps some costs as well) that accrue to individuals and societies. The concept has proven useful in the assessment of educational achievement, health outcomes, time use statistics, the growth of feminism, and geographical differences in happiness [47].

The Dissenters

Not all social scientists have jumped on the happiness bandwagon. Dissenters come in many stripes. If we try to classify the several streams of non-belief, there seem to be at least five avenues of resistance: the Big Brother argument, the General Bullmoose argument, the political bias argument, the evolutionary argument, and the pure-and-simple backlash to what is seen as just the latest fad.

The Big Brother argument has been made most strikingly by the contrarian blogger and journalist, Brendan O'Neill [48]. He claims that the politics of happiness is usually promoted by authoritarian regimes. He refers to the Communist posters of the Stalin era: "Glory to the Great Stalin: Constructor of Happiness." And former North Korean leader Kim Il Sung's promise "to ensure the prosperity of the motherland and the happiness of the people." He sees such regimes as seeking a placid, sedate populace, whose leaders use pseudo-scientific measurements of national wellbeing to prove that their subjects are "happy."

The General Bullmoose argument is made in the title of a book by the political economist, William Davies: "The Happiness Industry: How the Government and Big Business Sold Us Well-Being." [49]. He sees the happiness movement less as a science and more as an extension of hyper-capitalism. In his view, it has much to do with corporate interests and little to do with personal fulfillment. In support of this view, he cites the use of happiness research to develop strategies for businesses to get the most out of their already-overtaxed workers. He decries the increased surveillance of every nook and cranny of our lives that is inherent in the polling and data-gathering aspects of the social indicator movement.

The issue of political bias has been raised by Clifford Cobb, who is an otherwise firm supporter of the new economics. His thoughts appeared in a widely-circulated report put out by the San Francisco think-tank Redefining Progress in 2000. Redefining Progress is no longer extant, but it was an early participant in the social indicator movement. In the report, Cobb states that the ideological underpinnings of social indicators cannot be argued away. He sees social indicators as "moral statistics" that offer a "means of entering political debate over contentious issues," and that usually promote a particular vision of the good society. He notes that "even the driest and most statistical work has a value orientation," and that the very collection of a particular suite of data is an "implicit defense of the mission of the agency that collects them." In his opinion, social indicators cannot stand above the fray. They are politically relevant, and represent a commitment to a set of ideals [50].

The evolution argument has been made by the noted Harvard linguist, Steven Pinker. His point is that enduring satisfaction and permanent contentment, which seem to be the goals of the happiness movement, are not conducive to the survival of the species. He argues that under the tenets of natural selection: "It is in our interest, and in our genes to strive for more." [51] Erik Wilson, a professor of English Literature at Wake Forest University, seems to agree. In his book, "Against Happiness: In Praise of Melancholy," he holds that it is *unhappiness* that acts as the muse of great literature, art and music. He urges us to "throw off the shackles of positivity, and relish the blues that make us human." [52].

The backlash against the happiness movement comes largely against its self-help wing. In her book, "Self-Help, Inc.," the Fordham University sociologist, Micki McGee, sees happiness therapy as a worthless fad. She argues that the constant striving for happiness, and the incessant pressure to self-improve, is leading to much social dissatisfaction and societal stress [53].

Economics As If People Mattered

To put matters of this section into perspective, we turn to two of the most influential economists of all time, each one as different from the other as they could possibly be in terms of time and place, but perhaps brothers-in-arms for all that.

Adam Smith is, of course, the father of free-market capitalism, the author of the 1776 treatise on *The Wealth of Nations* that most economists accept as the founding bible of their field. Many of the basic ideas of economic thought have their birth in Adam Smith's work, and to some degree it is these ideas that are being re-examined and found wanting in the modern social indicators movement. It may therefore come as a bit of a surprise that Adam Smith himself held some of the same doubts. We are indebted to Russ Roberts, a Hoover Foundation economist at Stanford University, for rediscovering Adam Smith's other grand opus. In *The Theory of Moral Sentiments*, the patron saint of capitalism lays out the other side of the equation [54]. He differentiates between economic self-interest and economics in support of the greater good. He presents a system of moral thought which praises human values like sympathy, virtue, conscience, and the making of moral judgements. Not only that, but he specifically gives greater value to the respect of family and friends than to the pursuit of fame and fortune. It could be maintained that the traditional arguments, which place self-interest at the center of all economic decisions, and the revisionist arguments that rely on a more holistic approach, may have both emerged together, but unfortunately, only half the story was heard.

E.F. Schumacher, in contradistinction to Adam Smith, was a little-known economist working in relative obscurity as an advisor to the British National Coal Board when he burst onto the public radar with a fiercely-argued and elegantly-written screed against the economic status quo. His book, *Small is Beautiful: Economics As If People Mattered,* was published in 1973 and has been in print ever since [55]. It is best to let Schumacher speak for himself. "What is the meaning of democracy, freedom, human dignity, standard of living, self-realization, fulfilment?" he asks. "If economic thinking cannot get beyond its vast abstractions, the national income, the rate of growth, capital/output ratio, input-output analysis, labour mobility, capital accumulation; if it cannot get beyond all this and make contact with the human realities of poverty, frustration, alienation, despair, breakdown, crime, escapism, stress, congestion, ugliness, and spiritual death, then let us scrap economics and start afresh."

He was on the environmental bandwagon long before there was a bandwagon: "We find, therefore, that the idea of unlimited economic growth, more and more until everybody is saturated with wealth, needs to be seriously questioned on at least two counts: the availability of basic resources, and alternatively or additionally, the capacity of the environment to cope with the degree of interference implied."

The then-current economic thinking, he argued in a final salvo, is based on "a procedure by which the higher is reduced to the level of the lower and the priceless is given a price.... All it can do is lead to self-deception and the deception of others. . . .What is worse, and destructive of civilization, is the pretence that . . . money is the highest of all values."

References

1. Karabell, Zachary, *The Leading Indicators: A Short History of the Numbers that Rule Our World*, Simon and Schuster, 2014; Rogers, R. Mark, *Handbook of Key Economic Indicators*, McGraw Hill, 1998.
2. [foreignpolicy.com/gdp-a-brief-history]
3. Business Encyclopedia. *Gross Domestic Product GDP, Gross National Product GNP, and Gross National Income GNI, Explained*. [www.business-case-analysis.com/gross-domestic-product.html]
4. Friedman, Benjamin, *The Moral Consequences of Economic Growth*, Knopf, 2005.
5. Waring, Marilyn, *If Women Counted: A New Feminist Economics*, Harper and Row, 1988.
6. [www.bea.gov]
7. [www.worldbank.org/en/programs/icp]
8. [cid.econ.ucdavis.edu/pwt.html]
9. Constable, Simon and Robert E. Wright, *Wall Street Journal Guide to Fifty Economic Indicators that Really Matter*, Harper Business, 2011.
10. Definitions of the five semi-serious economic indicators described in these two paragraphs can be found at [www.investopedia.com] and [www.raptureready.com].
11. Firebaugh, Glenn, Inequality: What it is and how it is measured, *The New Geography of Global Income Inequality*, Harvard University Press, 2003; Okulicz-Kozaryn, A. and J.M. Mazelis, More unequal in income, more unequal in wellbeing, *Social Indicators Research*, 132(3), 953-975, 2017. See also [www.inequality.org].
12. Easterbrook, Gregg, *The Progress Paradox: How Life gets Better While People Feel Worse*, Random House, 2003.
13. Diener, E. and M.E.P Seligman, Beyond money: Toward an economy of well-being, *Psychological Science in the Public Interest*, 5(1), 3-31, 2004
14. Easterlin, R.A., Explaining happiness, *Proc. National Academy Sciences*, 100, 11176-11183, 2003.
15. Frey, B.S. and A. Stutzer, *Happiness and Economics: How the Economy and Institutions Affect Human Well-Being*, Princeton University Press, 2002; Helliwell, J.F., How's life? Combining individual and national variables to explain subjective well-being, *Economic Modeling*, 20, 331-360, 2003.
16. Michalos, A.C. and P.M. Hatch, Good societies, financial inequality and secrecy, and a good life: from Aristotle to Piketty, *Applied Research in Quality of Life,* 15(4), 1005-1054, 2020.
17. Seligman, Martin E.P. and M. Czikszentmihalyi, Positive psychology: An introduction, *American Psychologist*, 55(1),5-14, 2000.
18. Batker, David K. And John de Graaf, *What's the Economy for Anyway? Its Time to Stop Chasing Growth and Start Pursuing Happiness*, Bloomsburg Press, 2011.
19. Mishan, Edward J., *The Costs of Economic Growth*, Staples Press, 1967.
20. Meadows, D.H., D.L. Meadows, J. Randers and W.W. Behrens III, *The Limits to Growth: A Report for the Club of Rome's Project on the Predicament of Mankind*, Universe Books, 1972.
21. Cantril, Hadley, *The Pattern of Human Concerns*, Rutgers University Press, 1965.
22. Bauer, Raymond A., ed., *Social Indicators*, MIT Press, 1966.
23. Ogburn, W.F, *Recent Social Trends in the United States*, President's Committee on Social Trends, 1933; as described in Cobb, Clifford W. and Craig Rixford, *Lessons Learned from the History of Social Indicators*, Redefining Progress, 1998.

24. Andrews, Frank M. And Stephen B. Withey, *Social Indicators of Well-Being*, Plenum Press, 1976. See also: Campbell, A., P.E. Converse and W.I. Rodgers, *The Quality of American Life*, Russell Sage Foundation, 1976.
25. Drewnowski, Jan, *Studies in the Measurement of Levels of Living and Welfare*, United Nations Research Institute for Social Development, Report No 70.3, 1970.
26. Sen, A., *Commodities and Capabilities*, North-Holland/Elsevier, 1985; Sen, A., *Development as Freedom*, Oxford University Press, 2001.
27. Nussbaum, M., *Creating Capabilities: The Human Development Approach*, Harvard University Press, 2011. See also [en.wikipedia.org/wiki/Capability_approach]
28. Anand, Paul, G. Hunter and R. Smith, Capabilities and well-being: Evidence based on the Sen-Nussbaum approach to welfare, *Social Indicators Research*, 74(1), 9-55, 2005.
29. Frey, Bruno, *Happiness: A Revolution in Economics*, MIT Press, 2008; Bruni, L. and P.L. Porta, eds., *Handbook on the Economics of Happiness*, Edward Elgar Publishers, 2007; Weimann, J., A. Knabe and R. Schob, *Measuring Happiness: the Economics of Well-Being*, MIT Press, 2015.
30. [wikiprogress.org]
31. Innes, Judith E., *Knowledge and Public Policy: The Search for Meaningful Indicators*, Transactions Books, 1990.
32. Diener and Seligman, 2004, op. cit.
33. Diener, E., Subjective well-being: The science of happiness, and a proposal for a national index, *American Psychologist*, 55, 34-43, 2000; Diener, E., Guidelines for national indicators of subjective well-being and ill-being, *Journal of Happiness Studies*, 7(4), 397-404, 2005.
34. Kahneman, D. et al., Toward national well-being accounts, *American Economic Review*, 94(2), 429-434, 2004. See also: Pesto, B.J., M.A. McDaniel and S. Bertsch, Toward an index of well-being for the fifty U.S. states, *Intelligence*, 38(1), 160-168, 2010; and Antolini, F., The evolution of national accounting and new statistical information: Happiness and GDP: Can we measure it?, *Social Indicators Research*, 129(3), 1075-1092, 2016.
35. Beachy, B. and J. Zorn, *Twenty-First Century GDP: National Indicators for a New Era*, John F. Kennedy School of Government, Harvard University, 2012. [www.hks.harvard.edu]
36. [www.stateoftheusa.org]
37. Stiglitz, J.E., Amartya Sen and J-P Fitoussi, *Report by the Commission on the Measurement of Economic Performance and Social Progress*, 2009.
38. Michalos, A.C., What did Stiglitz, Sen and Fitoussi get right and what did they get wrong?, *Social Indicators Research*, 102(1), 117-129, 2011.
39. Webster's New Collegiate Dictionary
40. [www.forumforthefuture.org]
41. Putnam, Robert, *Bowling Alone: the Collapse and Revival of American Community*, Simon and Schuster, 2000.
42. Bjornskov, C. and K.M. Sanderskov, Is social capital a good concept?, *Social Indicators Research*, 114(3), 1225-1242, 2013.
43. [https://ropercenter.cornell.edu/2006-social-capital-community-benchmark-survey/]
44. *American Behavioral Scientist*, 53(5), 2010.
45. Grootaert, C. and T. Van Bastelaer, *Understanding and Measuring Social Capital: A Multidisciplinary Tool for Practitioners*, World Bank, 2002.
46. OECD, *The Well-Being of Nations: The Role of Human and Social Capital*, 2001.
47. Lin, N., *Social Capital*, Cambridge University Press, 2001.
48. O'Neill, Brendan, *Vancouver Sun*, April 15, 2011. Also available at [brendanoneill.co.uk/post/i-am-standing-up-for-the-right-to-be-unhappy]
49. Davies, William, *The Happiness Industry: How the Government and Big Business Sold Us Well-Being*, Verso, 2015.
50. Cobb, Clifford W., *Measurement Tools and the Quality of Life*, Redefining Progress, 2000.
51. Pinker, Steven, *How the Mind Works*, W.W. Norton, 1997.

52. Wilson, Erik G., *Against Happiness: In Praise of Melancholy*, Sarah Crichton Books, 2008. See also: Norem, Julie, *The Positive Power of Negative Thinking*, Basic Books, 2002; Burkman, Oliver, *The Antidote: Happiness for People Who Can't Stand Positive Thinking*, Penguin, 2013.
53. McGee, Micki, *Self-Help, Inc., Makeover Culture in American Life*, Oxford University Press, 2005. See also: Salerno, Steve, *SHAM: How the Self-Help Movement Made America Helpless*, Crown Forum, 2006; and Burnett, Simon, *The Happiness Agenda: A Modern Obsession*, Palgrave, 2012.
54. Roberts, Russ, *How Adam Smith Can Change Your Life*, Portfolio, 2014; Smith, Adam, *The Theory of Moral Sentiments*, Penguin Classics, 2010. (Reprint of original publication of 1759.)
55. Schumacher, E.F., *Small Is Beautiful, Economics As If People Mattered*, Harper and Row, 1973.

Chapter 4
The Sustainability Movement

The Environmental Externalities

Of all the externalities that are not considered by purely-economic indicators, it is the environmental ones that seem to rankle most. It is now widely accepted that there is a need to include the negative impacts of climate change, environmental degradation, and resource depletion in assessments of national wellbeing, and to develop socio-economic policies that will minimize these impacts. Lester Brown, pioneering environmentalist, founder of the Earth Policy Institute, and president of the Worldwatch Institute, has argued forcefully in his many books and publications that a global economy shaped solely by market forces fails to reflect the true costs of goods and services, and that it leads to an economy that is out of sync with the earth's ecosystem, thus destroying its own natural support system [1]. He has tried to convince policy makers that nothing less than an Environmental Revolution is needed, a paradigm shift that has an impact on society comparable to that engendered by the Agricultural Revolution and the Industrial Revolution in their day.

This viewpoint is affirmed by Bill McKibbon, the environmental author, and founder of the activist climate-change organization, 350.org, who writes that "a single-minded focus on increasing wealth has driven the planet's ecological systems to the brink of failure, without making us happier." [2] What is needed, both Brown and McKibbon argue, is an economic system that maintains and improves *both* human wellbeing and ecosystem wellbeing, not one at the expense of the other.

Yet, it must be recognized that there is something different in kind about the concerns we have about environmental matters, relative to the ones we have about the economy itself, or even those we have about the social fabric. Economic worries might involve such bottom-line issues as job security or rising home prices. Social worries might involve close-to-home issues like marriage breakdown or the availability of medical care. Economic and social indicators therefore tend to measure aspects of life that bear directly on personal happiness and wellbeing. The costs of a degrading environment are at best, once-removed. They are eudaimonic rather than

R. A. Freeze, *The Metrics of Happiness*, Social Indicators Research Series 86,
https://doi.org/10.1007/978-3-031-10913-3_4

hedonic, and they have more relevance to long-term communal wellbeing than to short-term personal happiness. Protection of the environment would seem to fit into the equation of wellbeing in the same way that charitable giving and volunteerism do, providing the deep-seated satisfaction that comes from contributing to the common good, rather than a jolt of immediate joy.

Of course, environmental externalities are not all negative. There are positive benefits to mankind in maintaining a healthy ecosystem. Many environmentalists do not accept the once-removed argument and instead draw a direct connection between the overall ecological health of the planet and the personal happiness of individuals. Such a position can certainly be supported by the pleasures of hiking, the joy that species diversity brings to nature lovers, or the rewards of family bonding on a back-to-nature vacation in one of our National Parks. There is also positive value in the availability of clean water to drink and fresh air to breathe. Furthermore, a clean and aesthetically-pleasing environment in which to live is conducive to positive states of physical and mental health. So, we can identify two strands of the environmental ethic; one in which ecosystem wellbeing has value on its own, and a second where the maintenance of the ecosystem has value because it contributes to human wellbeing. Whichever we choose, any set of meaningful environmental indicators will have to pay attention not only to the negative costs of environmental degradation but also to the positive benefits of environmental health.

Even if we accept the premise that a healthy environment brings much benefit to the current generation, it is still likely that the greatest value of environmental protection is not for those of us living today but for the benefit of future generations. Surely there is worth to a society to act as responsible stewards of the environment for our progeny. In fact, it can be argued that doing so is little different than passing on a healthy economic position to the next generation. And on that score, our current generation of voters, taxpayers, and legislators has not set a very good example. The growth of governmental debt, and the costs of servicing it, are routinely identified as a negative draw on the economic component of wellbeing. So, too, is the loss of environmental capital inherent in environmental degradation.

Sustainable Development

In the 1980s, a new catchphrase arrived on the socioeconomic horizon. It was in 1983 that the United Nations General Assembly asked Bro Harlem Brundtland, a former (and future) Prime Minister of Norway, to chair the World Commission on Environment and Development. The Commission produced its report in 1987 under the title, *Our Common Future* [3]. In that report, emphasis was placed on the fostering of a global economy that features *sustainable development*. The Brundtland report defined the term as "development that meets the needs of the present without compromising the ability of future generations to meet their own needs."

The Brundtland report led to the UN Conference on Environment and Development in Rio de Janeiro in 1992, commonly known as the first Earth Summit, where an action plan identified as Agenda 21 (for the twenty-first century) was laid out. This in turn led to the Millennium Summit in 2000, the World Summit on Sustainable Development in 2002, and eventually to a second Rio summit in 2012 where a series of Sustainable Development Goals (SDGs) were announced. The third listed goal (after "No Poverty," and "Zero Hunger") was "To Promote Good Health and Well-being for All."

The members of the Brundtland Commission were not the first to think about sustainability. As early as 1973, the ecovisionary, Herman Daly, now at the School of Public Policy at the University of Maryland, had been talking about something similar. His book *Toward a Steady State Economy* was among the first to question the viability of endless economic growth [4]. He defined a steady-state economy as one that has the ability to continue on a defined course indefinitely without depleting the planet's environmental capital. From 1988 to 1994 he labored valiantly in the stuffy confines of the World Bank, trying with limited success to get that organization onto the growing bandwagon of sustainable development. His 1996 book, *Beyond Growth: The Economics of Sustainable Development* remains a bible of the sustainability movement [5].

Daly's golden rules for his steady-state economy were as follows. For renewable resources, the rate of harvest should not exceed the rate of regeneration. For non-renewable resources, the rate of depletion should not exceed the rate of development of comparable renewable substitutes. And for pollution, the rates of waste generation should not exceed the assimilative capacity of the environment. Whether or not these mantras are attainable or not, they do represent desirable targets that can form the basis of meaningful environmental indicators.

Ecological Economics and Environmental Economics

The terms *ecological economics* and *environmental economics* sound like synonyms, but as we shall see in the next few paragraphs, that is not quite so. Both these terms involve attempts to couple human economics and natural ecosystems. The differences lie in whether the coupling is seen as bringing economic thought into a fundamentally ecologic view of the world; or bringing ecological thought into a fundamentally economic view of the world.

The foundational concept of *ecological economics* emphasizes the role that a healthy environment plays in allowing a productive economy to thrive. It is the ecology-centered version of the coupling. Courses in ecological economics are usually taught by economists based in environmental departments rather than traditional economics departments. In their world view, one of the reasons for protecting the terrasphere, the hydrosphere, the atmosphere, and the biosphere from degradation lies in the need to maintain the production of the goods and services that drives our economy. Agricultural land must be defended and soil fertility preserved in order to ensure adequate grain and vegetable production. Grazing lands must be protected against overuse to ensure the viability of meat production. Sustainable forestry is needed to ensure a continued supply of wood for construction. Pumping of groundwater at rates greater than the available safe yield of aquifers must be discouraged in order to guarantee long-term water supplies for both domestic use and in manufacturing processes. Contamination of water from manufacturing processes must be brought under control before the costs of remediation exceed the costs of production. Air pollution must be controlled to avoid runaway respiratory health care costs. The true costs of the various energy alternatives must be weighed, taking into consideration their full fuel cycles from extraction to waste disposal. Environmentalism is not just a fad for activists. It is an important and necessary aspect of the world economy. Healthy ecosystems are necessary for both the short-term functioning of the economy and the long-term survival of the human race.

On the other side of the coin, the environmental awakening of the 1960s and 1970s did not go unnoticed by mainstream economists. Many traditional university economics departments began offering courses and programs in what came to be known as *environmental economics*. However, this new sub-discipline did not fully escape its traditional moorings. According to the ecological economists, the environmental economists recognize the importance of environmental health, but they still tend to treat it as an economic good, a capital asset that can be assessed with traditional supply/demand theories. The ecological economists reject this monetarization of the earth's natural capital. They feel that traditional economic theories see the environment as simply one aspect of the economy, whereas they see the economy as just one aspect of the environment. In their view, the economy ought to be seen as embedded within the environmental system. Their philosophy emphasizes the earth's limited carrying capacity; it sees the value in preserving natural resources; it encourages the development of alternative energy sources, ecologically-integrated technologies, and sustainable agriculture; but all of this as an unarguable social good in its own right, not just as a term in a market-based economic analysis.

Ecological economists reject the utilitarian framework of traditional economic theory whereas environmental economists try to work within it. In the latter view, "intangible amenities such as a crime-free neighborhood, breathable air, or even the comfort that comes from knowing that fewer people are homeless . . . can still be easily understood within the framework of utilitarian theory." The ecological economists, on the other hand, feel that there are "many spheres of action (politics, public rituals, family, school, work, and elsewhere) that should be judged by a different set of norms and should be treated as incommensurable with the others." [6] These internecine disagreements probably seem somewhat anal to the non-academic, and indeed, like many of the other distinctions that have been drawn earlier, this one also has fuzzy boundaries. There is much crossover between the two groups and many economists are comfortable keeping one foot in each camp.

Both ecological and environmental economists favor the *precautionary principle*, which counsels caution in the face of uncertainty. If an activity raises threats of serious or irreversible environmental harm, precautionary measures should be taken even if the cause and effect relationships are not fully established. A lack of full scientific certainty shall not be used as a reason for postponing cost-effective measures to prevent irreversible environmental degradation. Or as mother used to say: "Better safe than sorry," and "Look before you leap."

Both groups also have much to say to consumers. McKibbon rails against what he calls "Wal-Mart Nation," the world of gigantic, globalized retailers who keep prices down by spending social and environmental capital. He favors a "Farmer's Market Nation" that features local, communitarian shops calibrated to human scale. This school of thought also recommends the support of green technologies, the development and use of renewable energy sources, the avoidance of overconsumption, and the practice of ethical consumerism. It is their contention that such eudaimonic actions lead to personal satisfaction and the wellbeing of society.

Lester Brown foresees an "eco-economic future" that will feature a slow but steady transition to an environmentally-sustainable and socially-just society. The purpose of the State of the World reports put out by his Worldwatch Institute, he says, is to inspire people to demand new policies, investment patterns, and lifestyle choices. He sees the cities of the future powered by solar cells and wind turbines, bicycle- and pedestrian-friendly, with rail-centered transport systems. He envisions smaller families, better health care, and reductions in per-capita consumption that lead to concomitant reductions in obesity, debt, time pressures, and the degradation of the environment [7].

Sustainable development and ecological economics now represent thriving new sub-genres in the economic community. Table 4.1 lists a sampling of research programs and private think tanks that emphasize ecological economics and/or sustainable development. An International Society for Ecological Economics was formed in 1989, with branches in Europe, Russia, Latin America, Australia/New-Zealand, Canada, India and the USA. The journal of the Society, *Ecological Economics*, promises to integrate "nature's household" (the environment) and "humankind's household" (the economy). There is also an International Society of Sustainable Professionals, and a phalanx of specialty journals that includes *Environment, Development and Sustainability,* the *Journal of Industrial Ecology,* and *Human Ecology Review*.

The Three Pillars

In the Brundtland Commission report, the authors placed the attainment of a sustainable-development ethos under the umbrella of *three pillars*: economic development, social development, and environmental protection; or more pithily, Prosperity, People, and Planet.

In all the subsequent efforts at international cooperation sponsored by the United Nations on this front - the Summits, Agenda 21, and the designation of the Sustainable Development Goals - the three pillars remained the rock on which further plans were built.

Table 4.1 A sampling of academic research centers and private institutes that focus on sustainable development and/or ecological economics

	Name	Location
Academic Research Centers	Earth Institute	Columbia University
	Green Economics Institute	Oxford University
	Sustainability Institute	Penn State University
	Bainbridge Graduate Institute	Seattle, WA
Private Institutes	Beijer Institute of Ecological Economics	Stockholm, Sweden
	Earth Economics	Tacoma, WA
	Worldwatch Institute	Washington, DC
	Third Way	Washington, DC
	International Institute for Environment and Development	London, UK
	International Institute for Sustainable Development	Winnipeg, MN, Canada
	Center for the Advancement of the Steady State Economy	Arlington, VA
	New Economics Foundation	London, UK
	Resources for the Future	Washington, DC
	Center for Sustainable Economy	Washington, DC
	Donella Meadows Institute	Norwich, VT
	SustainAsia	Hong Kong
	EcoSTEPS	Australia
	Center for Sustainable Production	Chile
	The Natural Step	New Zealand
	The Sustainability Consortium	USA
	Global Footprint Network	Oakland, CA
	Sustainable Scale Project	Lynden, ON, Canada

This triple bottom line of economy, society, and environment also forms a reasonable starting point for the consideration of the role of sustainability in the assessment of human wellbeing. It is clear that neither the Dow-Jones average nor the GDP model of wellbeing takes into consideration either of the two non-economic pillars. What seems clearer now than it did 30 years ago, or even 10 years ago, is that the unbridled pursuit of higher income, and the unprecedented accumulation of material wealth, has come at the expense of declining social and environmental capital. These losses directly affect our long-term wellbeing, and even our more-transitory happiness. Measures of wellbeing and happiness must include consideration of the social and environmental pillars as well as the economic.

On the social front, we have already seen in the earlier chapters that measures of wellbeing need to include the value of strong supportive relationships with family, friends, and colleagues. They need to include more meaningful consideration of quality-of-life indicators that reflect levels of workplace satisfaction, safety and security, and physical and mental health. They need to address issues of social justice and the societal rewards of ethical behavior. Part II of this book is rife with indicators and indexes that reflect the importance of the many aspects of the social development pillar.

On the environmental front, there are a host of issues that require consideration in any holistic assessment of societal wellbeing. Measurements are needed that track the path of climate change, the emission of greenhouse gases, the growth of population, air and water quality, biodiversity, energy consumption, disaster prevention, resource depletion, and many other measures of environmental health or degradation.

The question is how to select a meaningful set of environmental indicators. Take water quality, for example. Are we going to zero in on groundwater contamination, lake eutrophication, streamflow quality, ocean dumping, waste disposal practices, recycling percentages, pesticide use, and so on, one item at a time, or are we going to search for measures that integrate these widely-diverse issues in some sense? The assessment of resource depletion, as another example, would require indicators that reflect the sustainability of forest resources, fish stocks, agricultural production, and mining activity. Data for such indicators would have to come from a widely-disparate suite of sources.

In Chap. 8 we will look at some of the indexes that have been developed to chart environmental health or degradation. Some of them, like the Water Poverty Index, deal with just one aspect of the broad environmental spectrum, while others, like the Environmental Performance Index try to integrate all the environmental threads into a single number. Each of these indexes may utilize many individual environmental indicators. The Water Poverty Index, for example, considers five different measures; the Environmental Performance Index uses 16.

The Bellagio Principles

In November 1996, a group of sustainability experts met at a resort hotel in Bellagio, Italy, sponsored by the International Institute for Sustainable Development, an environmental think tank based in Winnipeg, Canada. The meeting was funded in part by the Rockefeller Foundation, and participants were there by invitation only. The purpose of the meeting was "to review progress toward achieving sustainability and to synthesize insights from practical ongoing efforts." One of the exercises, carried out by a subcommittee of 24 sustainability mavens from 13 countries, was to develop a set of principles, or guidelines, for assessing the world's progress toward a sustainable future [8]. Their guidelines are reproduced here as Table 4.2. Even a cursory perusal of the table suggests that they have relevance not just to sustainability but also to human-wellbeing as a whole.

Many of the points that appear on the table have already been made. The two bullets under "Holistic Perspective," for example, reiterate the three pillars, and the

Table 4.2 The Bellagio Principles: Guidelines for practical assessment of progress toward sustainability. (Adapted from the source material listed in [8])

Guiding vision	• Be guided by a clear vision and goals
Holistic perspective	• Consider the wellbeing of human, ecological, and economic subsystems, their component parts, and the interactions between parts • Consider both positive and negative impacts of human activity in a way that reflects the full costs and benefits to human and ecological systems, in monetary and non-monetary terms
Essential elements	• Consider equity and disparity within the current population, and between current and future generations • Include consideration of economic development that contributes to social wellbeing • Include consideration of the ecological conditions on which life depends
Adequate scope	• Adopt a time horizon that is long enough to capture both human and ecosystem time scales • Define a large enough scale of study to include both local and long-distance impacts on people and ecosystems • Build on historic and current conditions to anticipate future conditions
Practical focus	• Use an organizing framework with an explicit set of categories • Use a limited number of well-defined indicators and indices in each category • Be sure that results are related to targets, reference values, ranges, thresholds, and trends
Openness	• Make the methods, data and results accessible to all • Make explicit all assumptions and uncertainties in data and interpretation
Effective communication	• Aim for simplicity and use of clear, plain language • Design studies to meet the needs of anticipated users
Broad participation	• Grass-roots, social, professional and technical representation
Ongoing assessment	• Capacity for repeated measurements • Iterative and adaptive ability to adjust goals, framework, and indicators in response to complex, changing systems • Promote collective learning and feedback
Institutional capacity	• Ongoing support for data collection, maintenance and documentation

need to consider both positive and negative valuations of environmental capital. Among the "Essential Elements" is the need to consider inequalities within the current population, and between current and future generations. The recommendation under "Practical Focus" to use an organizing framework that includes explicit and well-defined categories, indexes, and indicators was foreshadowed by discussions back in Chap. 1.

There are, however, several principles that have not yet been emphasized in earlier discussions here. The suggestions under "Adequate Scope" to adopt a time horizon that is long enough to capture both human and ecosystem timescales, and an areal scale of study that is large enough to include both local and long-distance impacts, is good advice for assessments of all the components of wellbeing. The same is true for the several guidelines on Table 4.2 that have to do with practical matters of assessment: the need for openness, the importance of using clear concepts, the clarity that is achieved by relating results to pre-set targets or thresholds, the value of broad participation by all interested parties, and the requirements of ongoing institutional capacity.

Sustainable Development Goals

The United Nations Sustainable Development Goals mentioned at the start of this chapter are also worth looking at in more detail. There are 17 of them and they are listed on Table 4.3 [9]. The repeated usage of the terms "sustainable," "inclusive," and "resilient" throughout the SDGs emphasizes the importance that the authors

Table 4.3 United Nations Global Sustainable Development Goals. (Adapted from the source material listed in [9])

1.	**No poverty.** End poverty in all its forms everywhere
2.	**Zero hunger.** End hunger, achieve food security and improved nutrition, and promote sustainable agriculture
3.	**Good health and well-being.** Ensure healthy lives and promote well-being for all ages
4.	**Quality education.** Ensure inclusive and equitable quality education, and promote lifelong learning opportunities for all
5.	**Gender equality.** Achieve gender equality and empower all women and girls
6.	**Clean water and sanitation.** Ensure availability and sustainable management of clean water and sanitation for all
7.	**Affordable and clean energy.** Ensure access to affordable, reliable, sustainable and modern energy for all
8.	**Decent work and economic growth.** Promote sustained, inclusive economic growth, full productive employment, and decent work for all
9.	**Industry, innovation and infrastructure.** Build resilient infrastructure, promote inclusive and sustainable industrialization, and foster innovation
10.	**Reduced inequalities.** Reduce income inequality within and among countries
11.	**Sustainable cities and communities.** Make cities and human settlements inclusive, safe, resilient and sustainable
12.	**Responsible consumption and production.** Ensure sustainable consumption and production patterns
13.	**Climate action.** Take urgent action to combat climate change and its impacts by regulating emissions and promoting developments in renewable energy
14.	**Life below water.** Conserve and sustainably use the oceans, seas and marine resources for sustainable development
15.	**Life on land.** Protect, restore and promote sustainable use of terrestrial ecosystems, sustainably manage forests, combat desertification, halt and reverse land degradation, and halt biodiversity loss
16.	**Peace, justice, and strong institutions.** Promote peaceful and inclusive societies for sustainable development, provide access to justice for all, and build effective, accountable and inclusive institutions at all levels
17.	**Partnerships for the goals.** Strengthen the means of implementation, and revitalize global partnerships for sustainable development

attached to these concepts. The SDGs have particular relevance to assessments of wellbeing in underdeveloped or developing nations where the absence of poverty and hunger, the presence of educational opportunities and decent work, and the availability of clean water and sanitation, exert considerable influence on daily happiness and long-term wellbeing.

The SDGs also lay out the need for equitable justice, effective institutions, operative infrastructure, and affordable energy. These may look like motherhood statements to those of us lucky enough to take these issues for granted, but a failure to provide them in many countries of the world leads to much personal unhappiness and lack of community wellbeing.

IPAT and the Ecological Footprint

There are two very different measures of human impact on the environment that deserve our attention. The first is the simple equation, $I = P \cdot A \cdot T$, which is sometimes called the Ehrlich Identity, after its founder, Paul Ehrlich, the Stanford biologist best known for warning us about population growth in his 1968 book *The Population Bomb*. In the equation, I stands for environmental impact (usually thought of as resource depletion and/or waste accumulation), P is population, A is affluence (or level of consumption), and T is technology (the type of processes used to convert resources into goods and services) [10]. The two dots between the P, the A, and the T imply multiplication. However, the equation should not be viewed as one in which numerical values of P, A and T are inserted to produce a numerical value of I. It is a qualitative expression, not a quantitative one. It is meant to highlight the multiplicative interplay among these three factors. Increased environmental impact may be caused by increased population, increased consumption, or inefficient technology. The IPAT relationship also implies that there are multiple ways of reducing undesirable impacts. Rich countries might do so by reducing per capita consumption, for example, whereas poorer countries might do it by controlling population growth. In all economies, technologies that minimize waste production are favored over those that don't.

In principle, the IPAT concept can be applied to single-variable indicators of environmental impact like, say, greenhouse gas emissions, or to integrated multiple-indicator impacts like that represented by an across-the-board water quality index. Later researchers have run with the original IPAT formulation, suggesting different weightings for the three terms on the right hand side of the equation, and inventing modified versions under the acronyms STIRPAT and ImPACT [11].

The other clever conceptualization of environmental impact is the Ecological Footprint (EF). It is actually a media-friendly version of the older concept of "carrying capacity." This older term is defined as the maximum population that can survive indefinitely on the natural resources available in a given area. The EF turns this definition on its head. It is defined as the area of biologically-productive land that would be required to produce the natural resources consumed by a community of a given population, and to assimilate the wastes generated by the usage of those resources. It is usually measured on a population basis in units of hectares per capita. The concept was first coined in 1992 by William Rees and Mathis Wackernagel of the School of Community and Regional Planning at the University of British Columbia [12]. It has since been utilized and revised by the World Wildlife Federation and the environmental think tank, Redefining Progress. The Global Footprint Network maintains a set of National Footprint Accounts with the cooperation of over 100 partner organizations around the world. The whole operation is overseen by an international review committee.

The EF can be applied at the scale of communities, cities, nations, or humanity as a whole. In practice, the EF for a given jurisdiction is adjusted by a set of *yield factors* that take into account the differing crop yields in various jurisdictions (due to the levels of available technology and the sophistication of resource management skills), and a set of *equivalence factors* that take into account the differences in productivity from different land types (cropland, grazing land, forests, fishing grounds, and built-up lands). The approach uses data from UN sources to track the consumption of resources and the generation of wastes, together with reference to global land cover maps and maps of agro-ecological zones provided by the Food and Agriculture Organization (FAO).

As a final step, the ecological footprint is often compared to the actual available biocapacity (also reported as an area of land.) In the most recent calculations on a nation-wide basis, Canada's footprint was roughly equal to its biocapacity, but the United States footprint exceeded its capacity by a factor of five. As of 2012, according to the Global Footprint Network, humanity as a whole is using the earth's natural capital 1.6 times as fast as nature can renew it.

Like the IPAT equation, the ecological footprint probably has more value as a qualitative rather than a quantitative concept, serving to educate people about the earth's carrying capacity and the dangers of overconsumption. From our perspective, the IPAT equation and the ecological footprint are very useful in providing further direction as to the type of indicator variables that may have to be accessed in order to get a handle on the environmental contributions to happiness and wellbeing.

Time Horizon, Discount Rates, and Future Generations

One of the factors that make meaningful environmental protection so difficult to achieve is the differing views that are held with respect to *time horizons* and *discount rates*. Politicians in their consideration of possible legislation have a time horizon that seldom exceeds one election cycle, say 4–5 years. Private corporations and their shareholders make decisions in a somewhat longer timeframe, perhaps on the order of decades. Environmentalists who feel responsibility for future generations have a time horizon of hundreds of years or more. Positions that are taken and decisions that are made by these various actors with their differing views of time are a primary source of the conflict between short-term economic growth and long-term environmental protection [13].

Economic decisions that involve dollars spent or earned at different points in time require consideration of the time value of money. Every investor knows that the value of a dollar won or lost now is greater than the value of a dollar won or lost at some time in the future. A dollar won now can be put in the bank and with the interest gained on it will be worth more when it is withdrawn at some future date. If you were to put $100 in the bank now at 3% interest it would be worth $134 10 years from now. Or viewed from the other direction, the *net present value* of $134 gained or lost 10 years from now at a *discount rate* of 3% is $100. As the time horizon gets longer, or the discount rate gets larger, the net present value of a future gain or loss gets smaller, and plays less and less role in current cost-benefit decisions.

Many environmental risks, whether they involve the effects of climate change, or the possible failure of a nuclear waste facility, or the repercussions of deforestation, or whatever, don't come home to roost until sometime in the distant future. If the impacts of these future environmental costs on current decisions are small, bottom-line decision makers will not take them into account, and future generations will not be protected from the environmental carelessness of the current generation. Environmentalists therefore press for government action to force free-market developers to use longer time horizons and lower discount rates. In fact, many argue for essentially infinite time horizons and zero discount rates as the essence of a sustainably-developed future.

Interestingly, a recent study examined the relationship between subjective wellbeing and one's view of an appropriate discount rate. The author found that those who place greater value on the protection of future generations are happier, and report higher levels of life satisfaction, than those who don't [14].

The Skeptics

The positive societal benefits of environmental health, and the negative impacts of environmental degradation, are now accepted as gospel in most quarters. However, there is still a minority position that is skeptical about the relevance of environmental issues to the economy or, for that matter, to the assessment of communal wellbeing. The primary focus of most skeptics is the prediction of global warming by climate scientists, and the dire warnings that accompany this prediction. The writer, Michael Crichton, for example, author of such blockbusters as *The Andromeda Strain* and *Jurassic Park*, wrote a novel a few years before he died in 2008, called *State of Fear* that was a thinly-disguised polemic against the evidence for climate change. Donald Trump in his campaign for the Presidency in 2016 often took a skeptical stance. Some public figures on the right have even suggested that the whole thing is a left-wing plot to sabotage the free-market economy and replace it with statist controls. In fact, the whole issue of climate change seems to have somehow become a political rather than scientific issue. On the scientific front, only a tiny minority of climate specialists gives any credence to the skeptical position. Those with a tendency to move in that direction might want to read the statements of scientific support provided by such non-partisan organizations as the World Health Organization, Doctors Without Borders, or the World Economic Forum.

The darling of the anti-environmental movement is a Danish political scientist named Bjorn Lomborg who was at one time the Director of the Danish Environmental Assessment Institute in Copenhagen. His book *The Skeptical Environmentalist: Measuring the Real State of the World* was devised as an antidote to the annual *State of the World* reports put out by Lester Brown and his Worldwatch Institute [15]. In his book, Lomborg questions the importance of many environmental concerns, arguing that they are much less pressing than the bigger concerns of poverty and hunger. With respect to global warming, he does not question its existence, or even the role played by the burning of fossil fuels (in fact, he has even supported initiatives to remove fossil fuel subsidies because such subsidies lead to increased consumption that exacerbates global warming). Rather, he opposes government-sponsored control measures on the grounds that they impose huge costs on national economies and will have only minimal impact on the earth's rising temperatures. Opponents of Lomberg's views have accused him of distorting evidence and misrepresenting facts. He is a controversial and polarizing figure in the environmental world and likely to remain so.

References

1. Brown, Lester R., *Eco-Economy: Building an Economy for the Earth*, W.W. Norton, 2001.
2. McKibben, W.R., *Deep Economy: The Wealth of Communities and the Durable Future*, Times Books, Henry Holt and Company, 2007.
3. Bruntland, G.H., *Our Common Future*, Report of the World Commission on Environment and Development, Oxford University Press, 1987. For a qick definition of the three pillars, see [www.thwink.org].
4. Daly, Herman, *Toward a Steady State Economy*, W.H. Freeman, 1973
5. Daly, Herman, *Beyond Growth: The Economics of Sustainable Development,* Beacon Press, 1996.
6. These quotes are taken from: Cobb, Clifford W., *Measurement Tools and the Quality of Life*, Redefining Progress, 2000.
7. Brown, Lester, The eco-economic revolution, *The Futurist*, 23-32, March-April, 2002.
8. The material in this section was informed by discussions in Appendix 1 of: Prescott-Allen, Robert and Tony Hodge, *Report on British Columbia's Progress Toward Sustainability*, B.C. Commission on Resources and Environment, B.C. Ministry of Environment, Lands, and Parks, 1997.
9. [https://sustainabledevelopment.un.org]
10. Ehrlich, Paul R. and John P. Holden, Impact of population growth, *Science*, 171, 1212-1217, 1971.
11. York, R., E.A. Rosa and T. Dietz, STIRPAT, IPAT, and ImPACT: Analytic tools for unpacking the driving forces of environmental impacts, *Ecological Economics*, 46(3), 351-365, 2003.

12. M. Wackernagel and W. Rees, *Our Ecological Footprint: Reducing Human Impact on the Earth*, New Society Publishers, 1996.
13. The material in this section was informed by: Linstone, H.A., On discounting the future, *Technological Forecasting and Social Change*, 4, 335-338, 1973; and Freeze, R.A., *The Environmental Pendulum: A Quest for the Truth about Toxic Chemicals, Human Health, and Environmental Protection*, University of California Press, 2000.
14. Kennedy, J., Subjective wellbeing and the discount rate, *Journal of Happiness Studies*, 21, 635-658, 2020.
15. Lomberg, Bjorn, *The Skeptical Environmentalist: Measuring the Real State of the World*, Cambridge University Press, 2001.

Chapter 5
Happiness Studies in the Biological and Medical Sciences

Emotions, Moods and Temperament

Daniel Goleman in his widely-quoted treatise on *Emotional Intelligence* defines *emotion* as a feeling, together with its "distinctive thoughts, psychological and biological states, and range of propensities to act." [1] He identifies eight families of emotions: Anger, Sadness, Fear, Enjoyment, Love, Surprise, Disgust, and Shame. Under each of these familial headings he identifies over one hundred variations, mutations and nuances that together constitute our range of emotional response to life. "Happiness" appears under the rubric of "Enjoyment" along with joy, contentment, bliss, delight, amusement, sensual pleasure, rapture, satisfaction, euphoria and ecstasy. The "Love" family includes many positive emotions such as acceptance, friendliness, trust, kindness, devotion, adoration, and infatuation, all of which would also seem to have direct bearing on happiness and wellbeing.

Goleman differentiates between *emotions*, which are triggered by outside stimuli, and can be vehement and passionate, but also tend to be short-lived; *moods*, which are independent of outside stimuli, more muted, but last longer; and *temperament*, which is a personality trait that identifies a person's propensity to exhibit certain suites of emotion and mood. Emotions are not just mental constructs. There is a physiological response in the human body to each and every emotion [2]. Almost every one of the body's many physiological systems is triggered into action. There is certainly going to be activity in the brain and the central nervous system, but there are also important roles to be played by the heart and its circulatory system, and by hormonal releases from the glands and organs of the body's endocrine system. One possible route to the measurement of happiness and wellbeing lies in the assessment and monitoring of these aspects of the body's functional performance.

R. A. Freeze, *The Metrics of Happiness*, Social Indicators Research Series 86,
https://doi.org/10.1007/978-3-031-10913-3_5

Medical Research and Happiness

For many years now there have been a cadre of researchers based in widely-disparate subdisciplines of medical science who have attempted to use their specialized expertise to shed light on the physiology of happiness. Some come from the neurosciences where their work focuses directly on the brain and the central nervous system. Others come at the topic from their roots in biochemistry, endocrinology, genetics, or pharmacology. The highly-specialized studies that they produce appear under many generic names: cognitive psychology, cognitive neuroscience, neuropsychology, neurobiology, psychophysiology, and behavioral neuroscience. Many popular-science books have been published to bring the findings of these studies to the interested reader [3].

Table 5.1 provides a sampling of academic research centers and private institutes that focus on the science of happiness and wellbeing. The diversity of names is evident there too; we find the Social Neuroscience Laboratory at Stanford University, The Duke Center for Cognitive Neuroscience, and the University of Reading's Centre for Integrative Neuroscience and Neurodynamics. Some organizations go for a more layman-friendly title like the Mayo Clinic's Mind-Body Initiative. Others like the private Wellspring Institute in San Rafael, California, try to bridge the gap

Table 5.1 A sampling of academic research centers and private institutes that focus on the neuroscience of happiness and wellbeing

	Name	Location
Academic Research Centers	Social Neuroscience Laboratory	Stanford University
	Center for Cognitive Neuroscience	Duke University
	Waisman Laboratory for Brain Imaging and Behavior	University of Wisconsin
	Centre for Integrative Neuroscience and Neurodynamics	University of Reading, UK
	Mayo Clinic Mind-Body Initiative	Rochester, MN
	Brown Institute for Brain Science	Brown University
	Center for Brain Health	University Texas Dallas
	Brain and Creativity Institute	University Southern California
	Stevens Neuroimaging and Informatics Institute	University of Southern California
	Human Neuroimaging Laboratory	Virginia Tech Carillon Research Institute
	Semel Institute for Neuroscience and Human Behavior, and Cousins Center for Psychoneuroimmunology	UCLA
Private Institutes	Wellspring Institute for Neuroscience and Contemplative Wisdom	San Rafael, CA
	Laboratory of Neural Imaging	Massachusetts General Hospital

between the hard and soft sciences in their promise to integrate the Neurosciences and Contemplative Wisdom.

In the following sections of this Chapter, four aspects of medical science will be addressed: firstly, the human endocrine system and its plethora of hormones and neurotransmitters; secondly, the direct investigations of brain structure through neuroimaging studies; thirdly the genetics of happiness; and lastly the general physiological relationships that have been uncovered between good health and happiness.

Raging Hormones

We have all felt at one time or another the surge of adrenaline that courses through our body when we are faced with a sudden threat. The threat may be real, like the startling appearance of a wild animal in the woods; or it may be manufactured, like the emergence of the psychopathic villain from behind a dark curtain in a horror movie. It may even accompany a threat averted, like a narrowly-avoided traffic accident. In all these cases, one is likely to experience jangled nerves, a racing heart, and shortness of breath. An emotional sensation has led to a physiological response. Mind and body are attuned.

Adrenaline (which nowadays goes by its more-chemically-descriptive name, epinephrine) is a hormone. Hormones are chemical compounds that are produced in one or other of the 14 major glands that make up the body's endocrine system [4]. Hormones are secreted in their host gland, released into the bloodstream, and carried by the circulatory system to target receptors throughout the body. They act as messengers that carry chemical signals to the target cells to regulate physiology and behavior. When the adrenal glands release that extra shot of epinephrine, the message that goes out is one that leads to a spike in blood pressure, increased heart rates, and a boost in the supply of oxygen and glucose to the brain. Our body's endocrine system has alerted us to danger and in so doing has contributed to our wellbeing. In point of fact, epinephrine is not just released in negative "fight or flight" situations; it is also released under sudden positive excitement, say when your team scores an overtime goal, or your daughter nails her triple axel, in which case it contributes directly to our hedonic happiness.

The endocrine system produces many other specialized hormones that have significance to happiness and wellbeing. The thyroid gland, for example, produces two hormones known as T3 and T4, which control the body's metabolic functions, among them, breathing, heart rate, and body temperature. If one has too much T3 and T4 in one's body, it leads to anxiety, irritability and moodiness; if one has too little, it leads to fatigue and depression.

The pineal gland produces melatonin which helps control sleeping and waking cycles. Melatonin's role in support of a positive sleep cycle contributes to wellbeing by conserving energy and allowing one to live a full and satisfying lifestyle. The so-called Seasonal Affective Disorder (SAD), with its associated fatigue, drop in energy, and moodiness, is the result of insufficient melatonin production.

There are many more hormones of interest. Estrogen and testosterone contribute to the pleasures of sexual desire. Insulin protects against the ravages of diabetes. And so on. The point to be made is that the endocrine system is not just a hotbed of meaningless physiological activity. The physiological activity is triggered by feelings, emotions, and moods. Measures of the relevant hormone levels, and therapies to increase or decrease them, have a role to play in understanding and moderating human happiness.

Neurotransmitters: The Great Facilitators of Life

There is a second messaging system operating in our bodies that is even more tightly connected to emotion and mood. It is the neuro-endocrine system that operates within the brain itself, using neurotransmitters to pass information between neuronal cells. It is closely associated with the hormonal endocrine system, but certainly different in kind.

Neuroscientists have determined that the human brain has over 100 billion nerve cells (or neurons), and that each neuron can have thousands of connections with its adjacent cells [5]. These numbers boggle the mind of the lay person, especially when it turns out that each neuron is itself quite complex, consisting of the cell body (or soma), a long nerve-fiber extension of the cell body (the axon), and a set of thin filaments that extend from the cell body (called dendrites). Information arrives into the brain via stimuli from the sensory organs (skin, eyes, nose, tongue and ears) and is then transmitted through the brain from neuron to neuron, arriving in each cell via the dendrites and leaving via the axon. There is a small gap called a synapse that lies between the axon of one cell and the dendrites or soma of an adjacent cell, and it is across these synapses that communication must take place if the brain is to successfully process our emotions into an appropriate set of physiologic responses.

The necessary communication takes place with the help of neurotransmitters which are highly-specialized chemical compounds that are manufactured in the brain itself. They are stored in vesicles in the axon on the pre-synaptic side of the synapses, and then released to diffuse across the synaptic gap, where they bind to specific targeted receptors on the post-synaptic side.

Neurotransmission differ from hormonal messaging in several ways. Hormonal pathways are via the bloodstream in the body's circulatory system; neural pathways are across neuronal synapses and along nerve tracks of the central nervous system. Target receptors in hormonal signaling may be distant from the gland that secretes the hormone; target receptors in neuronal signaling are immediately adjacent to the source. Hormonal response times are on the order of seconds, minutes or hours; neural response occurs in milliseconds. Hormonal impact can be effective over considerable time periods; neural impact is short lived.

Perhaps the primary difference is that hormonal signals are purely chemical in nature whereas the synaptic signaling mechanism in the brain is a complex electrochemical process. Under neurotransmission, neurons receive, propagate, and transmit electrochemical impulses throughout the brain, sending their messages to that part of the brain that will forward the appropriate physiological instructions to the rest of the body.

Neurotransmitters mediate the brain's response to all emotions, be they negative ones like fear and anger, or positive ones like joy, love and happiness. Some neurotransmitters are excitatory in that they increase activity in the receptor neurons in response to positive emotions, while others are inhibitory in that they decrease activity in response to negative emotions. Neurotransmitters also play a role in maintaining many cognitive activities associated with happiness and wellbeing such as alertness, concentration, memory, appetite, sleep, and perceptions of pain [6].

The brain generates a large number of neurotransmitters, over 60 of them at least, each of them with specific signaling functions. The discussion here will be limited to four of them that are closely identified with happiness and wellbeing: the endorphins, dopamine, oxytocin, and serotonin.

The endorphins are a family of 20 or so slightly-different but closely associated, chemical compounds. The name comes from the fact that their production is *end*ogenous (generated within the body) and that their physiologic response is similar to that of exogenously-administered m*orphin*e (morphine that is introduced into the body from an outside source). They are in fact opioids, and have a similar chemical structure to opium and morphine. The most active member of the endorphin family is known as beta-endorphin. It is manufactured at several locations throughout the brain, as well as in other parts of the central nervous system, and in the pituitary gland. Beta-endorphin is an inhibitory neurotransmitter. It acts as an analgesic, inhibiting the transmission of pain signals, and diminishing the perception of pain. Its receptor cells are located in parts of the brain that have been identified as being responsible for the assessment and mitigation of pain. Like exogenous morphine, the endogenous endorphins act as more than just pain-killers; they can also produce feelings of great contentment. Vigorous aerobic exercise stimulates endorphin production and leads to the feeling of euphoria known as "runner's high." Endorphin production is also known to be enhanced by sexual stimulation, laughter, and spicy foods [7].

The dopamine system in the brain is made up of several distinct excitory neuronal pathways that taken together are responsible for the physiological responses that lead to pleasure, emotional arousal, joy, and euphoria. Dopamine plays a major role in developing cravings, and in motivating behavior that will lead to satisfaction and reward. It is generated in the nerve cells of the brain and finds its receptors elsewhere in the brain's complex structure, in neural clusters that are known sites of the pleasure response. Many addictive recreational drugs like cocaine and methamphetamines, create their high by stimulating the production of dopamine or deactivating the enzymes that break it down [8].

Oxytocin is often called the "love hormone' for the feelings of affection, connection, and contentment that it generates. It is known to facilitate trust between individuals and to encourage charity and generosity to others. Production of oxycontin increases in women during pregnancy and childbirth, and is thought to enhance the mother-child bond after birth. One academic treatise highlights oxytocin in their title as "the great facilitator of life." [9]

Serotonin is perhaps the best known of the happiness neurotransmitters [10]. Unlike most other neurotransmitters, 80–90% of the body's supply of serotonin is manufactured and stored in the gastrointestinal tract, and only 10–20% in the brain. The serotonin in the GI tract is linked to such bodily functions as bowel control, liver regeneration, breast-milk production, and bone growth. The serotonin that is generated in the brain is an excitory neurotransmitter. It helps control mood, appetite, sleep, and sexual desire. It is considered to be a direct contributor to human happiness and wellbeing. A deficit of serotonin is thought by many medical researchers to be one of the leading causes of clinical depression.

It is possible to measure serotonin levels in the bloodstream and dopamine levels in urine tests, and to enhance concentrations through medication and supplements if levels are thought to be too low. However, the relationship between the levels of these neurotransmitters in blood and urine and their activity levels in the brain are still unclear. Such measurements cannot yet be directly related to human happiness and wellbeing. Despite this caveat, the apparent unanimity of neuroscientists on the important role of serotonin, dopamine, oxytocin and the endorphins in mediating responses to incoming sensory stimuli has led to at least two popular self-help books that emphasize training your brain to boost and optimize the performance of these neurotransmitters as a route to happiness and wellbeing [11].

Uppers, Downers and All-Arounders

If we are going to fully examine the neuroscience of happiness we cannot avoid consideration of the plethora of psychoactive drugs that promise to deliver immediate joy and bliss. Some of them are legal prescription drugs; others are illicit offerings of the recreational drug trade. Most of them produce only a temporary dose of happiness. Almost all of them are either physiologically or psychologically addictive. The title of this section comes from the classic drug-treatment book of the same name [12].

The *uppers* of the section title are the anti-depressant drugs that activate the dopamine and serotonin systems in the brain. They include widely-imbibed everyday drugs like nicotine and caffeine; prescription drugs like Prozac, Zoloft, and Paxil; and recreational drugs like cocaine and methamphetamine. All of them act as physiological stimulants, raising body temperature, heart rate, and breathing. Methamphetamines cause extra dopamine to be released into the brain. Cocaine deactivates an enzyme that breaks down dopamine, causing a surfeit of dopamine to accumulate in the synapses. In the short term, they decrease fear and anxiety;

improve alertness, energy, and mood; and bring temporary contentment to the user. In the long run, because they activate the pleasure and reward centers of the brain, they have the potential to be highly addictive. Over 3% of the US population is thought to take some type of uppers on a regular basis.

Downers are inhibitory drugs that depress overwrought emotions and impulses, creating their brand of happiness through relaxation and reduced anxiety. They include the opioids, like heroin, oxycontin, and fentanyl; tranquilizers like Valium, Nembutal, and Xanax; and alcohol. Heroin activates the opioid transmission pathways in the brain and mimics the behavior of the endorphins. Most of the tranquilizers act directly on dopamine receptors.

All-arounders are hallucinogenic drugs that distort the user's perceptions of reality by manipulating the brain's interpretation of the senses, leading to feelings of expansiveness and transcendence. They include LSD, marijuana, the party drug Ecstasy, and the psychedelic extracts from the peyote cactus (mescaline) and so-called magic mushrooms (psilocybin). All of these recreational drugs are powerful releasers of serotonin and dopamine in the brain's neurotransmission pathways.

The search for happiness through pharmacological intervention has a long and muddy history. While these so-called "happy pills" can be of life-saving help to those few who really need them, they are more often the cause of a tragic downward spiral for those who don't.

Hedonic Hot Spots in the Brain

Neuroscientists have been producing ever-more-detailed maps of the structure of the brain for many decades now, and they have identified the functional role of many of the mapped structures. Most brain maps start with the threefold identification of the brainstem (which connects to the spinal cord and the rest of the central nervous system), the cerebellum (which lies above the brainstem at the base of the brain), and the cerebrum (which constitutes over 75% of the brain mass). There are two cerebral hemispheres with four lobes (frontal, temporal, parietal, and occipital) in each hemisphere. The outer layer of the cerebrum is known as the cerebral cortex. Moving past this first-level characterization has lead to a more-detailed mapping of many more neuronal sub-areas in each of the structures, hemispheres and lobes of the brain. A recent article in *Nature*, for example, identified 180 separate neuronal parcels in each hemisphere of the cerebral cortex [13]. A similar explosion of detail has emerged for all parts of the brain, triggered in part by the research funding provided by the National Institutes of Health in its Human Connectome Project (HCP) based at Washington University in St. Louis, Missouri. The HCP has as its primary focus "the elucidation of neural pathways that underlie brain function and behavior." [14]

Neuroscientists now have a very detailed understanding of the specific sites in the brain that control speech, hearing, vision, taste, touch, smell, facial recognition, motor control, balance, breathing, blood pressure, heart rate, language, memory, concentration, planning, and problem-solving. More to the point for our purposes, they have identified the parts of the brain that are activated by emotions, moods, and reward-based behavior. Morten Kringlebach, Kent Berridge and co-workers from the Department of Psychology at the University of Michigan have dubbed these neuron parcels as *hedonic hot spots*. They lie primarily in a portion of the brain known as the limbic system, which is located deep in the cerebrum below the cortex and above the cerebellum. The limbic area is known to be rich in serotonin, dopamine, and endorphin receptors. It includes the amygdula, thalamus, hypothalamus, hippocampus, nucleus accumbens, and pituitary gland [15]. It is less important for our purposes to know exactly where these pleasure receptors are located than it is to simply know that such hot spots exist in the brain. Their activity in response to pleasurable stimulation provides a means for the physiological measurement of personal happiness.

So how have neuroscientists been able to identify and examine these pleasure points? The earliest methods that were used to map out happiness pathways in the brain were carried out in laboratory animal studies. In one approach, drugs that promote the neuronal production of certain types of proteins were injected into the brains of animals. Later removal and slicing of the brains identified the locations of dark protein plumes that trailed away from the zones of local neuronal activation [16].

The earliest mappings on human subjects were carried out in the 1960s during brain surgery for epilepsy or other neurological disorders. It was discovered then that the limbic areas produced feelings of euphoria and wellbeing when stimulated [17]. Other studies zeroed in on the loss of specific emotional facility suffered by victims of lesions or other brain damage in particular portions of the brain.

Most modern inquiries of the neuroscience of happiness have been based on non-invasive brain imaging. Among the most widely-used scans are Positive Emission Tomography (PET) and functional Magnetic Resonance Imaging (fMRI). PET monitors the activity of neurotransmitters that have been tagged with a radioactive dye, while fMRI captures the increased blood flow that occurs in activated areas of the brain. A recent review summarized 15 studies that used one or other of these imaging techniques [18]. Participants in each study were prompted to recall happy memories from their past while being scanned by PET or fMRI imaging systems. Results confirmed the activation of hedonic hot spots that exhibit a high density of receptors for pleasure-based neurotransmitters.

Table 5.1 lists several of the best-known brain imaging institutes in America. Research at these institutes continues to develop ever-more-powerful imaging techniques, many of them offshoots of the original MRI systems, among them Diffusion Spectrum Magnetic Resonance Imaging (DSI), High-Angular Diffusion Imaging (HARDI), and Magnetoencephalography (MEG).

By far the most famous use of brain imaging in happiness circles was carried out by Richard Davidson, Director of the Waisman Laboratory for Brain Imaging at the University of Wisconsin. He carried out traditional MRI scans of a group of Tibetan monks. His hypothesis was that the contentment engendered by their meditative lifestyle would register as higher activity levels in those portions of the brain associated with positive emotions. The participant with the highest activity levels was a French biologist and philosopher named Matthieu Ricard who had given up academic life in Europe to seek solace as a Buddhist monk. When the story was covered by the British newspaper *The Independent*, Ricard was singled out as "the world's happiest man." Ricard took this appellation to heart and wrote a best-selling self-help book entitled *Happiness: A Guide to Developing Life's Most Important Skill* [19].

In another study, Davidson carried out MRI scans on two groups of participants, one group of cheerful temperament (ebullient, sociable, and self-confident), as determined from standard personality testing, and the other group dour and melancholy (prone to moodiness, suspicious, and fearful of lurking dangers). He found measurable differences in brain activity between the two groups, with the cheerful group showing much higher activity in the pleasure centers of the brain. His team at the Waisman Laboratory has also identified the neural parcels associated with improvements to happiness levels in depressed patients due to positive incentives, anti-depressant medications, and mindfulness training [20].

The Genetics of Happiness and Set-Point Theory

So how was Richard Davidson able to so easily put together two cohorts of subjects for his testing, one cheerful, and the other melancholy? What is that makes some of us full of beans and others of us dour and cantankerous? Is it genetics or is it life experience that controls our temperament? It is certainly not a new question. It seems like the nature versus nurture argument has been with us forever. In the mid-to-late twentieth century, behaviorist arguments dominated and genetics was downplayed. In more recent times, genetic arguments are back in vogue again. Yet, despite this greater recognition and acceptance of the role of inherited traits, the relationship between the *genotype* (a person's genetic makeup) and the *phenotype* (a person's observed personality traits) is "still quite elusive." [21]

From the perspective of this book, the personality traits that interest us are the ones that control optimism, contentment, and a sense of wellbeing. The question on the table is how much of a person's innate happiness and subjective wellbeing is controlled by genes, and how much by life experience? We are not the first to wonder, and many studies have come up with an estimate for the genetic component. One of the most widely-quoted studies found that 33% of the "overall variation in life satisfaction" could be ascribed to genetics [22]. Another study estimated that 44–52% of the "stable component of wellbeing" is determined genetically [23] Yet a third claimed 40–50% [24]. Many others have rounded things off to claim a roughly 50–50 split between the influences of genetics and environment. The noted psychologist, Sonja Lyubomirsky, has broken things down even further, claiming 50% genetics, 10% circumstances, and 40% one's own attitudes and actions [25]. In her popular writings, Lyubomirsky calls this partitioning the "happiness pie."

Despite the differences in these estimates, some happiness researchers claim that the genetically-controlled component of happiness represents a kind of "set point" on a person's scale of life satisfaction. This concept was first introduced in 1984 by Bruce Headey and colleagues at the University of Melbourne in Australia. They noted that people's subjective well-being tended to be very stable over time; that it seemed to remain in a kind of "dynamic equilibrium" through life's ups and downs [26]. Leaders in the positive psychology movement were quick to pick up, and began to monitor the world of genetic research and adapt the results they found there to their own needs [27]. Set-point theory recognizes that every individual experiences times of greater or lesser happiness, but it holds that no matter what form these events might take, most people will return to their mean. It is this set-point that controls temperament, and it is genetics that controls the set point. David Lykken and Auke Tellegen of the University of Minnesota may have said it best: "Transitory variations are largely due to fortune's favors, whereas the midpoint of these variations is determined by the great genetic lottery that occurs at conception." More provocatively, they argue that "trying to become happier is like trying to become taller." [28]

Set point theory is far from universally held. There are many studies that claim to show a permanent influence on an individual's base happiness levels in response to major life events, both positive and negative. Some people never recover from the loss of a loved one. Others are buoyed by life-changing circumstances such as a happy marriage or a financial windfall. One review of national-scale longitudinal panel studies in Germany, Britain and Australia indicated that a large minority of respondents (but not a majority) recorded substantial, lasting changes in life satisfaction after positive or negative life-changing events [29]. In 2010, this "discordant data" led Bruce Headey to pull back from his long-held support of set-point theory and to muse in print about the "serious flaws" that were coming to light [30].

Set-point theory has been described as "the elephant in the room" for psychologists. The issue is important because it has implications for the expected efficacy of therapeutic interventions on those who are less happy. If happiness cannot be improved, then all the research that is being carried out to determine its causes and effects is rendered somewhat moot. The demise of set-point theory would be a considerable boon to the psychotherapy community.

In their defense, psychotherapists and clinical psychologists point to their many successes as proof that the genetic set point can be overridden, and some support for the value of therapeutic intervention has come from the neuroscience community. A recent review paper put it as follows: "[The neural] circuits that have been implicated in wellbeing all exhibit plasticity, the ability to grow and change. Contextual influences induce plastic changes in brain function and structure that clearly impact our wellbeing. However, plasticity in these circuits could also be harnessed for intentional cultivation and shaping. Engaging in specific forms of training to cultivate wellbeing through psychotherapy, meditation, and other forms of mental training has been found to induce functional and structural changes in the brain and has also been found to benefit wellbeing." [31] All that can be said at this point is that the long-term stability of genetic set points remains a contentious issue in the study of happiness.

Twins

There are two distinct approaches to the assessment of the role of genetics in the development of personality traits. *Behavioral genetics* attempts to tease out the causative factors on the basis of questionnaires of subjective wellbeing, and from personality testing tools like the Minnesota Multiphasic Personality Inventory. Behavioral genetics remains closely related to the domain of positive psychology [32]. *Molecular genetics*, on the other hand, attempts to identify particular genes and their function in the human genome. It makes greater use of hard science, and in particular the brain imaging techniques that have been developed in recent decades. It lies in the domain of medical science [33]. Although the two approaches are very different from one another, they do have one thing in common. Their studies are usually carried out on cohorts of related family members, especially twins or siblings. The nature/nurture question is addressed by looking at the differences in personality traits that arise, and relating these to the genetic similarities and environmental differences experienced. The cohort that has the most to offer in this regard is a cohort of identical twins raised apart.

Twin studies are so important in genetic research that several academic institutions maintain a registry of twins for the sole purpose of providing subjects for study by genetic researchers. Among the best known in America are those housed at Michigan State University, Washington State University, the University of Minnesota, and Virginia Commonwealth University. Several European countries, among them Sweden, Denmark, Norway, Finland and the U.K., maintain twin registries, as do Australia and Sri Lanka. Registration on the part of twins is voluntary in all cases, and data are made freely available to any reputable research organization. Genetic research on twins is so widespread that there is even an International Society for Twin Studies. It publishes a journal *Twin Research and Human Genetics* that is already in its twentieth year of publication.

Living organisms reproduce themselves by transmitting genetic information to their progeny. Individual cells are the minimal self-reproducing unit, and all genetic information is stored in the DNA in each cell. As every schoolboy now knows, the structure of DNA is a complex double helix of nucleotides, as first uncovered by Francis Crick and James Watson in 1953. The ordering of the nucleotides in the double helix contains instructions for producing proteins, and each DNA molecule may contain the specification for thousands of proteins. In order to fit inside the cells, the DNA is tightly coiled into structures called chromosomes which consist of long strands of DNA on which thousands of genes are encoded. A gene is a distinct region of the DNA sequence corresponding to the instructions for a single protein. The region on the chromosome at which a particular gene is located is called the locus, and each locus contains one allele (or variant) of the gene. However, different people may have different alleles and hence a slightly different gene sequence. It is this random deployment of genetic variants that influences our personality, and determines whether our temperaments are cheerful or melancholy.

Every cell in our body contains the same DNA inherited from the moment of conception. We inherit 50% of our genes from the maternal side and 50% from the paternal side. At the locus of each gene on its chromosomal strand, each newborn has a 50% chance of getting a particular gene from one or other parent. Development of the genotype is a probabilistic game, and so therefore is the resulting phenotype that describes the set of personality traits that give each of us our individuality.

So why the emphasis on twins in genetic research? Identical twins share 100% of their genetic makeup. Their phenotypes should be much more alike than those of fraternal twins or siblings, which share only 50%. When identical twins are raised apart, the differences in personality that arise can therefore be ascribed to environmental influences and life experience. Over the years, twin researchers have investigated almost every aspect of personality. Their hypothesis of alikeness between twins raised apart seems to hold, but it is the *degree* of alikeness uncovered in these studies that leads to the estimates quoted earlier for the genetic set point of happiness and wellbeing [34].

In case this all sounds set in stone, it isn't. The new millennium has seen the emergence and growth of a new field called *epigenetics* which has shown that modifications of gene expression can occur without alterations to the DNA sequence itself; that is, there can be changes in phenotype without changes in genotype [35]. These changes are brought about by chemical modifications that occur within the double helix, apparently influenced by one's circumstances of life including diet, aging, lifestyle, and disease. These chemical modifications have the ability to activate or deactivate individual genes, acting as a kind of on/off switch. As a result, even identical twins raised together can be expected to show divergence in their personalities due to this "epigenetic drift." These new findings also provide further ammunition for those who argue that the set-point of human happiness is not as set as some would claim.

Genes and Alleles

The most widely-quoted paper in the study of the molecular genetics of happiness was published by an international team led by Jan-Emmanuel De Neve of Oxford University, with contributions from researchers at Harvard University, the University of California at San Diego, and the University of Basel, Switzerland [36]. De Neve is a professor of Economics and Strategy at the Said Business School at Oxford and is a co-editor of the World Happiness Report issued by the United Nations. The research team worked with a cohort of identical and fraternal twins taken mostly from the National Longitudinal Study of Adolescent Health (ADD Health). They compared different genetic variations of the gene 5-HTTLPR in their twins and related these findings to the phenotype information in the ADD Health database.

The 5-HTTLPR gene is one of the roughly 21,000 genes identified by the Human Genome Project. It is critical to the metabolism of serotonin in the brain, and as we have learned throughout this chapter, serotonin is one of the neurotransmitters that is intimately associated with the neurological response to emotions, including happiness. The 5-HTTLPR gene has two alleles (or variants), a short form and a long form, the long form being the more transciptionally-efficient variant of the genotype. The short form is linked to emotional depression, whereas the long form provides better protection against depression and seems to code for an increased tendency toward life satisfaction. It is the observed correlations between the alleles of 5-HTTPLR and the ADD Health measures of life satisfaction that led De Neve and his team to their estimate of 33% for the genetic component of happiness.

There are other "happiness genes" that have been identified by different research teams. Meike Bartels and Philipp Koellinger at Vrije Universiteit Amsterdam, working through the Europe-based Social Science Genetic Association Consortium, have zeroed in on the FAAH gene which makes a protein that affects feelings of pleasure and pain. People who have a particular allele of the FAAH gene seem to be identifiably happier than those who don't [37]. The internecine battles have also begun. A recent paper tried to confirm the correlations of the 5-HTTPLR and FAAH genes with country-wide happiness measures. National gene frequencies were taken from a Yale University database, and happiness measures were based on data from the World Values Survey. The study confirmed a positive correlation for the FAAH gene but not for the 5-HTTPLR gene [38].

Barbara Frederickson of the University of North Carolina leads a team that has looked at the CTRA gene set (an acronym for Conserved Transcriptional Response to Adversity). They have found that people with eudaimonic personality traits have CTRA gene profiles that are favorable for a healthy immune system, while those of a more hedonic nature have gene-profiles that are adverse [39].

Clearly, there are more than one or two genes that are coding for happiness and wellbeing, and we can expect many more to be identified as the detailed examination of the human genome continues. Just in the past couple of years, several research teams using the Genome-Wide Association Study (GWAS) approach have identified several additional candidate genes and alleles that appear to code for happiness and wellbeing. The use of gene identification as a measure of happiness is still in its infancy, but more can be expected on this front in the future.

Health and Happiness

Many studies have shown a strong correlation between good health and happiness. There is, however, one outstanding question: What is the direction of the causal arrow? Are we happier because we are healthy? Or are we healthier because we are happy?

The argument that a happy disposition breeds better health has been made primarily by positive psychologists and behavioral geneticists. It is their contention that happier people eat better, exercise more, are less stressed, and have stronger social connections. As a result of these positive life choices, they tend to have stronger immune systems, exhibit lower vulnerability to viral infections, are less prone to hypertension, recover more quickly from disease, and live longer [40].

One of the largest studies to examine the relationship between health and overall wellbeing is the National Longitudinal Study of Adolescent Health, which has already been highlighted as a source of twin data for De Neve's investigation of the 5-HTTPLR gene. The ADD Health study was hosted by the Eunice Kennedy Shriver National Institute of Child Health and Human Development based at the University of North Carolina. The program was originally mandated by the U.-S. Congress under the umbrella of the National Institutes of Health but over the years it has received funding from over 20 other federal agencies and private foundations [41].

ADD Health is the most comprehensive longitudinal study ever undertaken of adolescents as they mature into young adults. The program started in 1994 with 90,000 students in Grades 7–12 from 145 schools. It progressed in four "waves" from 1994 to 2008, at which time 15,000 of the original cohort were still in the mill. The program involved student and parent questionnaires, in-home interviews, and the development of databases on the communities in which the subjects lived. In the final wave, measurements of cardiovascular, metabolic, genetic, and immune function were carried out on a subset of the students. The questionnaires and interviews zeroed in on the forces that influence adolescent behavior in the years in which the subjects matured into their adult roles and responsibilities. Among the forces examined were the demographic characteristics of the respondents, their family dynamics, nutrition, academic expectations, extracurricular activities, peer networks, decision-making processes, employment experience, romantic partnerships, and risk profiles.

The ADD Health data has been used by over 30,000 researchers and has led to over 6000 research articles, reports, reviews and books. Many of these have reported on correlations between the various input variables and the health status of the subjects [42]. It is clear from these studies that positive health outcomes depend on many of the same drivers that also control the development of a cheerful temperament and subjective wellbeing.

More recently, the ADD Health results have been buttressed by the MIDUS program, a National Longitudinal Study of Health and Well-Being at Midlife. The goal of the program is "to investigate the role of behavioral, psychological, and social factors in accounting for age-related variations in health and wellbeing in a national sample of Americans." [43] It is based at the Institute on Aging at the University of Wisconsin. The selected cohort consists of over 7000 English-speaking, non-institutionalized subjects between the ages of 25 and 74. The database for each subject includes information on demographics, parents, childhood, living arrangements, occupational history, finances, spouse or partner, sexuality, children and parenting, health status, psychological profile, social participation, and spirituality, over 130 separate entries in all. Researchers working with the MIDUS data sets have confirmed many of the same relationships between health and happiness as have the ADD Health researchers, but with an older suite of subjects.

Not all health researchers are persuaded that a happy temperament leads to better health. Barbara Ehrenreich in her book "Bright-Sided: How the Relentless Promotion of Positive Thinking Has Undermined America," makes the case that health outcomes are independent of temperament [44]. Ehrenreich, herself a cancer survivor, takes particular umbrage with the popular notion that seriously-ill people have a better chance of recovery if they "get happy and think positive thoughts." She finds this concept insulting to victims of debilitating disease, akin to blaming the victim, and suggests that it often leads to feelings of guilt in patients who do not show signs of recovery.

Health-Related Quality of Life

There is a massive literature in medical circles on *health-related quality of life*, so much so that the acronym HRQOL will cause a Google search to spin for minutes. In fact, much of the original research on life satisfaction and wellbeing arose in the context of medical outcomes, and several of the journals which now treat a broader clientele started with contributions that came largely from the health sciences. Many of the indicators and indexes that will appear later in this book, especially those that reflect the influence of good health on happiness and wellbeing, come from these beginnings [45]. Having said all this, it will not be possible to dive full bore into this world. It is simply too great a detour from the main thrust of our mission. Discussion here will be limited to two HRQOL efforts that are probably the closest cousins to our investigations of wellbeing: the *Medical Outcomes Study* (MOS) carried out by RAND Health, and the concept of *Quality Adjusted Life Years* (QALYs).

RAND Health is a division of the RAND Corporation, based in Santa Monica CA, a well-known think tank that has been a leader in health policy research for many years. In the late 1980s they received funding to develop a set of "generic, coherent, and easily-administered health-related quality-of-life measures." This led to a two-year program known as the Medical Outcomes Study that was based on self-reports from over 20,000 chronically-ill patients. An MOS questionnaire was developed with 116 core questions covering physical condition and mobility, the effects and severity of pain, the level of cognitive and social function, the occurrence of psychological distress, and the limitations imposed by health conditions and/or emotional problems.

There were two important outcomes of the MOS study. The first was the realization that the questionnaire was too long, and the second that with minimal tweaking it could serve to assess the life satisfaction of healthy patients in a preventive mode just as easily as the chronically ill. The result was the 36-question short version, now ensconced in the HRQOL literature as SF-36 [46]. Since its emergence in the early 1990s, the SF-36 health survey (and also SF-20, SF-12, and SF-6D spinoffs) has become a standard tool, and its results inform the deliberations of health professionals, insurance providers, regulators, and policy makers. It has also found application in happiness and wellbeing studies. Among the 36 questions are those that ask respondents if they are "calm and peaceful," "full of pep," and "a happy person."

The EuroQol Research Foundation in Rotterdam, the Netherlands, has developed a European competitor of the SF-36, known as EQ-5D [47]. It is a "standardized non-disease-specific instrument to describe and value health-related quality of life." It does so in five domains (pain, mood, mobility, self-care, and daily activity), with sub-categories that allow for the differentiation of 243 separate identifiable states of health. Like the SF-36, it has also seen application in studies of broader wellbeing.

There are two aspects to one's ultimate future prospects: the expected length of one's life, and the quality of life during these years. The concept of a *quality-adjusted life year*, or QALY, combines the two [48]. One QALY is defined as 1 year of perfect health. At the other end of the spectrum, death is assigned zero QALYs. Values thus range between zero and one, per year. The method assumes that a set of alternative health states can be defined, and that zero-to-one quality-of-life weightings can be assigned to each. In Britain, the National Institute for Health and Clinical Excellence (NICE) uses the 234 health states defined by the EQ-5D metric, and has assigned a weighting to each based on the results of a widely-distributed questionnaire that asks respondents to reveal their preferences with respect to the occurrence of the various health states.

The QALY was originally developed as a measure of the value of health outcomes due to medical intervention. It was designed to provide a more objective comparison of competing medical treatments both at an individual level (to inform personal patient decisions), and at the administrative level (to prioritize patients for treatment, to evaluate intervention programs, to set priorities for future programs, and to make difficult resource-allocation decisions). However its potential application to a broader perspective of wellbeing has long been recognized and one often encounters the QALY concept in studies of personal happiness and communal wellbeing.

The QALY has been criticized in some circles on both ethical and operational grounds [49]. The most serious charge is that it is unfair to the elderly, who have less potential QALYs than more youthful subjects. It is held that the resulting bias might lead to social decisions that unfairly undervalue programs for the elderly. Recognition of this bias has led some agencies to invoke age corrections and future-discounting methods (similar to those used in cost-benefit analysis) into their QALY-based assessments.

References

1. Goleman, Daniel, *Emotional Intelligence*, 10th Anniversary Ed., Bantam Books, 2005.
2. Rickard, N.S. and D.A. Vella-Brodrick, Changes in well-being: Complementing a psychosocial approach with neurobiological insights, *Social Indicators Research*, 117(2), 437-457, 2014.

3. Nettle, Daniel, *Happiness: the Science Behind Your Smile*, Oxford University Press, 2005; Layard, Richard, *Happiness: Lessons from a New Science*, Penguin, 2005; Braun, Stephen, *The Science of Happiness: Unlocking the Mysteries of Mood*, John Wiley, 2000; Klein, Stefan, *The Science of Happiness: How Our Brains Make Us Happy and What We Can Do to Get Happier*, De Capo Press, 2006; Huppert, Felicia, N. Bayliss and B. Keverne, eds., *The Science of Well-Being*, Oxford Univ. Press, 2006; Edelman, Shimon, *The Happiness of Pursuit: What Neurosciences Can Teach Us About the Good Life*, Basic Books, 2012.
4. Gardner, David G. And Dolores Shoback, *Greenspan's Basic Clinical Endocrinology*, 10th Ed., McGraw Hill, 2017.
5. Kandel, E.R., J.H. Schwartz and T.M. Jessell, *Principles of Neural Science*, 4th ed., McGraw-Hill, 2000.
6. Webster, Roy, *Neurotransmitters, Drugs and Brain Function*, Wiley, 2001; Pokorski, M., *Neurotransmitter Interactions and Cognitive Function*, Springer, 2015.
7. [science.howstuffworks.com/life/endorphins]
8. Neve, K.A., *The Dopamine Receptors*, Springer, 2009; Beaulieu, J.M. and R.R. Gainetdinov, The physiology, signaling and pharmacology of dopamine receptors, *Pharmacological Reviews*, 63(1), 182-217, 2011; Schultz, W., Neuronal reward and decision signals: From theories to data, *Physiological Reviews*, 95(3), 853-951, 2015.
9. Lee, H.J., A.H. Macbeth, J. Pagani, and W.S. Young III, Oxytocin: The great facilitator of life, *Prog. Neurobiology*, 88(2), 127-151, 2009. See also: Ishtak, W.W, et al, Oxytocin's role in enhancing well-being: A literature review, *Journal of Affective Disorders*,130(1),1-9, 2011.
10. Muller, Christian P. and Barry L. Jacobs, *Handbook of the Behavioral Neurobiology of Serotonin*, Academic, 2009.
11. Breuning, L.G., *Habits of a Happy Brain: Retrain Your Brain to Boost Your Serotonin, Dopamine, Oxytocin and Endorphin Levels*, Adams Media, 2015; Lee, James, *Living through Neurochemistry: A Guide to the Optimization of Serotonin, Dopamine, and the Neurotransmitters that Color Your World*, CreateSpace Independent Publishing Platform, 2014.
12. Inaba, Darryl S. And William E. Cohen, *Uppers, Downers and All-Arounders: Physical and Mental Effects of Psychoactive Drugs*, 8th Ed., CNS Productions, 2014; See also: Herzberg, David, *Happy Pills in America: From Miltown to Proxac*, Johns Hopkins Univ. Press, 2008.
13. Glasser, M.F., et al., A multi-modal parcellation of the human cerebral cortex, *Nature*, 536, 171-182, Aug. 2016.
14. [www.humanconnectomeproject.org]
15. Kringlebach, Morten L. and Kent C. Berridge, *Pleasures of the Brain*, Oxford Univ. Press, 2010. See also: Davidson, R.J., Well-being and affective style: Neural substrates and biobehavioral correlates, Chapter 5, in Huppert, F., N. Bayliss and B. Keverne, Eds., *The Science of Well-Being*, Oxford University Press, 2006.
16. Pecina, S., K.S. Smith and K.C. Berridge, Hedonic hot spots in the brain, *Neuroscientist*, 12(6), 500-511, 2006.
17. Nettle, 2005, op. cit.
18. Suardi, A. et al., The neural correlates of happiness: A review of PET and fMRI studies using autobiographical recall methods, *Cognitive, Affective and Behavioral Neuroscience*, 16(3), 383-392, 2016.
19. Ricard, Matthieu, *Happiness: A Guide to Developing Life's Most Important Skill*, Little Brown, 2007.
20. Davidson, R.J. and B.S. Schuyler, Neuroscience of happiness, Chapter 5, *World Happiness Report*, 2015.
21. Nes, R.B. and E. Roysamb, The heritability of subjective well-being: Review and meta-analysis, Chapter 5, in Pleuss, Michael, ed., *Genetics Of Psychological Well-Being: The Role of Heritability and Genetics in Positive Psychology*, Oxford Univ. Press, 2015.
22. De Neve, J-E, N.A. Christakis, J.H. Fowler, and Bruno S. Frey, Genes, economics and happiness, *Journal of Neuroscience, Psychology and Economics*, 5, 193-211, 2012

23. Lykken, D. And A. Tellegen, Happiness is a stochastic phenomenon, *Psychological Science*, 7, 186-189, 1996.
24. Bartels, M. And D.I. Boomsma, Born to be happy? The etiology of subjective well-being, *Behavior Genetics*, 39(6), 605-615, 2009.
25. Lyubomirsky, Sonja, *The How of Happiness: A New Approach to Getting the Life You Want*, Penguin Books, 2008.
26. Headey, B.W., E.L.Holmstrom and A.J. Wearing, The impact of life events and changes in domain satisfaction on well-being, *Social Indicators Research*, 15, 203-227, 1984; Headey, B.W. and A.J. Wearing, Personality, life events, and subjective well-being: Toward a dynamic equilibrium model, *Journal of Personality and Social Psychology*, 57, 731-739, 1989.
27. Stones, M.J., A. Kozma, and J.K. McNeil, *Psychological Well-being in Later Life*, Butterworths, 1991; Myers, D.G. and E. Diener, Who is happy? Psychological Science, 6, 10-19,1995; Fujita, F. And E. Diener, Life satisfaction set point: Stability and change, *Journal of Personal and Social Psychology*, 88(1), 158-164, 2005; Cummins, R.A. et al., A demonstration of set points for subjective well-being, Journal of Happiness Studies, 15(1), 183-206, 2014.
28. Lykken and Tellegen, 1996, op. cit.
29. Sheldon, K.M. and R.E. Lucas, eds, *Stability of Happiness: Theories and Evidence on Whether Happiness Can Change*, Academic Press, 2014; Hentschel, S., M. Eid and T. Kutscher, The influence of major life events and personality traits on the stability of affective well-being, *Journal of Happiness Studies*, 18(3), 719-741, 2017.
30. Headey, B., The set-point theory of well-being has serious flaws: On the eve of a scientific revolution, *Social Indicators Research*, 97(1), 7-21, 2010;
31. Davidson and Schuyler, 2015, op. cit.
32. Plomin, Robert, *Behavioral Genetics*, 6th ed., Worth Publ., 2012; Kim, Y., ed., *Handbook of Behavioral Genetics*, Springer, 2009.
33. Bartels, M. And B.M.L. Baselmans, Molecular genetics of psychological well-being, Chapter 10, in Pleuss, Michael, ed., *Genetics Of Psychological Well-Being: The Role of Heritability and Genetics in Positive Psychology*, Oxford Univ. Press, 2015.
34. Bartels, M., Genetics of well-being and its components: satisfaction with life, happiness, and quality of life: A review and meta-analysis of heritability studies, *Behavior Genetics*, 45(2), 137-156, 2015; Nes, R.B., Happiness in behavior genetics: Findings and implications, *Journal of Happiness Studies*, 11(3), 369-381, 2010; Brown, N.J.L., et al., A critical reanalysis of the relationship between genomics and well-being, *Proc. Nat. Acad. Sci.*, 111(35), 12705-12709, 2014; Miller, Peter, A thing or two about twins, National Geographic, 22(1), 38-65, 2012.
35. Carey, Nessa, *The Epigenetics Revolution*, Columbia University Press, 2013.
36. De Neve et al., 2012, op.cit.
37. Bartels, M. and P. Koellinger, et al., Genetic variants associated with subjective well-being, depressive symptoms, and neuroticism identified through genome-wide analysis, *Nature Genetics*, 48, 624-633, 2016.
38. Minkov, M. and M.H. Bond, A genetic component to national differences in happiness, *Journal of Happiness Studies*, 18(2), 321-340, 2017.
39. Fredericksburg, B.L., et al., A functional genomic perspective on human well-being, *Proc. Nat. Acad. Sci.*, 110(33), 13684-13689, 2013.
40. Diener, E. and M.Y. Chan, Happy people live longer: Subjective well-being contributes to health and longevity, *Applied Psychophysiology*, 3(1), 1-43, 2011; Pressman, S.D. and S. Cohen, Does positive affect influence health?, *Psychological Bulletin*, 131(6), 925-971, 2005.
41. Harris, K.M., *The ADD Health Study: Design and Accomplishments*, 2013, [www.cpc.unc.edu/projects/addhealth/documentation/guides/DesignPaperWIIV.pdf].
42. Resnick, M.D. et al., Protecting adolescents from harm: Findings from the National Longitudinal Study of Adolescent Health, *Jour. Am. Med. Assoc.*, Sept. 10, 1997.

43. Brim, O.G., C.D. Ryff and R.C. Kessler, eds., *How Healthy Are We? A National Study of Well-Being at Midlife*, Univ. Chicago Press, 2004; [www.midus.wisc.edu]
44. Ehrenreich, Barbara, *Bright-Sided: How the Relentless Promotion of Positive Thinking Has Undermined America*, Picador, 2010.
45. Sirgy, M.J. et. al., The quality-of-life (QOL) research movement: past, present and future, *Social Indicators Research*, 76(3), 343-466, 2006.
46. [www.rand.org/health/surveys_tools/mos/36-item-short-form.html]; Stewart, A.L. and J.E. Ware, eds., *Measuring Function and Well-Being: The Medical Outcomes Study Approach*, Duke University Press, 1992.
47. [https://euroqol.org]
48. Weinstein, M.C., G. Torrance and G. McGuire, QALYs: The basics, *Value in Health*, 12, 55-59, 2009; Gold, M.R., D. Stevenson and D.G. Fryback, HALYs, QALYs and DALYs: Oh My: Similarities and differences in summary measures of population health, *Annual Reviews Public Health*, 23, 115-134, 2002; Garner, Sarah, The economics of health, at [https://plus.maths.org/content/economics-health]
49. Prieto, L. and J.A. Sacristan, Problems and solutions in calculating quality-adjusted life years (QALYs), *Health Quality Life Outcomes*, volume 1, article 80, 2003.

Part II
Eudaimetrics

Chapter 6
The Assessment of Personal Happiness and Life Satisfaction

Polls, Surveys and Questionnaires

The assessment of personal happiness of individual members of the general public is almost always carried out using self-reported subjective measures, based on polls, surveys, and questionnaires. Sometimes the emphasis is on hedonic happiness with inquiries into one's state of contentment "right now" or "at the present time." Alternatively, the survey questions may highlight eudaimonic happiness, often couched in terms of longer-term notions like wellbeing, life satisfaction, or quality of life.

Most surveys are *cross-sectional* in nature, that is, they sample a cohort of representative respondents from across the target population. If the survey is repeated on a yearly or multi-year schedule, the selected cohort for the later surveys would be equally representative but it would constitute a different set of randomly selected individuals. A *longitudinal survey*, on the other hand, follows the same cohort of individuals from survey to survey. Cross-sectional surveys provide a snapshot from a wide audience at a particular moment in time. Longitudinal surveys provide a long-running video but from a narrower audience.

Most of us are probably aware of the many online websites that provide happiness or life-satisfaction questionnaires, encouraging us to check our own state of wellbeing for our own edification. More salient to the purposes of this book are the surveys carried out by polling organizations on behalf of private think tanks, academic research projects, or government agencies, in order to gather statistical data on the overall level of happiness in communities, cities, and nations. These polls may be conducted online, or with paper questionnaires, or by telephone, or with face-to-face interviews. Table 6.1 lists some of the largest and most-widely-quoted of the national and international polling organizations that include questions on happiness and life satisfaction in their surveys and questionnaires.

The *Gallup World Poll* (GWP) is the current manifestation of the dreams of George Gallup (1901–1984) who founded the American Institute of Public Opinion

R. A. Freeze, *The Metrics of Happiness*, Social Indicators Research Series 86,
https://doi.org/10.1007/978-3-031-10913-3_6

Table 6.1 Sources of data on personal happiness from surveys and questionnaires

International Surveys	Gallup World Poll (GWP)	Gallup Organization	[www.gallup.com]
	International Social Survey Program (ISSP)	GESIS—Liebniz Institute for the Social Sciences, Mannheim, Germany	[www.issp.org]
	World Values Survey (WVS)	Vienna, Austria	[www.worldvaluessurvey.org]
	European Social Survey (ESS)	University of London, UK	[www.europeansocialsurvey.org]
	European Values Study (EVS)	Tilburg University, The Netherlands	[www.europeanvaluesstudy.eu]
	Eurobarometer	European Commission, Brussels, Belgium	[ec.europa.eu/publicopinion/index.cfm]
National Surveys	US General Social Survey (GSS)	NORC at the University of Chicago (formerly National Opinion Research Center)	[www.norc.org]
	Canadian General Social Survey (Can GSS)	Statistics Canada	[www.statcan.gc.ca]
	British Household Panel Survey (BHPS)	University of Essex Institute for Social and Economic Research	[www.iser.essex.ac.uk/bhps]
	Sozioekonomisches Panel (SOEP)	German Institute for Economic Research, Berlin	[www.diw.de/de/soep]
	Rand American Life Panel	The Rand Corporation	[https://alpdata.rand.org]
Archives	Interuniversity Consortium for Political and Social Research	Host: University of Michigan Institute for Social Research	[www.icpsr.umich.edu]
	World Database of Happiness	Ruut Veenhoven, Erasmus University, the Netherlands	[www.worlddatabaseofhappiness.eur.nl]

in 1935 and watched it morph into the leading private polling organization in the world. The Gallup Organization currently employs more than 2000 professionals in 30 offices around the world. The results of its surveys are used by the United Nations, the World Bank, the Organization for Economic Cooperation and Development, and many other national and international agencies. The Gallup World Poll was initiated in 2005. It is carried out in over 160 countries, home to over 98% of the world's population. It uses one-hour face-to-face interviews and/or 30-minute telephone interviews with 500–2000 respondents in each country. The GWP features numerous questions on over 100 crucial areas of concern including law and order, food and shelter, institutions and infrastructure, and more pertinent to our interests, happiness and wellbeing.

The *International Social Survey Programme* (ISSP) is a cross-national collaboration that conducts annual surveys on timely specific issues relevant to the social sciences. It was established in 1984 with four founding agencies: the British National Centre for Social Research in London, the Australian National University in Canberra, the National Opinion Research Center at the University of Chicago, and the Zentrum fur Umfragen, Methoden und Analysen in Mannheim, Germany (now a part of the GESIS program at the Liebniz Institute for the Social Sciences in Mannheim, where GESIS is an acronym for Gesellschaft Sozialwissenschaftlicher Infrastruktureinrichtungen). The ISSP archives reside with GESIS.

The *World Values Survey* (WVS) is carried out by a global network of social scientists who "study changing values and their impact on social and political life." It was founded in 1981 by Ronald Inglehart, a professor of political science at the University of Michigan. The WVS secretariat is based in Vienna, Austria, with archives in Madrid, Spain. The survey has been carried out in seven "waves" with ever-increasing international representation. Wave 7, conducted in 2017–2018, reached 400,000 respondents in almost 100 countries, making it the "largest non-commercial, cross-national, time-series investigation of human beliefs and values ever executed." The Wave 7 questionnaire has 290 questions in 14 thematic subsections, one of which is "societal wellbeing."

There are three European surveys listed on Table 6.1: the *European Social Survey* (ESS), the *European Values Study* (EVS), and the *Eurobarometer*. The ESS has carried out social surveys every 2 years since 2002 reaching over 45,000 people in 24 European countries. Its headquarters are in London, England, and its archives are housed at the Norwegian Centre for Research Data in Bergen, Norway. Its surveys provide "accurate data about the values, opinions, attitudes and beliefs of European citizens." Most of the data are collected in face-to-face interviews. The wellbeing module uses the WHO-5 questionnaire developed by the World Health Organization.

The EVS covers similar ground to that of the ESS. Their survey reaches respondents in 47 countries. It is based at Tilburg University in the Netherlands. It has been carried out in four waves since 1981, and is designed to assess how Europeans think about life, family, work, religion, politics, and society in general. Data are archived with GESIS.

The Eurobarometer is a public opinion survey carried out since 1974 on behalf of the European Commission. It is a cross-national, longitudinal study to "compare and gauge trends within the 28 member states of the EU." Results are based on at least 1000 face-to-face interviews in each country. The Eurobarometer has spawned similar efforts in other parts of the world leading to the development of an Afrobarometer, an Asiabarometer, an Americasbarometer, and a Latinobarometer.

Table 6.1 also lists four representative social surveys carried out at a national scale: the *US General Social Survey* (US GSS), the *Canadian General Social Survey* (Can GSS), the *British Household Panel Survey* (BHPS), also known as the *Understanding Society Survey*, and the German *Sozioeconomisches Panel* (SOEP), all of which include a happiness and/or wellbeing module in their questionnaires. Many other countries carry out similar programs, and almost all countries have a national census which often invites information from citizens that is pertinent to their quality of life.

The US GSS is administered by the National Opinion Research Center at the University of Chicago (now known as the NORC Center for Public Affairs Research). NORC is an independent social research organization funded in part by the National Science Foundation. It carries out opinion surveys and other data collection projects for a wide host of government agencies, non-profit organizations, and corporate clients, including the American Bar Association, the Centers for Disease Control and Prevention, NASA, CNN, the World Bank, and the US departments of Education, Energy, and Defense. The GSS has been operating since 1972. It provides a "clear unbiased perspective on what Americans are thinking and feeling" about such issues as national spending priorities, crime and punishment, race relations, and their own quality of life. The 2016 version of the US GSS questionnaire included a special module on hope and optimism. The US GSS program was one of the founding members of its international counterpart, the International Social Survey Programme (ISSP), described above. The questionnaires used by the GSS and the ISSP are coordinated so that data from the two surveys can be easily integrated.

The BHPS has been carried out in 18 waves starting in 1991. The program is based at the University of Essex Institute for Social and Economic Research. The most recent survey covered 9000 households in 250 separate areas of Great Britain. The use of the word "panel" in the name of a sociological survey (as in the British Household *Panel* Survey) implies that it follows the same "panel" of individual respondents from wave to wave, thus providing more meaningful longitudinal results than are available from cross-sectional surveys that select a different randomized sample for every wave.

The SOEP is also a panel survey. It has been operating since 1984. It currently interviews respondents in 12,000 German households. The SOEP questionnaire includes questions on all facets of life including, family, work, money, politics, and life satisfaction.

Almost all of the surveys listed on Table 6.1 are operated on a not-for-profit basis by government organizations or academic consortiums that provide their data freely to all interested users. Of interest then is the last-listed survey on the table, the *Rand American Life Panel* (ALP), which is offered as a business service by the US-based Rand Corporation. It has a 6000-member panel that is interviewed regularly online. There are core questions, including a module on life satisfaction, with additional questions provided by clients of the service. To date, over 450 separate surveys have been carried out.

The World Database of Happiness

The reader has already been introduced to two of the larger archival collections of data from surveys on happiness and wellbeing. *NORC at the University of Chicago* is the archival home not only to the US General Social Survey (US GSS) but also to many other academic, governmental, and privately funded studies. *GESIS at the*

Liebniz Institute for the Social Sciences in Mannheim, Germany, holds the data from both the International Social Survey Programme (ISSP) and the European Values Study (EVS).

Table 6.1 lists two archival centers that are even larger yet: *The International Consortium for Political and Social Research* (ICPSR), and the *World Database of Happiness* (WDH). The ICPSR is housed at the University of Michigan. It represents more than 750 academic institutions and research organizations. It was established in 1962, and is funded by a mix of government agencies and private foundations. The archives contain over 250,000 files of research results from the social and behavioral sciences. Of interest to us are the files of 2351 studies on wellbeing. The ICPSR is the North American home for data from the Eurobarometer. It also hosts data from the US Uniform Crime Reporting System, the US Census, several twin registries, and the National Longitudinal Study of Adolescent Health.

The granddaddy of all the happiness archives is the World Database of Happiness. The WDH is the brainchild of Ruut Veenhoven, the director of the Happiness Economics Research Organization at Erasmus University in Rotterdam, the Netherlands. Veenhoven was a founding editor of the Journal of Happiness Studies in 2011 and authored the first paper ever published in that journal. He has been called the "pope of happiness." [1] The World Database of Happiness was created by Veenhoven in 1985. It is a web-based compendium that summarizes the findings of over 11,000 scientific publications on happiness, and presents the results of every happiness survey carried out since 1945 in over 110 countries. Longitudinal results are available for 15 of these countries for 25 years or more. The WDH website is a monumental resource. It includes a bibliography of happiness studies, definitions of over 1000 published measures of happiness, and a suggested classification system for these measures. Every study and/or survey can be brought up as an individual page which lists the host and date of the study, the questionnaire on which results are based, the results themselves, and all reported correlations of the results with available demographic input. The WDH is a labor of love that deserves the gratitude of every happiness researcher the world over.

We Feel Fine

One of the most original attempts to discern the emotional state of the populace is the *We Feel Fine* (WFF) website, created by Jonathan Harris, an award-winning web designer, and Sep Kamvar, a professor of media arts and science at MIT [2]. The WFF website is driven by an app that searches the internet automatically every 10 min for expressions of human emotions. Any blog that contains sentences starting with "I feel ...." or "I am feeling ...." is flagged and the words that follow are compared with a pre-set list of 5000 identified feelings (cold, hot, happy, sad, depressed, guilty, sick, alone, loved, proud, bored, excited, etc.). There is no human involvement in the process; the system runs autonomously. Since the system was launched in 2006, almost 14 million feelings have been collected from 2.8

million unique bloggers. Because many of the bloggers provide personal demographic profiles on their websites, it is possible for the app to determine and report correlations. The primary finding is that blogging is a young person's game; 50% of all the recorded feelings come from people in the 20–29 age bracket, and only 1–2% come from bloggers over 40. The feelings that are reported are therefore young peoples' feelings. Apparently young people are not all that happy, as happiness accounts for only one-half of one percent of all the recorded emotions. However, this is enough for the WFF app to determine that the happiest state in the USA is Hawaii which runs at 32% above average. The New England States and the Sun Belt states follow close behind.

A similar effort is being undertaken by the University of Vermont Complex Systems Center. Their app automatically carries out a random sampling of 10% of the 50-million Twitter messages that go out across the blogosphere each day, with each one searched for more than 10,000 different words that are scored on a 10-point happiness scale (with 1 being the least happy and 10 the most). The integrated score for the USA bounces back and forth between 5.6 (around mass shootings, say) and 6.2 (Christmas) [3].

A psychologist at the University of Warwick in the UK has carried out a similar type of search, but this one a *historical analysis* of subjective wellbeing based on the language used in the British Library's digital catalog of millions of books published over the past 200 years. The results show the clear negative impacts of the European revolutions of 1848, the Great Depression, and World Wars I and II [4].

Core Questions, Likert Scales, and the Cantril Ladder of Life

The happiness and wellbeing modules that are used in social surveys can take many forms. Some ask only a single question; others several questions; and still others pages of questions. Many of them do not ask questions at all but instead provide statements that the respondent is asked to agree or disagree with. A questionnaire that follows the *question format* would provide the respondent with a set of possible answers to a question such as: "Taken altogether, how happy would you say you are these days?" The choices might be: Very Happy, Happy, Neither Happy nor Unhappy, Unhappy, and Very Unhappy. In *statement format*, the same idea would be expressed as a positive (or negative) declaration: "Taken altogether, I am very happy these days," and the respondent might be asked to choose between: Strongly Agree, Agree, Neither Agree nor Disagree, Disagree, and Strongly Disagree.

Lists of responses that take this form are known as *Likert Scales*, named after the psychologist Rensis Likert who developed his ideas on scales in 1932 while working for the US Department of Agriculture Survey Program. He later went on to become one of the founding members of the Institute for Social Research, the archival center at the University of Michigan that hosts the Interuniversity Consortium for Political and Social Research. Almost every questionnaire-based survey of personal happiness that one encounters uses Likert-scale responses, sometimes offering a 5-point choice as Likert originally recommended, sometimes offering as few as three or as many as 11. It was Likert who first argued that the response scales on social science questionnaires ought to be symmetric, bipolar, and set up so that the psychological distances between each of the scale points are equal [5].

One of the most influential life-satisfaction scales ever devised is the *Cantril Ladder of Life* (also called the Self-Anchoring Striving Scale) [6]. It was developed in 1965 by Hadley Cantril, the Princeton psychologist whose book on *The Pattern of Human Concerns* has already been highlighted in Chap. 3. The Ladder of Life uses a particularly-unique 11-point Likert scale. Respondents are asked to imagine a ladder with steps numbered from zero at the bottom to ten at the top. Then: "Suppose we say that the top of the ladder represents the best possible life for you and the bottom step of the ladder represents the worst possible life for you. On which step of the ladder do you feel you personally stand at the present time?" The Ladder of Life is widely used in many happiness questionnaires including that of the World Gallup Poll.

Regardless of whether a survey uses a single-question or multiple-question approach in its happiness or life-satisfaction module, there is usually a single *core question* that attempts to elicit an overall judgment from the responder. Table 6.2 lists a random sample of 15 such core questions (or statements) used in subjective questionnaires of happiness and life satisfaction. It is worth noting that these 15 represent the tip of a very large iceberg. On the World Database of Happiness, Ruut Veenhoven identifies hundreds of unique forms that such a question might take.

On Table 6.2, the first four quotes are from three influential academic studies that were among the earliest to use questionnaire-based happiness surveys in their research; the next six quotes identify the core questions from four of the international surveys highlighted on Table 6.1; and the last five are miscellaneous examples from the World Database of Happiness.

The three academic studies listed on Table 6.2 represent a kind of modern-era starting point, but they are not the earliest questionnaire-based happiness surveys. As early as 1930, Goodwin Watson, a professor of education at Columbia University Teachers College polled 388 adult students of education on their "general level of happiness." [7] He asked his respondents to complete four different tasks: (1) a self-rating of their happiness; (2) selection of a single-sentence description that best captured their attitude toward life (from a list of ten provided to them); (3) selection of one or more adjectives that they believed could fairly be applied to themselves (from a list of 50 provided to them); and (4) instructions to write a sentence or two "which will most truly describe your own general happiness in life." All of these techniques remain in the arsenal of current happiness researchers.

The earliest study listed on Table 6.2 is that of Gerald Gurin and his coworkers at the University of Michigan Institute for Social Research in 1960 [8]. Their survey involved face-to-face interviews with 2460 adults drawn from across the nation. Their report was titled *Americans View Their Mental Health: A Nationwide Interview Survey*. It is often credited with being the first large-scale, nationwide, social-science survey of the modern era. For the happiness question listed on Table 6.2,

Table 6.2 Some examples of single "core questions" used in subjective questionnaires of happiness and life satisfaction

Source	Question or statement	Number of scale divisions	Highest scale descriptor	Lowest scale descriptor
Gurin et al (1960)	"Taken altogether, how would you say things are these days?"	3	Very happy.	Not too happy.
Neugarten et al (1961)	"I've got pretty much what I expected out of life."	3	Agree.	Disagree.
	"How satisfied would you say you are with your way of life?"	3	Very satisfied.	Not very satisfied.
Andrews and Withey (1976)	"Taking everything into account about what has happened in the last year and what you expect in the near future, how do you feel about your life as a whole?"	7	Delighted.	Terrible.
Gallup World Poll	"On which step of the Cantril Ladder of Life do you feel you personally stand at the present time?"	11	Best possible life.	Worst possible life.
	"All things considered, how satisfied are you with your life as a whole these days?"	10	Completely satisfied.	Completely dissatisfied.
World Values Survey	"Taking all things together, would you say you are:"	4	Very happy.	Not at all happy.
Eurobarometer	"On the whole, how satisfied are you with the life you lead?"	4	Very satisfied.	Not at all satisfied.
European Social	"Taking all things together, how happy would you say you are?	10	Extremely happy.	Extremely unhappy.
Survey	"All things considered, how satisfied are you with your life as a whole these days?"	10	Extremely satisfied.	Extremely dissatisfied.
Miscellaneous Examples from the World	"In general, how happy or unhappy do you usually feel?"	10	Complete elation, rapturous joy, soaring ecstasy.	Utter depression and gloom, completely down.
Database of Happiness	"On the whole, my life is close to how I would like it to be."	5	Strongly agree.	Strongly disagree.
	"Generally speaking, Are you a happy person?"	7	Very happy.	Very unhappy.
	"How would you rate yourself as to how successful you have been in terms of	10	Completely successful.	Entirely unsuccessful.

(continued)

Table 6.2 (continued)

Source	Question or statement	Number of scale divisions	Highest scale descriptor	Lowest scale descriptor
	achieving your own goals and aims in life?"			
	"In getting the things you want out of life, how would you say you are doing right now?"	3	Very well.	Not too well.

respondents were given only three Likert scale divisions to choose from (very happy, pretty happy, and not too happy).

In 1961 Herbert Neugarten, a gerontologist with the Harvard University Psychological Clinic and his coworkers developed a survey that produced two Life Satisfaction Indexes. Index A was based on 20 *statements* like the first one listed on Table 6.2, and Index B was based on 12 *questions* like the second one listed there [9].

Yet another contribution from the University of Michigan Institute for Social Research came with the publication of the 1976 book by Frank Andrews and Stephen Withey on *Social Indicators of Well-being* (which has already been highlighted back in Chap. 3) [10]. They used the results of surveys to inform their text. One of their innovations was a highly original 7-point suite of Likert-scale responses to their life satisfaction question: "How do you feel about life as a whole?" Respondents were given their choice among: delighted/pleased/mostly-satisfied/mixed/mostly-unsatisfied/unhappy/terrible. Ever since, this suite of responses has been known as the Andrews and Withey Delighted/Terrible Scale.

Looking at the suite of questions and statements on Table 6.2, it is clear that some of them are inquiring about hedonic happiness (as indicated by phrases like "these days," "at the present time," and "right now"), while others refer to eudaimonic happiness or life satisfaction (as indicated by phrases like "way of life," life as a whole," and "the life you lead"). Almost all of them request the respondent to think broadly (by prefacing the questions with such qualifiers as "all things considered," "in general," "on the whole," or "taking all things together").

Multiple-Question Scales and Questionnaires

There are hundreds of multiple-question scales and questionnaires that allow individual respondents to subjectively assess their own personal happiness or level of life satisfaction. Table 6.3 lists a representative suite of 18 of the best-known and most-widely-quoted ones. They are listed in order by the number of questions or statements that are included in the exercise. These 18 can be considered the cream of the crop in the sense that they were all developed by leading researchers working at

Table 6.3 Some of the best-known multiple-question scales used in subjective assessments of happiness and life satisfaction

Name of scale	Primary developer	Number of questions or statements	Number of scale divisions
Happiness measures	Michael Fordyce, Edison Community College, Fort Myers, Florida	2 Questions	11 3
Subjective happiness scale	Sonya Lyubomirsky, University California, Riverside	2 Statements, 2 Questions	7
Satisfaction with life scale	Ed Diener, University of Illinois	5 Statements	7
WHO-5 well-being index	World Health Organization	5 Statements	6
Personal well-being index	Robert Cummins, Deakin University, Melbourne, Australia	7 Questions	11
Meaning in life questionnaire	Michael Steger, Colorado State University	10 Statements	7
Pursuit-of-happiness project	Mark Setton, University of Bridgeport	4 Questions, 9 Statements	5
Warwick-Edinburgh mental well-being scale	Ruth Tennant, University of Warwick, UK	14 Statements	5
Scales of psychological well-being	Carol Ryff, University of Wisconsin	18 Statements	6
Orientations to happiness scale	Christopher Peterson, University of Michigan	18 Statements	5
Questionnaire for Eudaimonic well-being	Alan Waterman, The College of New Jersey	21 Statements	5
Pemberton happiness index	G. Hervas and C. Vasquez, Complutense University, Madrid Spain	21 Statements	11
Meaningful life measure	Jessica Morgan, Kingston University, UK	23 Statements	7
Authentic happiness inventory questionnaire	Martin Seligman, University of Pennsylvania	24 Statements	5
Oxford happiness inventory	Michael Argyle and Peter Hills, Oxford University, UK	29 Statements	6
The happiness index	Laura Musikanski, Happiness Alliance, Seattle, WA	31 Questions 19 Statements	5
Multiple discrepancies theory	Alex Michalos, University Northern British Columbia, Canada	96 Questions	7
Gross National Happiness Survey	Centre for Bhutan Studies and GNH Research	148 Questions	10

institutions with specialized programs in happiness studies: the *Happiness Measures* [11] developed by Michael Fordyce, the *Subjective Happiness Scale* [12] by Sonja Lyubomirsky, the *Satisfaction with Life Scale* [13] by Ed Diener, the *WHO-5 Well-Being Index* [14] developed by the World Health Organization; the *Personal Well-Being Index* [15] by Robert Cummins, the *Meaning in Life Questionnaire* [16] by Michael Steger, the *Pursuit of Happiness Project* [17] by Mark Setton, the *Warwick-Edinburgh Mental Well-Being Scale* [18] by Ruth Tennant, the *Scales of Psychological Well-Being* [19] by Carol Ryff, the *Orientations to Happiness Scale* [20] by Christopher Peterson, the *Questionnaire for Eudaimonic Well-Being* [21] by Alan Waterman, the *Pemberton Happiness Index* [22] by Gonzalo Hervas and Carmelo Vazquez, the *Meaningful Life Measure* [23] by Jessica Morgan, the *Authentic Happiness Inventory Questionnaire* [24] by Martin Seligman, the *Oxford Happiness Inventory* [25] by Michael Argyle and Peter Hills, the *Happiness Index* [26] by Laura Musikanski, the *Multiple Discrepancies Theory* [27] by Alex Michalos, and the *Gross National Happiness Survey* [28] by the Centre for Bhutan Studies and GNH Research.

Perusal of Table 6.3 shows that most of these questionnaires use the statement format, one or two use the question format, and a couple are mixed. The number of questions or statements can be as few as two or as many as 148. The number of scale divisions in each response suite varies from 5 to 11.

There seems little value in looking at all 16 of these questionnaires in detail. The interested reader can easily locate detailed descriptions in the manuals or websites highlighted for each one in the Notes and References. The discussions here will be limited to just a few of them.

The shortest questionnaire has just two questions (and is touted as the "sixty-second happiness scale"). It was developed by Michael Fordyce, a pioneering happiness researcher who gained renown despite working out of a small community college in Florida. The first question asks respondents how happy they are and gives them an 11-point scale from which to choose (from "extremely unhappy, utterly depressed, completely down" at the bottom of the scale to "extremely happy, ecstatic, joyous, fantastic" at the top). The second question asks respondents to estimate what percent of their time is spent, on average, in a happy, neutral, or unhappy mood. With just the two questions Fordyce claims to address both the intensity and frequency of happiness.

Table 6.4 lists the full questionnaires for each of the next three shortest multiple-statement questionnaires listed on Table 6.3. These three are among the most widely-used happiness-measurement tools, perhaps *because* they are short and sweet. Each one can be completed in a matter of minutes.

The Satisfaction With Life Scale (SWLS) developed by Ed Diener and coworkers features five very-general positive statements. Respondent chooses from a 7-point agree/disagree scale for each statement, and adds the five scores together to get his or her overall life-satisfaction score. An interpretation of the overall score is included in the upper-right-hand box on Table 6.4. The WHO-5 Well-Being Index developed by the World Health Organization presents the respondent with five positive statements and asks him or her to use a 6-point scale to estimate the percentage of the time over

Table 6.4 Three multiple-statement questionnaires. (Adapted from the source materials listed in [12–14])

Scale	Statements	Scale divisions	Interpretation
Diener Satisfaction With Life Scale	1. In most ways, my life is close to my ideal. 2. The conditions of my life are excellent. 3. I am completely satisfied with my life. 4. So far, I have gotten the most important things I want in life. 5. If I could live my life over, I would change nothing.	For each statement: 7 = Strongly agree. 6 = Agree. 5 = Slightly agree. 4 = Neither agree nor disagree. 3 = Slightly disagree. 2 = Disagree. 1 = Strongly disagree.	Add five scores: 5–9 Extremely dissatisfied with life. 10–14 Dissatisfied with life. 15–19 Slightly dissatisfied with life. 20 Neutral life satisfaction. 21–25 Slightly satisfied with life. 26–30 Satisfied with life. 30–35 Extremely satisfied with life.
WHO-5 Well-Being Index	Over the past 2 weeks: 1. I have felt cheerful and in good spirits. 2. I have felt calm and relaxed. 3. I have felt active and vigorous. 4. I woke up feeling fresh and rested. 5. My daily life has been filled with things that interest me.	For each statement; 5 = All the time. 4 = Most of the time. 3 = More than half the time. 2 = Less than half the time. 1 = Some of the time. 0 = At no time.	Add five scores and multiply by four: 0. Worst possible level of well-being. 100 Best possible level of well-being.
Lyubomirsky subjective happiness scale	1. In general, I consider myself: 2. Compared with most of my peers, I consider myself: 3. Some people are generally very happy. They enjoy life regardless of what is going on, getting the most out of everything. To what extent does this characterization describe you? 4. Some people are not very happy. Although they are not depressed, they never seem as happy as they might be. To what extent does this characterization describe you?	7 = A very happy person. → 7 = More happy. → 7 = A great deal. → 7 = Not at all. →	1 = Not a very happy person. 1 = Less happy. 1 = Not at all. 1 = A great deal.

the past 2 weeks that each statement has held true. An overall score is determined by adding the five scores together and multiplying the total by four to produce a range of 0–100. The Lyubomirsky Subjective Happiness Scale (LSHS) uses two statements and two questions, three of them worded positively and one negatively. Each one has its own 7-point Likert scale. Overall scores run from 4 to 28. In all three questionnaires, low overall scores are indicative of low levels of happiness and life satisfaction, and high scores are indicative of high levels. The SWLS is really the only one of the three that provides a detailed quantitative interpretation of overall scores. The WHO-5 and LSHS leave it to the respondent to interpret their own scores. Presumably, if Likert-style thinking prevails, the midpoint (50 in the WHO-5, and 14 in the LSHS) represents the boundary between happiness and unhappiness, or satisfactory and unsatisfactory quality of life.

The primary observation that arises from Table 6.4 is how unique each one of these three happiness measurement tools is, and how different they are from one another. It gives more credence to Veenhoven's claim on the World Database of Happiness that there are hundreds of identifiably different measures of happiness, a claim which originally may have seemed excessive, and now may seem more defensible.

As an example of a longer questionnaire, consider the Oxford Happiness Inventory, which is summarized here in Table 6.5. There are 29 statements, 17 of them worded positively, and 12 negatively. Respondents use a 6-point agree/disagree scale, which is reversed for the negative questions. An overall score is determined by adding up the 29 scores and dividing by 29, leading to a range of 1–6, and interpretations from "not happy" to "very happy." The longer suite of statements allows for finer distinctions and greater coverage. Among the issues that are addressed by the Oxford questionnaire on Table 6.5 that do not appear on any of the shorter questionnaires from Table 6.4 are questions of optimism, commitment, attractiveness, decision-making, health, and memories of the past.

The Theory of Multiple Discrepancies developed by the Canadian political scientist Alex Michalos holds that happiness and life satisfaction are controlled by the perceived gaps between what one has and what one wants; what one has relative to what others have; and what one has had in the past relative to what one expects in the future. The intensity of these discrepancies is measured with a questionnaire that uses the 7-point terrible-delightful scale on eight questions in each of 12 domains (health/financial/security/family/employment/friendships/housing/areas lived in/recreation/religion/self-esteem/transportation/education). A recent paper calls the dissatisfaction that some people feel because of what they have not yet acquired as the "monkey trap" because it prevents them from enjoying what they already have [29].

Some of the other longer questionnaires also divide their questions or statements into modules that allow for the separation of happiness or life satisfaction scores into individual domains or component parts. The 18 statements on Ryff's Scale of Psychological Well-Being, for example, are divided into six modules representing six different components of wellbeing: positive relations with others, self-acceptance, autonomy, personal growth, environmental mastery, and purpose in life. The 23 statements of the Meaningful Life Measure are divided into five

Table 6.5 Template of questions used in the Oxford Happiness Inventory. (Adapted from the source materials from listed in [25])

1. I don't feel particularly pleased with the way I am.* 2. I am intensely interested in other people. 3. I feel that life is very rewarding. 4. I have warm feelings towards almost everyone. 5. I rarely wake up feeling rested.* 6. I am not particularly optimistic about the future.* 7. I find most things amusing. 8. I am always committed and involved. 9. Life is good. 10. I do not think that the world is a good place.* 11. I laugh a lot. 12. I am well satisfied about everything in my life. 13. I don't think I look attractive.* 14. There is a gap between what I would like to do and what I have done.*	15. I am very happy. 16. I find beauty in some things. 17. I always have a cheerful effect on others. 18. I can fit in (find time for) everything I want to. 19. I feel that I am not especially in control of my life.* 20. I feel able to take anything on. 21. I feel fully mentally alert. 22. I often experience joy and elation. 23. I don't find it easy to make decisions.* 24. I don't have a particular sense of meaning and purpose in my life.* 25. I feel I have a great deal of energy. 26. I usually have a good influence on events. 27. I don't have fun with other people.* 28. I don't feel particularly healthy.* 29. I don't have particularly happy memories of the past.*

For 17 positively-worded statements:	For 12 negatively-worded statements (marked with an *):	Add 29 numbers. Divide by 29
6 = Strongly agree. 5 = Moderately agree. 4 = Slightly agree. 3 = Slightly disagree. 2 = Moderately disagree. 1 = Strongly disagree.	1 = Strongly agree. 2 = Moderately agree. 3 = Slightly agree. 4 = Slightly disagree. 5 = Moderately disagree. 6 = Strongly disagree.	1–2 Not happy. 2–3 Somewhat happy. 3–4 Not particularly happy or unhappy. 4 Somewhat happy, moderately happy. 4–5 Rather happy, pretty happy. 5–6 Very happy.

sub-scales: the purposeful life, the valued life, the accomplished life, the principled life, and the exciting life. The Orientations to Happiness Scale is broken into three modules: life of pleasure (hedonia), life of meaning (eudaimonia), and life of engagement (flow). These breakdowns are meant to give the self-responder some indication of his or her strengths and weaknesses.

Most of the scales listed on Table 6.3 can be found on the PsyToolkit website, a "free-to-use toolkit for demonstrating, programming, and running cognitive-psychological experiments and surveys" maintained by the British psychologist Gijsbert Stoet [30]. The PsyToolkit also lists many other specialized scales for some of the secondary contributions to happiness and life satisfaction including the Emmons *Gratitude Scale* [31] (6 statements, 7-point scale), the Goleman *Emotional Intelligence Scale* [32] (33 statements, 5-point scale), the Baron-Cohen *Empathy Quotient* [33] (40 statements, 4-point scale), the Rosenberg *Self-Esteem Scale* [34] (10 statements, 4-point scale), the Rempel *Trust Scale* [35] (17 statements, 7-point scale), and several scales that measure optimism and resilience.

There are also scaled questionnaires directed to particular subsets of responders, for example, the *Multidimensional Students Life Satisfaction Scale* [36], the *Satisfaction with Relationships Status Scale* [37], the *Marital Happiness Scale* [38], and the *CASP-19 Scale* [39], which deals with wellbeing in later life. Others that deal with particular issues or domains include the *Living Conditions Index* [40], the *Index of Ethnic Diversity* [41], and the *Socioemotional Well-Being* Index [42]. There are at least three indexes that record gender inequity: the *Gender Gap Index* [43] put out by the World Economic Forum, the *Gender Equity Index* [44] by Social Watch, and the *Gender Inequality Measure* [45] by the UN Development Programme.

There is one more personal-happiness index worthy of note. The *Global Person Generated Index* [46], developed by a group of Oxford-based health researchers, is unique in that it allows the respondent to identify the five "areas of your life that are most important to you," and then answer questions on "how you felt about these areas over the past month. An 11-point scale runs from "exactly how you would like it to be" to "the worst you could imagine."

In 1991, John Robinson, a noted sociologist from the University of Maryland, was the lead editor on a handbook on *Measures of Personality and Social Psychological Attitudes*. It includes full descriptions and scoring instructions for over 100 scales developed by sociologists and psychologists to that date. Each scale allows for the detailed subjective assessment of a specific personality trait, many of which have significance in happiness studies, including personal values, purpose in life, self-esteem, morale, interpersonal trust, attitudes toward authority, social desirability, shyness, loneliness, anxiety, alienation, and depression [47].

Measures of Affect

Psychologists differentiate between two types of learning and decision-making: cognitive and affective. The *cognitive* part of the process is the rational, reasoned, and deliberative consideration that most of us use as our primary approach to life. The *affective* part leads to the more spontaneous reactions that are based on our emotions, feelings and moods. Happiness falls more into the affective than the cognitive side of life, and this has led some happiness researchers to try to measure personal happiness and life satisfaction through the use of questionnaires based on affect.

The most widely used tool of this type is the *Positive and Negative Affect Schedule* (PANAS) [48] developed in 1988 by David Watson, a professor of psychology at Southern Methodist University (and later at the University of Iowa) and Auke Tellegen, one of the original founders of the Minnesota Multiphasic Personality Inventory. As indicated on Table 6.6, PANAS respondents must examine a list of 20 adjectives (ten of them positive, and ten negative) and indicate the extent to which each of these adjectives matches the way that they have felt over the previous week (or day, or month, or year, or in general). A 1-to-5 Likert scale is used and the individual scores are totaled separately for the positive and negative affects,

Table 6.6 Positive and negative affect schedule (PANAS). (Adapted from the source materials listed in [48])

Positive affect	Negative affect	Scale and interpretation
Indicate the extent you have felt this way over the past week.	Indicate the extent you have felt this way over the past week.	
Active Alert Attentive Determined Enthusiastic Excited Inspired Interested Proud Strong	Afraid Ashamed Distressed Guilty Hostile Irritable Jittery Nervous Scared Upset	1 = Very slightly or not at all. 2 = A little. 3 = Moderately 4 = Quite a bit 5 = Extremely. Add positive affect scores. Range 10–50 Add negative affect scores. Range 10–50

giving a range of 10–50 for each. In the original study of 660 American undergraduate students, the positive score was 29.7 and the negative score was 14.8, indicating a considerable degree of happiness in this cohort. Later observers have suggested that the negative score be subtracted from the positive score to determine a single-valued result having a range of −40 to +40, with zero as the dividing line between happiness and unhappiness. Others have developed shorter (PANAS-SF) and longer (PANAS-X) versions, as well as a version for children (PANAS-C).

PANAS was not the first affect schedule. That honor goes to Norman Bradburn and coworkers at The National Opinion Research Center (NORC) at the University of Chicago. Their *Affect Balance Scale* was published in 1965 [49]. Nor is it the only one in common use. A research team from New Zealand produced a 96-item affect scale (later shortened to 40) that they call the *Affectometer* [50]. Ed Diener and co-workers produced the *Scale of Positive and Negative Experience* (SPANE) in 2010 [51].

Daily Record Methods

One of the obvious shortcomings of a one-time questionnaire or interview is that the respondent may have been caught at a particular bad moment, in which case the respondent's answers may underestimate his or her usual levels of happiness and life satisfaction (or conversely, at a very good moment, in which case the opposite is true). To get around this problem, there has always been interest in collecting a time series of responses from the same subject over a period long enough to smooth out the effects of short-lived circumstances and moods.

Use of daily record methods in the modern era can be dated to the late 1970s, but there were earlier precursors. In 1940, Hornell Hart used his "euphorimeter" to take measurements of happiness from individual respondents at regular intervals and plotted these as a time series to create a "chart for happiness." Respondents were asked on each occasion to estimate their level of happiness on a scale that went from −700 to +700, where 0 was the dividing line between happiness and unhappiness, and +100 was pegged as the happiness level of an average respondent. Values between 0 and 100 identified a respondent who is happy, but not as happy as the average person [52]. Values below 0 identified an unhappy respondent. In his original work, Hart prepared happiness charts for several subjects, including two young men, one who was falling in love and one whose mother was dying. The smitten subject showed wild swings about his mean throughout the courtship depending on his day-by-day perceptions of his likely success in gaining the affections of his heart's desire. The subject whose mother fell ill went from his apparent set point of a very happy +600 to the depths of despair at −700, then back up to +500, over the course of a month or so.

The modern era has seen the development of two daily record methods: the *Experience Sampling Method* (ESM) and the *Day Reconstruction Method* (DRM). The ESM approach was introduced by Mihaly Czikszentmihalyi and coworkers in a 1977 paper on "the ecology of adolescent activity and experience." In this study, a group of adolescents were provided with pagers programmed to beep at randomly selected moments during waking hours. At these moments, respondents were expected to carry out a self-observation task by recording their answers to a short questionnaire identifying their location, their current activities, the people with whom they were interacting at the time, their emotional states, and the possible motives for these states [53]. ESM is an "at-the-moment" approach. It records feelings "right then, not later" and "right there, not elsewhere." It links emotions like happiness with situations and circumstances, and is not influenced by memory biases. In the early 1980s, Herman Brandstatter and coworkers at the University of Linz in Austria used an ESM approach (which they called the *Time Sampling Diary* or TSD) to study a wide variety of cohorts including university students, faculty members, housewives, elderly citizens, and members of military units; and in 1994 Stone and Shiffman introduced a similar approach in behavioral medicine circles (where it is known as Ecological Momentary Assessment or EMA) [54]. In more recent years, the beeper has become passé, and ESM, TSD, or EMA studies can be carried out using smartphone platforms and specially designed apps such as iHabit, MetricWise, and BeepMe.

The Experience Sampling Method has been subjected to considerable testing to clarify its strengths and weaknesses [55]. Among the latter are worries that the very act of repetitive reporting might influence responses, and concerns that the method emphasizes the frequency of feelings but not necessarily their intensity. The method also places a heavy demand on subjects, perhaps biasing the results toward highly conscientious responders. Lastly, ESM is expensive to run and requires an enterprising organizational capacity on the part of the measurement team.

The Day Reconstruction Method addresses these last concerns by providing a simpler approach that has been shown to efficiently approximate the results of the more demanding Experience Sampling Method [56]. Developed by Daniel Kahneman and coworkers at Princeton University, the DRM asks respondents to complete a diary of meaningful events that occurred on the preceding day. Such an approach is much easier to administer, and it is felt that the memory bias over such a short interval will be limited. Respondents use checklists on their smartphones to record the timing of the events, where they were during each event, and who they were with. The subjects are also provided with a list of affective adjectives (such as happy, worried or angry, much like in a PANAS questionnaire), and requested to record the intensity of their feelings with respect to each adjective for each event on a 6-point Likert scale (from "not at all" to "very much").

The relative merits of the "remembered wellbeing" of the DRM, with its retrospective evaluations of happiness, vis-a-vis the "experienced wellbeing" of the ESM, with its real-time assessments, remains a topic of considerable interest and contention in the personal happiness literature. So, too, does the more basic question of the relative worth of either of the daily record methods (DRM or ESM) vis-a-vis the more traditional subjective questionnaires. A recent review paper summarizes the strengths and weaknesses of each, and concludes that a multi-method assessment that uses the best features of each technique represents the optimal approach [57].

In recent years, happiness researchers have tried to piggy-back onto the *American Time Use Survey* (ATUS) [58] carried out by the US Census Bureau on behalf of the Bureau of Labor Statistics. Starting in 2010, the ATUS questionnaire included a subjective-wellbeing module that not only asked respondents what they were doing at specific times but also how they felt about it on a 7-point scale. A separate question addressed their overall level of life satisfaction using the Cantril Ladder. Results from the ATUS surveys provide a much larger sample than could ever be put together for more specialized social surveys.

The OECD Guidelines

In 2013, the Organization for Economic Cooperation and Development (OECD), recognizing that many of its member countries were investigating the use of social indicators and/or measures of "gross national happiness" to buttress their more-traditional economic indicators, decided to issue a set of guidelines on measuring subjective wellbeing, in hopes of bringing some sense of uniformity to this burgeoning enterprise [59]. These OECD guidelines provide a kind of closure for much of the material covered thus far in this chapter.

The guidelines recommend the use of six modules; Module A—*Core Measures*, Module B—*Life Evaluation*, Module C—*Affect*, Module D—*Eudaimonic Well-Being*, Module E—*Domain Evaluation*, and Module F—*Experienced Well-Being*. All of the modules contain a set of specific questions or statements that must be addressed using a 0–10 Likert scale. The Core Measures module includes five questions that allow respondents to record their happiness and life satisfaction "these days." The wording of the questions is taken from the World Values Survey, the European Social Survey, and the Gallup World Poll. The Life Evaluation module asks the respondents to consider their life "as a whole." It has nine items that includes the Cantril Ladder of Life and Diener's five-statement Satisfaction With Life Scale. The Affect module requires the subjects to rate their intensity of feeling "yesterday" with respect to a list of ten provided adjectives (calm, worried, sad happy, etc.). The Eudaimonic Well-Being module presents nine statements taken from the European Social Survey and Diener's Flourishing Scale. The Domain Evaluation module asks the respondent how satisfied they are with each of ten areas of life: standard of living, health, achievement, personal relationships, safety and security, being part of their community, time management, quality of their local environment, and job satisfaction. The Experienced Well-Being module uses the Day Reconstruction Method, asking subjects to identify any meaningful episodes during the previous day and rating them with respect to a sixfold affect list (happy, calm, angry, sad, pained, and tired).

Issues and Problems with Polls and Questionnaires

The tasks associated with the design of a questionnaire and its use in a poll of suitable respondents is not as straightforward as it might first appear. Critics have identified many potential issues and problems, and the avoidance of these pitfalls is the subject of many textbooks, guides and manuals. There are academic research centers such as the Blaustein Center for Survey Research at Rutgers University that deal solely with these issues. There is also an association of polling organizations, the National Council on Public Polls established in 1969, that sets professional standards for polls and promotes better understanding among the media and general public on how polls are conducted and how to interpret results.

One of the first issues that may be raised is the question of representativeness of the sampled cohort. David Morse, a former senior editor of the Gallup World Poll, notes in his book *The Opinion Makers* [60] that more than 80% of those approached to participate in a poll refuse, so that results are biased toward the views of those few who are willing to take part. If telephone interviews are used, the sample must be drawn from the ever-shrinking pool of people who have land-line home phones. If the internet is used, samples are skewed toward young urban males.

Assuming a representative sample can be obtained, many questions remain with respect to the validity and reliability of a poll and its constituent questionnaire. In the world of public opinion surveys, the term *validity* is concerned with the extent to which a poll measures what it is intended to measure, while *reliability* is concerned with the internal consistency, stability, and repeatability of poll results. It is safe to say that every one of the multiple-question scales highlighted on Table 6.3 has been assessed for validity and reliability by its creators (reported in most cases in the papers referenced for each one).

Validity is not a simple concept. The National Business Research Institute actually lists 12 different types of validity [61], among them: *construct validity* (the extent to which a poll truly measures the desired issues of greatest importance), *content validity* (the extent to which the questions on a questionnaire cover a sufficiently representative subset of the full behavior domain under investigation), *criterion validity* (the extent to which the subjective poll results correspond to any available objective criterion), *statistical validity* (the extent to which adequate sampling procedures, reliable measurement methods, and appropriate statistical analysis have been used), *internal validity* (the degree to which causal relationships can be determined from poll results), *external validity* (the extent to which internally-valid results are transferable to different cohorts, places or times), and *ecological validity* (the extent to which research results can be applied to real-life situations).

Validity concerns can arise from gamesmanship on the part of respondents, effects of the wording and order of questions on a questionnaire, issues related to the interpretation of the scales used to answer questions, and situational biases.

Gamesmanship may be intended or unintended, but either way it leads to biased answers on questionnaires. For example, respondents may give responses that reflect how happy they think they should be, not how happy they are. They may overstate their happiness as a kind of ego-defense, or understate it to garner sympathy. They may show stronger agreement with statements as presented than they actually feel in an eagerness to please the interviewer. They may give answers to make a political point or to push a hidden agenda. They may feel obligated to give answers to questions on issues for which they have no opinion or do not care about (possibly in response to coaching or cajoling on the part of the interviewer).

The specific wording of questions on a questionnaire can influence results [62]. A request to the respondent to agree or disagree with a positively-worded statement (I am happy) generally garners a higher score than the inverse score of a negatively-worded statement (I am unhappy). Questions can be biased by the presence of lengthy preambles that appear to be soliciting a particular answer. Statements that refer to some theory or fact as "so-called" will bias respondents in a negative direction. Poll designers must beware of leading questions and loaded words. In one poll, a question that asked: "Are we spending too little on *welfare*?" received only 17% support, but: "Are we spending too little on *assistance to the poor*? got 62% [63].

The order of the questions can also be important. In one instance, famous in polling circles, the Gallup-Healthways Well-Being Index recorded its largest ever one-day jump on April 6, 2009, apparently because the order of several questions was changed [64].

When it comes to numeric scales, the number of options, or the labels on the available options (recall the delighted/terrible scale), can affect results. It has been reported that ten-point scales produce lower mean scores than five- or seven-point scales. Apparently, scales with the highest number (and the most-positive label) on the left-hand side tend to produce higher scores than when it is on the right-hand side. Horizontal layouts produce higher scores than vertical layouts. Bipolar scales (-5 to $+5$) tend to produce higher scores than unipolar scales (0 to 10) [65].

Situational conditions can also affect results. Daily record researchers have reported that happiness scores vary significantly with both time of day and day of the week. Even the weather may affect how respondents react to questions; scores are usually higher on nicer days [66]. In-person interviews may elicit more thoughtful responses than anonymous telephone calls or impersonal internet formats. The style of the interviewer can also affect responses. One study found that an interviewer in a wheelchair stimulated higher life satisfaction scores on the part of respondents than were obtained by an able-bodied interviewer [67].

Concerns over the *reliability* or *internal consistency* of poll results are usually assessed using test/retest procedures. Even when the same question is asked at two different points in the same interview, respondents do not always give the same answer. In studies where re-interviews were carried out 2 weeks after the original survey, test/retest correlations showed a range of 0.59 to 0.77, implying significant changes in respondents' answers over time, perhaps in response to changing moods or other situational factors [68].

Despite all this hand-wringing, most leading happiness researchers do not feel that the long list of possible pitfalls has any serious negative impacts on the overall value of their survey results. Ruut Veenhoven has led the defense, using data from his World Database of Happiness to "debunk" these "classic qualms." [69] He has tested many of the critic's hypotheses statistically and has concluded that they do not have merit. He belittles the charge that many responders may have no interest in their own levels of happiness, by quoting data indicating that 8 out of 10 Americans think about their life style at least once a week, and that less than 1% of responders offer no opinion on such questions. To answer charges that respondents might inflate their level of happiness out of ego-defense or social desirability, he quotes studies that specifically address potential response distortion and conclude that it is rare. He is not impressed by the main argument of the doubters, the fact that well over 50% of respondents think that they are happier than average, arguing that this is just further evidence of the true happiness of most respondents. All in all, he concludes that while many of the suggested pitfalls might bias an individual result, these random fluctuations will tend to balance out over sample populations, and it is the population statistics that are under increasing consideration for use in policy evaluation.

Ed Diener and coworkers also present several arguments which they feel indicate that scales of happiness, life satisfaction, and subjective wellbeing "validly reflect the quality of respondents' lives." They note that: (1) differences in life satisfaction between nations are associated with differences in objective conditions in those countries; (2) differences between groups who live in the same country or community but under different circumstances are also accurately reflected in survey results; (3) self-reported happiness is highly correlated with objective, non-self-reported measures; (4) survey results are in keeping with genetic and physiological predictors of happiness; (5) longitudinal surveys show systemic patterns of change before, during, and after significant life events; and (6) life satisfaction scores have been shown to be relatively reliable predictors of the future behavior of individual respondents [70].

We will give the final word on the subject to Alan Kreuger of Princeton and David Schkade of the University of California at San Diego who carried out a meta-analysis of various measures of wellbeing and concluded that "reliability figures for subjective wellbeing measures are lower than those typically found for education, income, and many other microeconomic variables, but they are probably sufficiently high to support much of the research that is currently being undertaken." [71].

So How Happy Are We?

The main thrust of this book is on the methods of measurement of happiness rather than the results obtained or the interpretations of those findings. Nevertheless, it is recognized that readers would like to see some discussion of the levels of happiness extant in the population and the correlations and connections that have been uncovered by happiness researchers. It is hoped that this section and the three that follow satisfy these expectations.

The first point to make with respect to overall societal happiness is that respondents to subjective questionnaires apparently do not differentiate very much between happiness, wellbeing, life satisfaction, and quality of life. While researchers jump through hoops to carefully define hedonic and eudaimonic components of happiness, and to differentiate between at-the-moment happiness and on-the-whole life satisfaction, the public seems blissfully unaware of such niceties. The results that are obtained from polls tend to track along together regardless of the wording.

This is helpful in that it allows us to place all of the studies under one umbrella. Regardless of which of the core questions from Table 6.2 were highlighted in a particular study, it seems that the results can be mixed in a single pot. When we do so, at least in the western democracies, it is clear that Ed Diener got it right in the title of his 1996 paper: "Most people are happy." [72] This was true before he wrote his paper and it has held true since. Referring to the two earliest studies highlighted at the top of Table 6.2, Gurin and coworkers found 89% of Americans to be "pretty happy" or "very happy" in 1960. Andrews and Withey identified 84% of the population as "above neutral" and only 5% "below neutral" in 1976. Brandstatter's experience sampling in 1991 determined that people are "in a positive emotional state" 68% of the time. In 2000, Robert Cummins reported that the "average level of life satisfaction" in the western democracies was 75% ± 2.5% [73]. In an analysis of life satisfaction for the UK based on the 2006 wave of the European Social Survey, the average level of satisfaction was 7.2 on a ten-point scale, with only 10% of the population falling below the neutral score of 5. On the same scale, many studies have shown the average happiness factor for the USA and Canada to lie in the range 7.0 to 8.0, (in the "happy" to "very happy" range), with Canada usually a half a point or so higher than the US.

One can also turn to the daily tracking of wellbeing carried out by the Gallup Organization in the US. On the randomly-picked day of June 26, 2017, 52% of respondents reported that their standard of living was "getting better," only 27% that it was "getting worse;" while 46% reported their mood as "happy," only 10% as "stressed." On two other questions, responses were still largely positive, but the percentages of negative responses were more significant. On life-as-a-whole, 57% said their life was "thriving," but 40% reported themselves as "struggling." On personal health, 52% reported that their health as "energized," but 37% were "ailing [74].

One interesting finding from these various meta-analyses is that when respondents are asked to rate themselves relative to an "average" for the cohort, most of them believe that they are above average in most major domains of their life. The Australian researchers Bruce Heady and Alexander Wearing quote results from three waves of a panel study in which a large majority of panel members believed that they were above average in meeting their job requirements (85.9%), as a parent (78.3%), as a spouse (77.9%), and as a friend (76.1%). They quote earlier studies that show that most respondents believe that they are "healthier, will live longer, and are more considerate, honest and creative than others." Headey and Wearing claim that this "sense of relative superiority" is central to wellbeing and a major contributor in the enhancement of one's self-esteem [75].

Many people today feel that societal happiness is on the wane, but that is not borne out by polling results. Ruut Veenhoven identified 199 time series of happiness from 67 countries with lengths of record from 10 to 40 years from the World Database of Happiness. Most of these time series show a remarkable stability through the years right up to the present day. Overall, he found a slight *increase* in worldwide happiness of 0.012 per year on a ten-point scale (or one full scale division every 83 years) [76]. In their 2019 review article, well-known quality-of-life researchers, Robert Estes and Joseph Sirgy, spoke to "transformative changes in the human condition" since 1950. They cite improved health outcomes, increased life expectancy, stronger levels of educational attainment, reduced rates of extreme poverty, and greater efficiencies in food production and distribution. They do temper their optimism by noting that these gains are not distributed evenly, and that progress in participatory forms of government in developing countries is often thwarted by government corruption, loss of press freedom, and setbacks in political rights and civil liberties [77].

Correlations and Connections

In 1994, Ruut Veenhoven wrote a report with the title: "Correlations of happiness: 7837 findings from 603 studies in 69 nations, 1911–1994." [78] It is hard to believe that there are over 7000 *different* correlates of happiness, so presumably some of the findings must be confirming earlier results, or perhaps contesting them. Nevertheless, these are a lot of findings, and one must consider that Veenhoven's analysis only included studies carried out prior to 1994. Since 1994 the number of happiness studies has exploded. Furthermore, the great majority of these studies are *designed* to provide correlative explanations of personal happiness and wellbeing, so further findings abound. The point is that it would take a multi-volume treatise to summarize and reference all this work, quoting original sources, and examining all the detailed findings, opinions, and points of view. Fortunately for all of us, at least two such efforts have already been made. Ed Diener is the lead editor of the free, online, *Handbook of Well-Being*, a 997-page compendium of 68 review articles authored by many of the leading lights in the field [79]. Even more encompassing is the *Encyclopedia of Quality of Life and Well-Being Research* a massive anthology edited by Alex Michalos, the Canadian-based quality-of-life researcher, and the long-time editor of the journal *Social Indicators Research.* It is a monumental effort, constituting 7347 pages, in 12 volumes, with over 2000 articles, and 661 illustrations. It was put together with the support of an editorial board of 155 members from 32 countries, and 1300 contributors from 58 countries. It cost $7050 US for the print version when it was first released [80].

Clearly the brief coverage here is not going to compete with this work of a lifetime. Rather, the reader is directed to Table 6.7 (in two pages), which summarizes the apparent consensus viewpoint on the relationship between happiness and 17 widely-recognized correlates. These include demographic identifiers like age, gender, marital status, parental status, and educational attainment; internal characteristics like temperament, personality, intelligence, spirituality, and health; external influences like good governance, equality of opportunity, and environmental protection; time-balance issues like job satisfaction and leisure activities; and the presence of strong relationships with family and friends.

The consensus views on Table 6.7 are based on summaries of the various correlates that have appeared in review papers over the years in the happiness literature. Among the most detailed early reviews are those by Veenhoven in 1984, Argyle in 1999, Diener and Seligman in 2004, Kahneman and Krueger in 2006, Huppert et al. in 2006, and Sirgy et al. in 2006 [81]. Among the more recent reviews are those by Kapteyn et al. in 2015, Veenhoven in 2015, Eger and Maridal in 2015, and Clark et al. in 2017 [82]. Attention is also drawn to three other influential collections: the *Oxford Handbook of Happiness*, the *Handbook of Social Indicators and Quality of Life Research*, and the six-volume set entitled *Well-Being: A Complete Reference Guide* [83]. The interested reader will find references to all the original papers in one or more of these quoted meta-studies.

Perhaps the most contentious issue with respect to many of the correlations indicated on Table 6.7 is the direction of the causal arrow. Correlations are exactly what they claim to be. They identify a relationship between two variables. They do not indicate the direction of the causal arrow. Does good health cause happiness? Or does the very act of being happy lead to better health? Does marriage make people happier? Or do happy people tend to sustain good marriages? Do good relationships with family and friends generate happiness, or do happy people tend to develop healthy relationships? The happiness literature is filled with strong opinions, claims and counter-claims, and studies ostensibly designed to ferret out the cause-and-effect truths. Unfortunately, or perhaps fortunately, those truths remain elusive.

The cause-and-effect question is closely related to that of genetic set-points, and arguments over the direction of causal arrows tend to bring out the same players. It

Table 6.7 Correlates of happiness and life satisfaction

Correlates	Consensus view on relationship to happiness and life satisfaction
Gender	No consensus. Some studies claim women are happier than men. Some find men are happier than women. All agree that the differences are small. Women are generally more sensitive to interpersonal relationships than men. Women are more prone to anxiety and depression. Men are more prone to alcoholism. Working fathers are happier than non-working fathers. Working mothers are less happy than non-working mothers.
Age	Cross-sectional studies show a U-shaped curve, with happiness highest in youth and old age, lower in middle age. Men bottom out at 56, women at 45. A minority viewpoint holds that cross-sectional data are misleading, and that longitudinal studies indicate slightly-decreasing happiness with age, presumably due to declining health. Many studies show a strong positive correlation between life satisfaction and retirement.
Intelligence	No significant correlations are reported between intelligence and happiness.
Temperament and personality	It is widely held that temperament and personality account for much more of the variance in life satisfaction than do life circumstances. Sociability, extraversion, cheerfulness, optimism and self-esteem are all positively correlated with happiness. Neuroticism is negatively correlated. Personality traits tend to remain fairly stable over a lifetime due to genetically-controlled set points (although set-point theory remains controversial among many happiness researchers).
Marriage or life partnership	It is a consistent finding that those who are married or have a close partner are significantly happier than those who do not. Researchers who support the set-point theory find that people are happiest right after marriage, and then slowly decline to their set point. They find people are least happy preceding and during divorce, then rise to their set point afterwards. Widowed women are identifiably less happy than others, as are single parents, and others who live alone.
Having children	The question of children is perhaps the most contentious issue in the field of happiness research. Some studies show a lifelong happiness dividend from parenting. Others show that very young children and adolescents lead to much parental stress and anxiety. The consensus view is probably "more joy than misery." The so-called empty-nest syndrome is not widespread. There is a strong two-way correlation between happy parents and happy children.
Physical health	Good physical health is strongly correlated with high levels of happiness and life satisfaction. Disease, disability, and chronic pain are strongly correlated with low levels of happiness and life satisfaction. A happy disposition is strongly correlated with longevity. There is some evidence that happy people are less susceptible to disease, but claims that a happy, optimistic outlook leads to better outcomes in ill people is not widely held. Exercise, fitness, good nutrition, non-smoking, and moderation of alcohol intake all improve health and happiness.
Mental health	Mental disorders are among the strongest correlates with low levels of happiness and life satisfaction. They are more negatively correlated than are physical diseases. Mental illness in a family member has a strong negative influence on the happiness of parents, siblings and spouses. Rates of occurrence have been increasing in recent decades.

(continued)

Table 6.7 (continued)

Correlates	Consensus view on relationship to happiness and life satisfaction
Education	Happiness levels are higher in highly-educated countries than in less-educated countries. Within countries, life satisfaction is positively correlated with years of schooling.
Job satisfaction	Managers and self-employed professionals are happier than salaried workers. Among salaried workers, good relations at work, fair and approachable bosses, and recognition of work well done, are more important than pay and benefits. There is a slight positive correlation with job status. Voluntary workers have greater job satisfaction than paid workers. Unhappiness of the unemployed is due as least as much to loss in pride as to financial hardship. Job loss leads to a greater fall in level of happiness than divorce.
Religiosity and spirituality	Active involvement in organized religion is positively correlated with life satisfaction, but not strongly. Prayer increases existential wellbeing in believers. There is much discussion in the literature, but no consensus, on whether the benefits of church attendance reported by church members are due to "believing or belonging."
Relationships	The strength of one's relationships with friends and family constitutes the single strongest correlate with happiness and life satisfaction. There is need for both a few close relationships and a network of secondary ones. Happiness is "contagious" in that it spreads effectively through social networks. Happiness is highest in communities where "social capital" is highest (where people trust one another and are mutually helpful through the giving and receiving of social support). Being in love and a healthy sex life are both strongly correlated with happiness.
Leisure activities	Life satisfaction is enhanced by club memberships, involvement in team sports, voluntary activities, cultural explorations, and travel.
Environment	There is considerable evidence that life satisfaction is positively correlated with good air quality, pristine waterways, well-maintained parklands, and other features of good environmental management. A few studies have correlated happiness with time spent outdoors. Hikers, campers, hunters, and fishermen all report enhanced nature-related life satisfaction.
Weather	Shorter days and lack of sunshine in winter lead to seasonal affective disorder and lower levels of happiness. In moderate climates, lower temperatures and lower humidity are positively correlated with happiness, while higher temperatures, higher humidity, and rain are negatively correlated.
Governance	Levels of life satisfaction are higher in countries with trustworthy governance, political stability, effective rule of law, freedom of the press, strong human rights records, and low levels of corruption. Happiness is more-highly correlated with *economic* freedom in poor nations, and with *political* freedom in wealthy nations.
Equality	Levels of happiness are higher in countries and communities where gender equality and minority rights are recognized.

must be recognized, of course, that happiness researchers have a conflict of interest when assessing these issues. If increased happiness does not lead to better health, better marriages, and better parenting, then what is the value of interventions that are designed to improve happiness? If the set-point controls the end-points of the causal arrows, then the *raison d'être* of the whole happiness mission somehow seems less important. It is not surprising that the psychology community, especially its self-help wing, is not enamored of set points or causal arrows that do not allow for the value of therapeutic intervention.

Does Money Buy Happiness?

The astute reader will have noticed that there is a major potential correlate of happiness and wellbeing missing from Table 6.7. The question of money, income, and wealth, and its correlation with happiness is sufficiently complex, and sufficiently contentious, to deserve its own section.

The source of contention is the so-called *Easterlin paradox*, coined in 1974 by the University of Southern California economist, Richard Easterlin, and reiterated by him many times since [84]. The paradox, first described back in Chap. 3, can be stated as follows: At any point in time, in comparisons between nations, or in studies within nations, happiness varies directly with average income, but over time, in both cases, happiness does not appear to increase with increased income. As a measure of average income, Easterlin used per capita gross domestic product. Over the years he has taken his happiness measures from a variety of sources including the original Cantril ladder study, and several "Gallup Poll type" core questions from the World Values Study, the Eurobarometer, and other international happiness surveys. If true, the Easterlin paradox calls into question the value of economic growth, which is the bedrock belief on which most of the economic policies of the free world rest.

Contention over the second half of the paradox has often muddied the waters with respect to the first part. Easterlin did not say, as some people seem to think, that wealth and income are not correlated with happiness. He only claimed that *increases* in wealth and income do not lead to *increases* in happiness. In point of fact, it has been proven time and time again that citizens of richer countries are much happier than those in poor countries. Within countries, too, the rich are happier than the poor. The correlation is not as strong within countries as it is between countries, but it is relatively robust. In this sense, then, it can be argued that money does buy happiness.

This should not come as any great surprise. In addition to their ability to live in better homes and amass more material goods, those who are better-off have access to better nutrition and medical care. They are likely to receive societal deference that bolsters their own self-esteem. They have the resources to fulfill personal goals. They have a better chance of avoiding regrettable events and keeping in control of life's turns. People who are less well-off are constantly under the yoke of a fragile financial position, possible debt, constraints on their borrowing power, and a lack of resources to ameliorate the impact of negative events in their life. Personal wealth and income are a very important element in the maintenance of subjective wellbeing, especially for the poor.

So what about the second half of the paradox; that increases in wealth and income do not lead to increases in happiness? There is certainly data to support this claim at the higher end of the economic scale. Many studies in the richer developed countries of the world, note that there are diminishing returns on happiness at higher incomes, perhaps even a threshold income above which little improvement in happiness is likely to accrue. In the USA in 2010, this threshold was estimated to occur at an income of about $75,000 per year [85]. It can also be argued that overall wealth (which may be inherited, or earned) is more important than annual income, and here too, there seem to be threshold levels of wealth above which increases in life satisfaction are unlikely to occur even as additional wealth is gained. In this sense then, the Easterlin paradox is confirmed.

There are, however, significant objections. The most obvious and well-founded objection is that while increased income *above* some threshold may not lead to increased happiness, it certainly does *below* the threshold, and the great majority of the world is below that threshold. More money definitely enhances subjective wellbeing when it allows people to escape poverty. In this light, the Easterlin paradox is seen to be a first-world issue, and of little import to the rest of the world.

The most common dissent is not so much an objection as an explanation. Many happiness researchers support the *rank income hypothesis* wherein it is argued that it is not absolute income that drives happiness but income relative to one's peers, friends, neighbors and co-workers. As income rises so too do desires for more material goods to keep up with the Joneses. Under this scenario, happiness depends more on the gap between income and material aspirations than on income itself, and neither your happiness nor that of the Joneses will rise with rising income. If this behavior is widespread, overall happiness in a (well-off) country won't necessarily go up as the economy grows [86].

Yet another explanation is offered by Daniel Kahneman and Angus Deaton, both Nobel Prize winners in economics. They differentiate, as was done in an earlier section of this chapter, between cognitive and affective reasoning, where it is cognitive thinking that assesses our life-as-a-whole eudaimonic quality of life, and affective thinking that assesses our emotional, experienced happiness. They conclude that cognitive life satisfaction rises steadily with increasing income for well-off people, whereas affective happiness rises only until a threshold is reached and then flattens out. For the poor, rising incomes increase both cognitive and affective happiness [87]. Ed Diener and coworkers summarize this duality of well being in the title of a 2010 paper: "Material prosperity predicts life evaluation, while psychosocial prosperity predicts positive feeling." [88]

A 2008 study based on data from the World Values Study gave credence to both the absolute and relative camps, concluding that both absolute income and relative income are positively and significantly correlated with happiness, but that *changes* in relative income have much larger effects on happiness than do changes in absolute income [89].

Is Happiness Relative?

The rank income hypothesis put forward in the previous section is one strand of a broader argument that holds that all happiness tends to be relative. Under this hypothesis, it is not absolute income, or specific health status, or the actuality of career success, per se, that controls personal happiness, but rather one's comparative situation *relative to one's own aspirations*, and *relative to the success of others*. Happiness is controlled by the perceived gaps, on the one hand, between what one has and what one wants, and on the other hand, between what one has and what one's neighbor has. This might explain why many people who most of us would consider to be in dire straits (say, refugees from civil wars in their home countries) can summon up positive responses on happiness questionnaires (because they are comparing themselves against those still left in their war-torn homeland). The high reported levels of happiness among many elderly people may be the result of comparison of their life situation with other seniors rather than with their own youthful selves.

Relativity is the prime feature of a psychological school of thought known as *social comparison theory*. It was originated back in the 1950s by the renowned MIT psychologist, Leon Festinger [90]. He argued that human beings are "creatures of comparison," and that most of us carry out a continuing process of self-evaluation through comparison with others. The most likely candidates for comparison are coworkers from the same occupational group, neighbors and friends who live in the same community, and others who are perceived to co-share one or more distinctive characteristics. When done with appropriate cohorts, social comparisons can help drive self-improvement and satisfy normal competitive urges, but overly-frequent comparisons with those who are much better off than ourselves (in some sense) can lead to happiness-sapping envy, and frustration over our inability to reach unrealistically high standards. The issue arises not just with respect to wealth and income, but also in such diverse aspects of life satisfaction as body image and athletic prowess.

The second thrust of the relativity argument relates to the concepts of adaptation and habituation (which are themselves related to the earlier-discussed set-point theory of happiness). Perhaps the most famous study in this genre dealt with the long-term happiness of those who experienced massive instantaneous changes in their life situation, either positively through the euphoric joy of winning the lottery, or negatively through the crushing blow of a crippling car accident [91]. The authors concluded that such events initially cause a huge upward or downward spike in happiness, but that as time goes on, these fortunate (or star-crossed) individuals adapt and become habituated to their new life situations. A new baseline is established against which subsequent events are judged. The lottery winners become "so accustomed to the additional pleasures made possible by their new wealth, that such events no longer contribute to their general happiness." As the accident victims proceed through the rehabilitation process, they may grow to thank their lucky stars that they did not suffer an even worse fate. In both cases, their levels of happiness are still based on relative comparisons with others, but now with new cohorts of others.

Once again, it is left to Ruut Veenhoven to provide the counterpoint· He argues that while relativity might apply to some of the contributing domains of happiness such as health status or level of job satisfaction, it does not apply to overall, life-as-a-whole, life satisfaction. He contends that overall happiness results primarily from the "gratification of basic bio-psychological needs," and to the extent that happiness depends on this component, it is not relative. Furthermore, he holds that habituation is far from universal, and that most people who experience a rise in their standard of living also record a permanent increase in their level of happiness. In a 2010 paper, Veenhoven was moved to conclude that "the theory that happiness is relative is simply wrong," but by 2015, after admitting that expectations and habituation may play some role for some people, he used the softer language that "happiness . . . is not *wholly* relative." [92]

Interventions and Prescriptions for Personal Happiness

There is no question within the happiness research community, or within the broader self-help industry that it has spawned, that personal happiness and overall life satisfaction are regarded as malleable, changeable, and open to improvement. The genetic factors that control personality traits are accepted as one component of happiness, perhaps accounting for half the total; unalterable life circumstances account for a few percent more; but the rest, maybe as much as 40%, remain under our own personal control and amenable to intentional activities. Set-point theory is accepted as an indicator of where one's average happiness level might lie, but not as an immutable impediment to the success of intervention therapy.

One of the earliest intervention programs was developed by the pioneering happiness researcher, Michael Fordyce, whose Happiness Measures were highlighted on Table 6.3. His Happiness Training Program, first developed in the late 1970s, later morphed into a widely-used online platform. It features the enhancement of 14 fundamentals (e.g. focus on the present, be organized, develop an optimistic mindset, keep busy, socialize more, use positive thinking, etc.). In one carefully-controlled clinical test, he claimed that all treatment groups demonstrated significant gains in happiness, and that such gains were still evident 9–28 months after participants had completed the program [93].

Michael Frisch of Baylor University has also reported success with his Quality of Life Inventory (QOLI), which can be used in intervention planning, and his Quality of Life Therapy, which is a book-length treatment that provides step-by-step instructions for putting the principles of positive psychology into practice in a therapeutic setting. The approach focuses on enhancing life-management skills, setting goals, developing self esteem, and improving relationships. There is also much attention paid to maintenance of good habits and the prevention of relapse [94].

Two New Zealand researchers have developed the Happiness-Enhancing Activities and Positive Practices Inventory (HAPPI). It is a questionnaire that helps people determine which types of interventions are likely to have the greatest impact on their wellbeing. There are 22 questions divided into four subscales (self-concordant work, personal recreation and people, spiritual and thought-related, and goal-focused activities). Once a participant's happiness deficits are identified, he or she can then choose from the many suggested interventions to select the ones that would be most likely to set things right. Studies with the HAPPI program suggest that about 10% of a person's happiness is due to self-motivated intentional activities [95].

The most complete assessment of the value of therapeutic intervention was carried out by Sonja Lyubomirsky and colleagues at the University of California Riverside in 2009. They reviewed 51 treatment programs reported in the literature that were aimed at "cultivating positive feelings, positive behaviors, or positive cognitions." Among the treatment approaches reviewed were hope therapy, mindfulness, life review therapy, positive reminiscence, cultivating sacred moments, goal setting, and those that fostered optimism, gratitude, and forgiveness. Among the happiness measures used in the various studies were Diener's Satisfaction With Life Scale, Ryff's Scales of Psychological Well-Being, Lyubomirsky's Subjective Happiness Scale, Fordyce's Happiness Measures, and many others. They found that individual therapy was more effective than group therapy, that volunteers benefited more than those randomly selected from a population, that depressed people benefited more than the non-depressed, that the success of intervention increased with the age of participants, that using multiple modes of intervention worked better than any single one, and that longer intervention programs were more effective than shorter ones [96].

The most common form of happiness enhancement probably doesn't involve intervention at all. The myriad self-help happiness books listed back in Tables 1.1 and 1.2 in Chap. 1 offer a form of "bibliotherapy" that is cheaper and perhaps just as effective. A paper in the Journal of Happiness Studies entitled "Do self-help books help?" examined 57 best-sellers and concluded that "the messages fit fairly well with observed conditions for happiness" (which is perhaps not all that surprising given that so many of them were written by the very researchers who identified the "conditions for happiness" in the first place). The author also notes that self-help books are undoubtedly "the most important (although not always the most reliable) channel through which psychological insights find their way to a general audience." [97].

So what are the "psychological insights" on happiness and wellbeing that these myriad self-help books bring to the public discourse? Table 6.8 provides our summary of the most common prescriptions for the attainment of personal happiness gleaned from these many works (or at least from their book jackets, Amazon.com blurbs, table-of-contents, indexes, reviews, and concluding chapters). The list is not full of surprises, but it probably represents a pretty good summary of the discussions of this chapter.

Table 6.8 Self-help prescriptions for increasing personal happiness

Attitude toward life	• Develop a sense of meaning and purpose in life. • Get into the flow. Do things with passion. • Be optimistic. Stay positive. Make use of humor. Laugh. • Develop your own sense of self-esteem. • Be open to new ideas. Seek out challenging experiences.
Money and material wellbeing	• Pursue wellbeing, not being well off. • Limit your desires for material goods. Ignore the consumer culture. Avoid the hedonic treadmill. • Control your finances. Avoid excessive or unnecessary debt. • Be prepared to ride out economic downturns. • Give to charity. Do good with your wealth. • Beware setting too-high expectations that are a setup for self-defeating perceptions of failure. • Beware making economic comparisons with others that lead to misplaced envy and dissatisfaction.
Relationships	• Nurture connections with family and friends. • Spend time with people you love. Play with your kids. • Respect your spouse. Try to promote marital harmony. • Use the internet to connect with distant friends. • Seek out happy people; happiness is contagious. • Minimize conflict in your life.
Health	• Age gracefully. Respect your body. • Eat lots of fish, fruit, veggies, and whole grains. Avoid sugar and fast food. Use a small plate. Stay hydrated. • Avoid stimulants like sugar, salt, caffeine, and alcohol that increase anxiety. • Exercise regularly. Keep fit. Run. Walk. Swim. Cycle. Stretch. • Get enough sleep.
Workplace	• Try to find work that challenges and engages you. • Focus on your strengths to become more energetic, productive, and successful. • Do not give in to status envy. • Avoid petty politics in the workplace. • Control your work/leisure time-use balance.
Gratitude and forgiveness	• Keep a gratitude journal. • Thank someone who has touched your life. • Say a grace of thanks at dinner every day. • Forgive others their failings. Leave revenge and resentment behind. • Be generous. Share your time and wealth with those less fortunate. • Be concerned for the happiness of others, not just yourself
Leisure time	• Develop a hobby that brings social contact with others. • Volunteer. • Gain an enhanced sense of community by joining a garden group, a service club, or a sports team.
Spirituality	• Reclaim your spirituality. • Quiet your mind. Read. Meditate. Listen to music. Gaze at the stars.
Environment	• Fill your home with happy memories, pictures of loved ones, art that means something to you. • Make connections to nature. Spend more time outdoors.

References

1. Veenhoven, R., The four qualities of life: Ordering concepts and measures of the good life, *Journal of Happiness Studies*, 1(1), 1-39,2011.See also: Veenhoven, R., Life is getting better: Social evolution and fit with human nature, *Social Indicators Research*, 97(1), 105-122, 2010. For biographical info on Ruut Veenhoven, see: Michalos, A.C., ed., The Pope of Happiness: A Festschrift for Ruut Veenhoven, *Social Indicators Research Series* 82, Springer Nature, 2021.
2. [www.wefeelfine.org]; Kamvar, Sep and Jonathan Harris, *We Feel Fine: An Almanac of Human Emotion*, Scribner, 2009.
3. [hedonometer.org]
4. Hills, T. et al, Historical analysis of national subjective wellbeing using millions of digitized books, *Nature and Human Behaviour*, 3, 1271-1275, 2019.
5. Likert, Rensis, A technique for the measurement of attitudes, *Archives of Psychology*, 140, 1-55, 1932.
6. Cantril, Hadley, *The Pattern of Human Concerns*, Rutgers University Press, 1965.
7. Watson, Goodwin, Happiness among adult students of education, *Journal of Educational Psychology*, 21(2), 79-109, 1930. The description of Watson's work is based on: Angner, Erik, The evolution of eupathics: The historical roots of subjective measures of wellbeing, *International Journal of Wellbeing*, 1(1), 4-41, 2011.
8. Gurin, G., J. Veroof and S. Feld, *Americans View Their Mental Health: A Nationwide Interview Survey*, Basic Books, 1960.
9. Neugarten, B.L. et al, The measurement of life satisfaction, *Journal of Gerontology*, 16(2), 134-143, 1961.
10. Andrews, Frank M. And Stephen B. Withey, *Social Indicators of Well-Being*, Plenum Press, 1976.
11. Fordyce, M.W., A review of research on the Happiness Measures: A sixty-second index of happiness and mental health, *Social Indicators Research*, 20(4), 355-381, 1988
12. [www.sonyalyubomirsky.com/subjective-happiness-scale-shs/]; Lyubomirsky, S. and H. Lepper, A measure of subjective happiness: Preliminary reliability and construct validation, *Social Indicators Research*, 46, 137-155, 1999.
13. [http://internal.psychology.illinois.edu/~ediener/SWLS.html]; Diener, E., R.A. Emmons, R.J. Larson and S. Griffin, The satisfaction with life scale, *Journal of Personality Assessment*, 49, 71-75, 1985; Pavot, W. And E. Diener, Review of the Satisfaction With Life Scale, *Psychological Assessment*, 5, 164-172, 1993.
14. [www.who.int]; The WHO-5 website: [www.psykiatri-region.dk/who-5]
15. Cummins, R.A., *Personal Well-Being Index (PWI) Manual*, 5th ed., 2013.
16. Steger, M.F., P. Frazier, S. Oishi, and M. Kaler, The meaning in life questionnaire: Assessing the presence of and search for meaning in life, *Journal of Counseling Psychology*, 53, 80-93, 2006.
17. [www.pursuit-of-happiness.org]
18. Tennant, R. et al., The Warwick-Edinburgh Mental Well-Being Scale (WEMWBS): Development and UK validation, *Health and Quality of Life Outcomes*, 5, 63, 2007.
19. Ryff, C.D. and C.L.M. Keyes, The structure of psychological well-being revisited, *Personal and Social Psychology*, 69, 719-727, 1995; Ryff, C.D. and B. Singer, The contours of positive human health, *Pschological Inquiry*, 9, 1-28, 1998.
20. Peterson, C., N. Park, and M.E.P. Seligman, Orientations to happiness and life satisfaction: The full life versus the empty life, *Journal of Happiness Studies*, 6, 25-41, 2005.
21. Waterman, A.S. et al., The questionnaire for eudaemonic well-being: Psychometric properties, demographic comparisons, and evidence of validity, *Journal of Positive Psychology*, 5(1), 41-61, 2010.
22. Hervas, G. And C. Vazquez, Construction and validation of a measure of integrative well-being in seven languages: The Pemberton Happiness Index, *Health and Quality of Life Outcomes*, 11, 66, 2013.

23. Morgan, J. And T. Farsides, Measuring meaning in life, *Journal of Happiness Studies*, 10, 197-214, 2009.
24. [www.authentichappiness.sas.upenn.edu]; Seligman, Martin E.P., *Authentic Happiness: Using the New Positive Psychology to Realize Your Potential for Lasting Fulfillment*, Free Press, 2002.
25. [www.new.meaningandhappiness.com/oxford-happiness-questionnaire/214/]; Hills, P. and M. Argyle, The Oxford happiness questionnaire: A compact scale for the measurement of psychological well-being, *Personality and Individual Differences*, 33, 1073-1082, 2002.
26. Musikanski, L. et al, Happiness Index methodology, *Journal of Social Change*, 9(1), 4-31, 2017
27. Michalos, A.C., Multiple discrepancies theory, *Social Indicators Research*, 16, 347-413, 1985.
28. [www.grossnationalhappiness.com/survey-results/questionnaire]
29. Keller, T., Caught in the monkey trap: Elaborating the hypothesis for why income aspiration decreases life satisfaction, *Journal of Happiness Studies*, 20, 829-840, 2019.
30. [www.psytoolkit.org/survey-library]
31. McCullough, M.E, R.A. Emmons, and J. Tsang, The grateful disposition: A conceptual and empirical topography, *Journal of Personality and Social Psychology*, 82, 112-127,2002.
32. Schutte, N.S. et al., Development and validation of a measure of emotional intelligence, *Personality and Individual Differences*, 25, 167-177,1998.
33. Lawrence, E.J. et al., Measuring empathy: Reliability and validity of the Empathy Quotient, *Psychological Medicine*, 34, 911-919, 2004.
34. Rosenberg, M., *Society and the Adolescent Self-Image*, Princeton University Press, 1965. Revised edition: Wesleyan University Press, 1989.
35. Rempel, J.K., J.G. Holmes and M.P. Zanna, Trust in close relationships, *Journal of Personality and Social Psychology*, 49, 95-112, 1985.
36. Huebner, Scott, *Manual for Multidemensional Student Life Satisfaction Scale*, 2001.
37. Lehman, V. Et al., Satisfaction With Relationship Status Scale: Development of a new scale and the role in predicting well-being, *Journal of Happiness Studies*, 16(1), 169-184, 2015.
38. Azrin, N.H. B.J. Naster and R. Jones, Reciprocity counseling: A rapid learning-based procedure for marital counselling, *Behavior Research and Therapy*, 11, 365-382, 1973.
39. Hyde, M. et al., A decade of research using the CASP scale: Key findings and future directions, *Aging and Mental Health*, 19(7), 571-575, 2015.
40. Krishnan, V., Development of a multidimensional living conditions index, *Social Indicators Research*, 120(2), 455-481, 2015.
41. Balakrishnan, T.R. and G.K. Jarvis, Socioeconomic differentiation in urban Canada, *Reviews Canadian Sociology and Anthropology*, 13(2), 204-216, 1976.
42. Bericat, E., The socioemotional well-being index (SEWBI): Theoretical framework and empirical operationalisation, *Social Indicators Research*, 119(2), 599-626, 2014.
43. [reports.weforum.org/global-gender-gap-report-2016]
44. [www.socialwatch.org]
45. [hdr.undp.org/en/content/gender-inequality-index-gii]
46. Martin, F., L. Camfield and D. Ruta, The Global Person-Generated Index (GPGI), in Preedy, V.R. and R.R. Watson, eds, *Handbook of Disease Burdens and Quality of Life Measures*, Springer, 2009.
47. Robinson, J.P., P.R. Shaver and L.S. Wrightsman, eds., *Measures of Personality and Social Psychological Attitudes*, Academic, 1991.
48. Watson, D., L.A. Clark and A. Tellegen, Development and validation of brief measures of positive and negative affect: the PANAS scales, *Journal of Personality and Social Psychology*, 54(6), 1063-1070, 1988. See also: [en.wikipedia.org/wiki/Positive_and_Negative_Affect_Schedule].
49. Bradburn, N.M. and D. Caplovitz, Reports on Happiness: *A Pilot Study of Behavior Related to Mental Health*, Aldine Publ., 1965; Bradburn, N.M., *The Structure of Psychological Well-Being*, Aldine Publ., 1969.
50. Kamman, R. And R. Flett, Affectometer 2: A scale to measure current level of general happiness, *Australian Journal of Psychology*, 35(2), 259-265, 1983.

51. Diener, E. et al., New well-being measures: Short scales to assess flourishing and positive and negative feelings, *Social Indicators Research*, 97, 143-156, 2010.
52. Hart, Hornell, *Chart for Happiness*, Macmillan, 1940; as reported in Angner, Erik, The evolution of eupathics: The historical roots of subjective measures of wellbeing, *International Journal of Wellbeing*, 1(1), 4-41, 2011.
53. Czikszentmihalyi, M., R. Larson and S. Prescott, The ecology of adolescent activity and experience, *Journal of Youth and Adolescence*, 6, 281-294, 1977.
54. Brandstatter, H., Emotions in everyday life situations: Time sampling of subjective experience, in *Subjective Well-Being: An Interdisciplinary Perspective*, 173-192, 1991; Stone, A.A. and S. Shiffman, Ecological momentary assessment in behavioral medicine, *Annals of Behavioral Medicine*, 24, 236-243, 1994.
55. Czikszentmihalyi, M. and R. Larson, Validity and reliability of the Experience Sampling Method, *Journal of Nervous and Mental Disease*, 175(9), 526-536, 1987; Scollon, C.N., C. Kim-Prieto and E. Diener, Experience Sampling: Promises and pitfalls, strengths and weaknesses, *Journal of Happiness Studies*, 4, 5-34, 2003.
56. Kahneman, D. et al., A survey method for characterizing daily life experience: The Day Reconstruction Method, *Science*, 306, 1776-1780, 2004.
57. Tay, L., D. Chan and E. Diener, The metrics of societal happiness, *Social Indicators Research*, 117(2), 577-600, 2014.
58. Stone, A.A. and C. Mackie, The Subjective well-Being Module of the American Time Use Survey: Assessment for its continuation, in Stone, A.A. and C. Mackie, eds, *Subjective Well-Being: Measuring Happiness, Suffering, and Other Dimensions of Experience*, Appendix B, National Academies Press, 2013.
59. Organization for Economic Cooperation and Development, *OECD Guidelines on Measuring Subjective Well-Being*, OECD Publishing, 2013.
60. Moore, David W., *The Opinion Makers: An Insider Exposes the Truth Behind the Polls* Beacon Press, 2008.
61. [www.nbrii.com]; See also: Diener, E., R.F. Inglehart and L. Tay, Theory and validity of life satisfaction scales, *Social Indicators Research*, 112(3), 497-527, 2013.
62. Schwartz, M., Self-reports: How questions shape the answers, *American Psychology*, 54(2), 93-105, 1999.
63. Bradburn, N.M., S.Sudman and B. Wansink, *Asking Questions: The Definitive Guide to Questionnaire Design: For Market Research, Political Polls, and Social and Health Questionnaires*, Jodey-Bass, 2004.
64. Weimann, J., A. Knabe and R. Schob, *Measuring Happiness: the Economics of Well-Being*, MIT Press, 2015.
65. DeJonge, T., R. Veenhoven and L. Arends, "Very happy" is not always equally happy on the meaning of verbal response options in survey questions, *Journal of Happiness Studies*, 16(1), 77-101, 2015. See also: [www.relevantinsights.com/validity-and-reliability].
66. Smith, T.W., Happiness, time trends, seasonal variations, intersurvey differences, and other mysteries, *Social Psychology Quarterly*, 42, 18-30, 1979; Kampfer, S. and M. Mutz, On the sunny side of life: sunshine effects on life satisfaction, *Social Indicators Research*, 110(2), 579-595, 2013; Schmiedeberg, C. and J. Schroder, Does weather really influence the measure of life satisfaction? *Social Indicators Research*, 117(2), 387-399, 2014.
67. Schwarz, N. And N. Strack, Evaluating one's life: A judgement model of subjective well-being, in Strack, N. et al., eds, *Subjective Well-Being*, 27-48, Pergamon Press, 1991.
68. Kahneman and Krueger, 2006, op. cit.; Lucas, R.E. and M.B. Donnellan, Estimating the reliability of single-item life-satisfaction measures: Results from four national panel studies, *Social Indicators Research*, 105, 323-331, 2011.
69. Veenhoven, R., What we have learnt about happiness, Classic qualms in the light of recent research, in *A Life Dedicated to Quality of Life*, Social Indicators Research Book Series, vol. 60, 151-170, 2015.
70. Diener, Inglehart and Tay, 2013, op. cit.

71. Krueger, A.B. and D.A. Schkade, The reliability of subjective well-being measures, *Journal of Public Economics*, 92, 1833-1845, 2008.
72. Diener, E. and C. Diener, Most people are happy, *Psychological Science*, 7, 181-185, 1996.
73. Cummins, R.A., Personal income and subjective well-being: A review, *Journal of Happiness Studies*, 1(2), 133-158, 2000.
74. [www.wbfinder.com]
75. Headey, B.W. and A.J. Wearing, The sense of relative superiority – central to well-being, Social Indicators Research, 20, 497-516, 1988.
76. Veenhoven, R., Greater happiness for a greater number: Did the promise of enlightenment come true? *Social Indicators Research*, 130(1), 9-25, 2017.
77. Estes, R.J. and M.J. Sirgy, Global advances in quality of life and well-being: Past, present, and future, *Social Indicators Research*, 141, 1137-1164, 2019.
78. Veenhoven, R., *Correlates of happiness: 7837 findings from 603 studies in 69 nations 1911-1994*, vols. 1-3, Erasmus University, Rotterdam, The Netherlands, 1994.
79. Diener, E., S. Oishi and L. Tay, Eds., *Handbook of Well-Being*, DEF Publishers, 2018. [nobascholar.com]
80. Michalos, A.C., *Encyclopedia of Quality of Life and Well-Being Research*, in 12 volumes, Springer, 2014.
81. Veenhoven, R., *Conditions of Happiness*, Reidel Publ. Co., 1984; Argyle, M., Causes and correlates of happiness, Chapter 18, in Kahneman, D., E. Diener and N. Schwarz, eds., *The Foundations of Hedonic Psychology*, Russell Sage, 1999; Diener, E. and M.E.P. Seligman, Beyond money: Toward an economy of well-being, *Psychological Science in the Public Interest*, 5(1), 1-31, 2004; Kahneman and Krueger, 2006, op. cit.; Huppert, F., N. Bayliss and B. Keverne, eds., *The Science of Well-Being*, Oxford University Press, 2006; Sirgy, M.J. et al., The quality of life research movement: Past, present, and future, *Social Indicators Research*, 76(3), 343-466, 2006.
82. Kapteyn, A., et al., Dimensions of subjective well-being, *Social Indicators Research*, 123(3), 625-660, 2015; Veenhoven, R., Social conditions for human happiness: A review of research, *International Journal of Psychology*, 50(5), 379-391, 2015; Eger, R.J. and J.H. Maridal, A statistical meta-analysis of the well-being literature, *International Journal of Well-Being*, 5(2), 45-74, 2015; Clark, A.E. et al., The key determinants of happiness and misery, Chapter 5, in Helliwell, J., R. Layard and J. Sachs, *World Happiness Report*, Sustainable Development Solutions Network, 2017; Clarke, A.E. et al, *The Origins of Happiness: The Science of Well-Being Over the Life Course*, Princeton University Press, 2018.
83. Land K.C., A.C. Michalos and M.J. Sirgy, eds., *Handbook of Social Indicators and Quality of Life Research*, Springer, 2012; Boniwell, I., S. David and A.C. Ayers, eds., *The Oxford Handbook of Happiness*, Oxford University Press, 2013; Cooper, C.L., *Well-Being: A Complete Reference Guide*, 6-volume set, 3226 pp, Wiley-Blackwell, 2014..
84. Easterlin, R.A., Explaining happiness, *Proc. National Academy Sciences*, 100, 11176-11183, 2003; Easterlin, R.A., et al., The happiness-income paradox revisited, *Proc. National Academy of Sciences*, 107, 22463-22468, 2010; See also: Cummins, R.A., Personal income and subjective well-being: A review, *Journal of Happiness Studies*, 1(2), 133-158, 2000; Frank, R.H., Does money buy happiness? Chapter 18, in Huppert, Bayliss and Keverne, eds., 2006, op. cit.; Bruni, L. and P.L. Porta, eds., *Handbook on the Economics of Happiness*, Edward Elgar Publishers, 2007; Zuzanek, J., Does being well-off make us happier? Problems of measurement, *Journal of Happiness Studies*, 14(3), 795-815, 2013; Pereira, M.C. and F. Coelho, Untangling the relationship between income and subjective well-being: The role of perceived income adequacy and borrowing constraints, *Journal of Happiness Studies*, 14(3), 985-1005, 2013.
85. Kahneman, D. and A. Deaton, High income improves evaluation of life but not emotional well-being, *Proc. National Academy of Sciences*, 107, 16489-16493, 2010. See also: Headey, B., R. Muffels and M. Wooden, Money does not buy happiness: Or does it? A reassessment based on the combined effects of wealth, income, and consumption, *Social Indicators Research*,

87(1), 65-82, 2008; Fischer, C.S., What wealth-happiness paradox? A short note on the American case, *Journal of Happiness Studies*, 9(2), 219-226, 2008.
86. Diener, E. and R. Biswas-Diener, Will money increase subjective well-being? *Social Indicators Research*, 57(2), 119-169, 2008.
87. Kahneman and Deaton, 2010, op. cit.
88. Diener, E. et al., Wealth and happiness across the world: Material prosperity predicts life evaluation, while psychosocial prosperity predicts positive feeling, *Journal of Personality and Social Psychology*, 97, 143-156, 2010.
89. Ball, R. And K. Chernova, Absolute income, relative income, and happiness, *Social Indicators Research*, 88, 497-529, 2008. For a user-friendly discussion of these matters, see: Graham, Carol, *Happiness Around the World: The Paradox of Happy Peasants and Miserable Millionaires*, Oxford University Press, 2009.
90. Festinger, L., A theory of social comparison processes, *Human relations*, 7(2), 117-140, 1954. For a more up to date treatment, see: Fujita, Frank, The frequency of social comparison and its relation to subjective well-being, in Eid, M. and R. Larsen, eds., *The Science of Well-Being: A Tribute to Ed Diener*, Guilford Publ., 2008.
91. Brickman, P., D. Coates, and R. Janoff-Bulman, Lottery winners and accident victims: Is happiness relative?, *Journal of Personality and Social Psychology*, 36(8), 917-927, 1978.
92. Veenhoven, R., Is happiness relative?, *Social Indicators Research*, 24, 1-34, 1991; Veenhoven, 2010, op.cit.; Veenhoven, 2015, op.cit.
93. Fordyce, M.W., A program to increase happiness: Further studies, *Journal of Counselling Psychology*, 4, 483-498, 1983.
94. Frisch, M.B. et al., Clinical validation of the Quality of Life Inventory: A measure of life satisfaction for use in treatment planning and outcome assessment, *Psychological Assessment*, 4, 92-101,1992; Frisch, M.B., *Quality of Life Therapy: Applying a Life Satisfaction Approach to Positive Psychology and Cognitive Therapy*, John Wiley and Sons, 2006.
95. Hendricksen, A. and C. Stephens, The happiness-enhancing activities and positive practices inventory (HAPPI): Development and validation, *Journal of Happiness Studies*, 14(1), 81-98, 2013.
96. Sin and S. Lyubomirsky, Enhancing well-being and alleviating depressive symptoms with positive psychology interventions: A practice-friendly meta-analysis, *Journal of Clinical Research*, 65, 467-487, 2009; Boehm, J.K. and S. Lyubomirsky, The promise of sustainable happiness, in *Oxford Handbook of Positive Psychology*, 2nd ed., 2012.
97. Bergsma, A., Do self-help books help? *Journal of Happiness Studies*, 9(3), 341-360, 2008.

Chapter 7
The Dimensions of Communal Wellbeing

How Many Dimensions?

This chapter begins the transition from the measurement of happiness on a personal level to the measurement of wellbeing on a communal or societal level. Of course, from one perspective, a community is nothing more than a consortium of individuals, and wellbeing at the communal level is simply the sum of the happiness levels of the individuals who make up the community. However, there is an argument to be made that this approach somehow belittles "the quality of collective life," that it neglects the positive impacts of neighborly interactions and the negative impacts of social inequalities [1]. Furthermore, the methods of measurement of communal wellbeing tend to be different in kind from those for personal happiness. On the one hand, as seen in Chapter Six, the assessment of personal happiness is usually carried out with subjective polls and questionnaires directed at individual respondents. On the other, the assessment of wellbeing on a societal scale is usually based on objective measures that can be gleaned from publically available databases. The next few chapters deal with these objective approaches to measuring communal wellbeing and societal quality of life.

The question to be answered in this chapter is this: If you wanted to specify a suite of measurements to be used in an objective assessment of communal wellbeing, just how many areas of life experience are you going to look at? There is already one suggestion on the table: the *three pillars* of the Brundtland Commission highlighted economic, social, and environmental dimensions [2]. Do you feel that these three sufficiently cover the waterfront? Can you easily include all the questions you might want to ask, or all the indicators you might want to look up, under these three headings?

Most of the researchers who work in the wellbeing game have concluded that these three are not enough. They tend to want to define more domains of interest. Sometimes they call these organizational elements *pillars*, sometimes *domains*, or

R. A. Freeze, *The Metrics of Happiness*, Social Indicators Research Series 86,
https://doi.org/10.1007/978-3-031-10913-3_7

Table 7.1 Dimensions of wellbeing

Brundtland Report	UN Human Development Index	Happy Planet Index	GNH Index: International Institute of Management	Canadian Index of Wellbeing	Sarkozy Commission
3	3	4	7	8	8
Economic Social Environmental	Life expectancy Education Income	Life expectancy Level of wellbeing Inequality of outcomes Ecological footprint	Mental Physical Workplace Social Economic Environmental Political	Community vitality Democratic engagement Education Environment Health Leisure and culture Living standards Time Use	Material living standards Health Education Activities and work Political voice and governance Social relationships Environment Security
GNH Index: GNH Centre, Bhutan	**The Economist Quality of Life Index**	**Legatum Institute Prosperity Index**	**Good Society Framework**	**OECD Better Life Index**	**Calvert-Henderson Quality of Life Indicators**
9	9	9	9	11	12
Psychological wellbeing Health Time use Education Cultural diversity and resilience Good governance Community vitality Ecological diversity and resilience Living standards	Material wellbeing Health Political stability Family life Community life Climate and geography Job security Political freedom Gender equality	Business environment Economic quality Education Governance Health Natural environment Personal freedom Safety and security Social capital	Relationships Economy Environment and infrastructure Health Peace and security Culture and leisure Spirituality, religion and philosophy Education Governance	Housing Income Jobs Community Education Environment Civic engagement Health Life Satisfaction Public safety Work/life Balance	Education Employment Energy Environment Health Human Rights Income Infrastructure National security Public safety Recreation Shelter

sectors, or *targets*, or *building blocks*, or *areas of interest*. Here they will be called *dimensions*.

Table 7.1 outlines 12 different attempts to answer the question of how many dimensions are needed. Each column on the table represents the organizational structure of one multi-dimensional assessment of wellbeing. Each of these dimensional structures has been developed by a specific set of authors, teams, or institutes, at different points in time, possibly for somewhat different purposes, although all of them are designed to ultimately provide a comprehensive evaluation of communal wellbeing. They are ordered on the table from the least number of dimensions (3) to the greatest (12).

First of all, let us clarify why some efforts at developing an organizational taxonomy of wellbeing have *not* been included in Table 7.1. Back in Chap. 2 three attempts to outline what their authors termed the *foundations of wellbeing* were introduced. There was Martin Seligman's five pillars of PERMA, Todd Kashdan's sevenfold organization, and Rick Hanson's 12 basic elements organized under his four-R's. While these classifications bring many concepts onto a single page, they are not truly multi-dimensional. If the three pillars (economic, social, and environmental) are used as a framework, then all of the concepts in Seligman's, Kashdan's, and Hanson's lists fit under the social dimension. There is little consideration of the economic or environmental pillars and their possible contributions to communal wellbeing. This is not to denigrate the importance of these works in helping to clarify the social dimension. It is simply an explanation of why they appear in Chap. 2 and not on Table 7.1.

Eight of the twelve columns on Table 7.1 represent the dimensional structure of individual quality-of-life indexes used to assess communal wellbeing at the scale of cities, states, or nations. Some of them have already been mentioned in earlier chapters. The concept of *Gross National Happiness* which originated in the Kingdom of Bhutan gets two columns on the table, one for the GNH Index developed by the Bhutanese, and one for a GNH-based Index developed in the USA. The original version of the Bhutanese index was based on only four dimensions, but a later version highlighted on Table 7.1 has nine [3]. The American-based *GNH Index* put out by the International Institute of Management in Las Vegas is organized under seven dimensions [4].

The other index-based columns on Table 7.1 include the *United Nations Human Development Index* (three dimensions) [5], the *Canadian Index of Wellbeing* (eight dimensions) [6], the *Better Life Index* of the Organization for Economic Development and Cooperation (11 dimensions) [7], and three indexes developed by London-based think tanks: the New Economics Foundation's *Happy Planet Index* (four dimensions) [8], the Economist Intelligence Unit's *Quality of Life Index* (nine dimensions) [9], and the Legatum Institute's *Prosperity Index* (nine dimensions) [10].

These eight indexes are introduced here solely for this exercise in counting dimensions. All of them are exceedingly important in the more-encompassing desire to shed light on the methodologies of measurement of communal wellbeing, and all of them will receive more-detailed attention in later chapters, particularly in Chap. 9.

There are four columns on Table 7.1 that come from studies that were not intended to develop a specific communal index of wellbeing. The *Brundtland Commission* report with its three-dimensional structure was the output from a UN-sponsored international conference. The report of the *Sarkozy Commission*, which was highlighted in Chap. 3, was a call-to-arms to look for alternatives to the GDP in measuring the wellbeing of nations. Their report features an analysis carried out using eight dimensions [11]. The *Good Society Framework* is notable in that it was developed solely as a self-standing intellectual exercise. Its nine-dimensional classification was developed by Patrick W. Jordon, a noted British business consultant who has written widely on such diverse topics as engineering design, ergonomics, and positive psychology [12]. The *Calvert-Henderson Indicators* were developed by Hazel Henderson, an independent author, futurist, and television producer, based in Fort Lauderdale, FL, in concert with the Calvert Investment Group, an asset-management firm in Bethesda, MD. Both Henderson and the Calvert Group are leaders in "socially-responsible investment" circles, and their indicators were originally developed to aid the Calvert Group in identifying suitable investment vehicles for their clients. In recent years the widespread interest shown in the Calvert-Henderson approach by those on the wellbeing circuit has led the founders to take a broader perspective, and the program is now supported by an advisory team of scholars and practitioners from universities, government agencies, and private think tanks [13].

Perusal of Table 7.1 reveals many recurring themes. Almost every organizational structure listed there includes an *economic dimension*, either directly, or in terms of "material wellbeing," "living standards," "income," or "basic necessities." Almost all include an *environmental dimension*, either directly, or as an "ecological footprint," or "ecological vitality," or subsumed in a broader category like "climate and geography." Almost all include a *health dimension*, some of them simply in the form of "life expectancy," others differentiating between physical health and mental health. The *social dimension* appears under many names: "social relationships," "social capital," "family life," "community vitality," and "cultural diversity." A dimension that includes *public safety* and/or *national security* occurs regularly throughout the lists, as does a *governance dimension*, sometimes identified as "political voice," "political freedom," or "political stability," sometimes as "democratic or civic engagement," and at least once as "human rights." An *education dimension* figures in 8 of the 12 lists. A *workplace dimension* also appears in several of the lists, often emphasizing "work/life balance" and "time use," or "employment" and "job security."

Perhaps the most original dimensional count comes from the Spanish economist Luis Herrero-Prieto. He suggests using the seven deadly sins to set the dimensional structure of a multi-dimensional wellbeing index [14]. The *Greed* dimension would capture the level of concentration of wealth in a nation or community. *Gluttony* relates to the sustainable use of resources. *Wrath* reflects safety and security issues. *Sloth* is a labor market issue. And *Pride, Envy* and *Lust* are facets of communal social structure.

An Eight-Dimensional Template

For the purposes of this book, an eight-dimensional template seems appropriate. The eight dimensions listed on Table 7.2 appear to cover the waterfront in terms of the areas of life experience that have some bearing on communal wellbeing: Economy,

Table 7.2 The eight dimensions of personal happiness and communal wellbeing used in this book

Economy	Basic needs/food/housing Cost of living/inflation Personal income/debt Personal wealth Job satisfaction Stock market performance Unemployment rates Government debt/deficit	Governance	Political freedom Enfranchisement and empowerment Civil liberties and human rights Transparency/corruption Freedom of the press
Environment	Livability of cities Air and water quality Land and natural resource use Ecosystem health/habitat Climate change Sustainability	Security and safety	From external wars From civil war From terrorism From crime Effective policing Fair justice
Social relationships	Marriage, parenthood, family Friendship and romance In groups, teams, clubs At educational institutions In the workplace In the military Arts and cultural activities Attitudes to diversity Religiosity and spirituality	Education	Quality of schools Access to education Educational outcomes Job training Intellectual development
Health	Longevity Physical health Mental health Access to medical care Fitness and recreation Work/leisure balance	Infrastructure and technology	Energy delivery Water supply Waste management Transportation and traffic Communications and Internet accessibility Technology innovation

Environment, Social Relationships, Health, Governance, Security and Safety, Education, and Infrastructure and Technology. This selection is made solely for the purposes of presentation, in order to bring some structure to the discussions in this chapter and those that follow. It has no other significance. When specific indexes of wellbeing are being analyzed, the analysis will be carried out using whatever dimensions are utilized in that index.

Table 7.2 also provides a first pass at listing some of the major component issues that fall under each dimension, the sub-dimensions if you will. The development of this table was helpfully informed by Patrick Jordon's Good Society Framework. If one looks at the sub-dimensions under the *Economy* dimension, for example, one sees such issues as cost-of-living, inflation, stock market performance, unemployment, and government debt. Objective communal data on all of these items are easily obtained from publically-available databases. So too for many of the other sub-dimensions listed on Table 7.2, like life expectancy, educational attainment levels, crime statistics, environmental quality, and so on. In fact, in the Appendix at the end of this book, Table A.1 provides an in-depth listing of the wide variety of sources that can be mined for data for each of the eight dimensions, both in an international context and for the USA alone. There will be reason to direct the reader to Table A.1 on many occasions in future chapters.

As in earlier chapters, the lines between personal and communal wellbeing, and between subjective and objective ways to measure them, are not carved in stone. Some of the sub-dimensions on Table 7.2 might appear to have more direct bearing on personal happiness than on communal wellbeing. Issues like the need for a sufficient level of personal income, or the need for adequate housing, are certainly pertinent to individual happiness. However, these issues also have resonance at the communal level, but now in a statistical sense, where the variations in personal income, and the availability of suitable housing, are aggregated over the whole population. Databases on these types of communal statistics are widely available.

The results of subjective polls can also be aggregated into objective communal databases. Referring again to some of the sub-dimensions listed on Table 7.2, one can imagine that overall community statistics can be gleaned from poll results on such issues as attitudes to diversity, participation in group activities, levels of religiosity, work/leisure balance, internet use, and many others. In this sense, subjective and objective approaches need not be seen as antithetical. Many researchers in the world of happiness studies hold that assessments of communal wellbeing ought to include both objective information from publically-maintained archival databases and subjective information from statistical databases developed from polling of the populace. Archival databases ought to provide a factual picture of the communal status of a particular issue, whereas polling statistics are more a reflection of public perceptions. In an electoral democracy, there is little question that perceptions are at least as important as cold, impersonal facts in determining policy.

The Question of Perspective

Some of the issues highlighted on Table 7.2 have greater resonance in the developed nations of the world, others in the less-developed nations. It is the widely-recognized difference between *needs* and *wants*. In the economic domain, there are many countries in the world where the basic needs of food and housing are at the forefront, and the performance of the stock market will have little traction. The *Governance* and *Safety and Security* dimensions probably have greater relevance in the less-developed nations of the world. Those of us in the more-affluent parts of the world often take democracy, freedom of the press, and freedom from war and terrorism for granted, whereas for those in strife-torn parts of the world, the presence or absence of these conditions bears directly on their happiness or wellbeing. Sadly, in recent years, the issue of terrorism has become globalized, and there are few places left where it does not represent a negative influence on both personal and community happiness.

If one looks at Table 7.2 from the perspective of more-developed nations like Canada and the United States, one sees the influence of "first-world issues" on happiness and wellbeing, things like access to fitness and recreation facilities, concern over traffic congestion, and demands for better internet accessibility. These issues may not resonate in less-developed parts of the world.

There are also questions of time and space. Some of the issues on the table, like one's social relationships with family and friends, are close to home. Others, like climate change, are of worldwide scope. It often seems in surveys of happiness and life satisfaction that the close-to-home issues resonate more clearly to most people than do the long-term, big-picture issues. In elections, the most contentious debates often revolve around short-term issues that have a direct effect on the pocketbook of individual voters. One of the greatest challenges in the measurement of communal wellbeing is how to be sure that the long-term worldwide threats to humanity get a suitable hearing. According to Lester Brown, in his State of the World assessments, the greatest threats to human wellbeing do not lie in the local issues but in the global ones: poverty, terrorism, and climate change [15].

Composite Indexes

In the introductory material in Chap. 1, an *indicator* was defined as a numerical or statistical measure of a single variable that changes its value over time, and that is thought to reveal some underlying aspect of happiness and wellbeing. An *index* involves the integration of several indicators into a single measure of greater breadth. Indexes may be *single-dimensional* or *multi-dimensional*, depending on whether they involve indicators that all come from one dimension, or whether they integrate across many dimensions. There are literally thousands, if not tens of thousands, of possible indicators that could be used in the calculation of either type of index. Most multi-dimensional indexes utilize tens, or even hundreds of specific indicators. Looking at three of the multi-dimensional indexes highlighted on Table 7.1: The Better Life Index uses 20 indicators spread over its 11 dimensions; the Canadian Index of Wellbeing uses 64 indicators over 8 dimensions; and the Prosperity Index uses 104 indicators over 9 dimensions.

Even a single-dimensional index may require many indicators to cover all its sub-dimensions. Take the Environmental Performance Index, for example, which provides a measure of environmental health and uses indicators that all come from within the environmental dimension. Even though it is single-dimensional, its developers need to cover some or all of the sub-dimensions listed under the Environment on Table 7.2. They will have to decide whether to include consideration of such diverse topics as water quality, climate change, and ecosystem health. For any one of them, say ecosystem health, for example, there are many, many possible indicators. Should they zero in on the animal kingdom or the plant kingdom? If the focus is to be on wildlife, which species deserve their attention? Will primary consideration be given to land, sea, or air? Wetland preservation, ocean habitat, or air pollution concerns? The data for each of these elements of the biosphere will probably come in different form, from different agencies.

In fact, even the sub-dimensions listed on Table 7.2 under each dimension may themselves require several indicators. Consider the sub-dimension *access to medical care* which appears under the Health dimension. Indicator data may be needed for such diverse issues as hospital capacities, doctor-to-population ratios, waiting times for operations, quality of senior care homes, and the availability of physiotherapy services. The *access to education* sub-dimension under the Education dimension might require data on participation rates and/or graduation rates for pre-school, elementary-school, high-school, and college education. In short, significant complexity can be anticipated in trying to integrate data, not just *across* dimensions, but also with respect to the wide spectrum of issues that appear *within* a single dimension or even within a single sub-dimension.

In the quality-of-life literature, any index, regardless of whether it is single-dimensional or multi-dimensional, is known as a *composite index* if it includes a number of different indicators which are integrated across the dimensions or sub-dimensions to produce a single-valued outcome. The area of research that promotes composite indexes is a rich one with much cooperation and much competition among the agencies that generate such indexes. In 2016, the European Union (EU), through its Joint Research Centre (JRC) in Ispra, Italy, launched its *Competence Centre on Composite Indicators and Scoreboards*. It offers member nations an audit service for new indexes. At last count the various EU countries were using 130 composite indexes, over half of them with JRC guidance. The JRC also hosts an annual 5-day convention where agencies can "showcase their capacity to inform policies through the use of indicator systems that summarize multi-dimensional concepts." Research teams are encouraged to discuss state-of-the-art methods, what level of faith to put in the results, how to avoid pitfalls, how to reach a broader public, and how to better inform policy [16].

The discussions in this book tend to be descriptive and practical, but there is also a highly-specialized quantitative wing to the wellbeing movement. Those readers who would like to see their indexes presented in full mathematical flower are directed to two academic treatises that follow this route [17].

A Ten-Step Scenario for Developing a Composite Index

In the chapters that follow the reader will be introduced to many composite indexes. Although it is unlikely that readers of this book are going to be setting up their own indexes, it still seems appropriate to look at how such indexes are designed and structured, and to review the steps and decisions that go into their genesis. If nothing else, such information ought to guide the reader in what to expect, and what to look for, in the descriptions of the various indexes.

As it turns out, the Organization for Economic Cooperation and Development (OECD) has produced a thorough guidance document in their *Handbook on Constructing Composite Indicators: Methodology and User Guide* [18]. On Table 7.3 their recommendations have been adapted into a ten-step scenario for the development of a composite index.

In Step One, the designer defines the purpose of the index, using what OECD calls the fitness-for-purpose principle. The primary decisions to be made at this early stage revolve around which dimensions need to be addressed, and which of the many available sub-dimensions need to be included under each dimension. The approach that is followed will depend in large part on the goals of the developer and the intended audience for the results. First-world and third world indexes may involve very different dimensions. Those developed by conservative think tanks will differ from those developed by poverty activists. Those developed for application in the workplace, or in the educational milieu, will differ from those with a broader societal perspective. Those developed for cities or communities will differ from those designed for application at the national or worldwide scales.

Step Two suggests setting guidelines for the selection of indicators, or at least making reference to one of the many sets of guidelines that have already been

Table 7.3 A ten-step scenario for the development of a composite index. (Adapted from source materials listed in Reference [18])

1. Define the purpose of the index, and determine the number of dimensions and sub-dimensions to be included.
2. Identify the selection criteria for the individual indicators.
3. Select the indicators on the basis of the selection criteria, identifying proxy indicators where needed.
4. Define a functional form for the indicator variables, where needed.
5. Identify data sources, and the quality and completeness of the available records.
6. Choose a methodology for the imputation of missing records.
7. Carry out an analysis to check for correlated interrelationships and possible redundancy among indicators.
8. Choose a technique for scaling and normalization of the data, including a method of directionality correction if needed.
9. Select the aggregation rules to be used in the aggregation of results across the dimensions or sub-dimensions.
10. Select a weighting scheme to reflect the relative importance of the various dimensions or sub-dimensions.

Table 7.4 Selection criteria for indicators of community wellbeing. (Adapted from source materials listed in Reference [19])

Purpose	The indicator is both meaningful for community understanding and useful for community planning and decision making.
Importance	The indicator measures an aspect of wellbeing that a diverse group of citizens in the community would agree is important.
Validity and accuracy	An indicator should be chosen only if a diverse group of citizens in the community would agree that an increase or decline in its value indicates improving or declining wellbeing.
Relevance	The indicator measures an aspect of wellbeing that the community can improve through public decision making.
Responsiveness	The indicator responds to real changes in the quality of life.
Anticipation	The indicator anticipates future trends rather than reacting to past trends.
Understandability	The indicator measures an aspect of the community's wellbeing in a way that can be easily understood by the citizens of the community.
Availability and timeliness	Data for the indicator are readily available and affordably accessible from a credible source.
Stability and reliability	Data for the indicator are collected, compiled, and calculated in a consistent manner over time.
Scale	The indicator is reported for a geographic area that is appropriate for the purposes at hand.
Clarity	The indicator uses inflation-corrected data, on a per-capita basis, and filters out any other extraneous factors.
Representativeness	Taken together, the indicators reflect the major dimensions of the community's wellbeing.

developed. An earlier discussion of this issue back in Chap. 3 highlighted the suggestions of Judith Innes, a well-known urban-planning specialist from the University of California at Berkeley. A more complete set of selection criteria is provided on Table 7.4. It is based in part on the suggestions of the Jacksonville Florida Community Council [19]. This local organization set up a wellbeing index for the city of Jacksonville that has become a model for many other American cities. The details of the Jacksonville index will be highlighted in Chap. 10, along with many other local indexes designed to assess and help improve the livability of cities.

Here, our interest lies more in the indicator-selection guidelines than the index itself. Let us go through Table 7.4 with respect to a specific example. Suppose you are trying to set up an index to measure the status of health care in a given jurisdiction. It will be a single-dimension index but it will have to cover several sub-dimensions, presumably including both physical and mental health. A possible starting point might be to define an indicator that reflects longevity in the community, perhaps using data on *life expectancy at birth*. Reference to Table 7.4 would show that such an indicator is well-suited to the *purpose, importance*, and *relevance* of the task at hand. According to the definitions on the table, its *validity, accuracy*, and *responsiveness* should not be in question, nor its *understandability* among the populace. Data on life expectancy is easily found in credible government databases, so that *availability, timeliness, stability,* and *reliability* are insured. It should also be possible to meet the *scale, clarity,* and *representativeness* criteria.

It will not always be so easy to confirm the appropriateness of an indicator that is under consideration, but the general admonitions of Table 7.4 provide some direction. The following chapters delve into the details of a variety of happiness and wellbeing indexes, and the reader is encouraged to cast a critical eye on whether the selected indicators pass the tests put forward in Table 7.4.

Step Three of the index-development scenario on Table 7.3 involves the actual selection of the specific indicators to be used for each dimension or sub-dimension. As noted in the previous section of this chapter, there may be hundreds of candidates and in most cases only a few can be selected without introducing unacceptable levels of complexity into the index. It must be recognized that the selected indicators are often acting as simplified representative proxies for a much more complex reality.

Step Four raises the issue of a functional form for the selected indicator variables. In most cases the raw data for each indicator is used directly in the index calculations without modification. In this approach higher values of the indicator variable will translate into higher wellbeing scores and they will do so on a linear scale. This is appropriate if changes in the indicator value have equal impact at all levels of wellbeing. However, if it is clear that changes in indicator values have different impacts at different levels of wellbeing, it may be more appropriate to transform the raw data by squaring them or taking them to an even higher power. Take GDP per capita, for example. An increase of $1000 would have far greater impact on jurisdictions at the lower level of this indicator than on those at a higher level. The relationship is logarithmic rather than linear. For this reason, this widely-used economic indicator is often taken to the second or third power before aggregating it with other indicators.

Step Five involves the identification of available databases for the selected indicators, and an assessment of the quality and completeness of the available records. In practice, Steps Two through Five are carried out interactively, because one of the most important criteria in the selection process revolves around the availability of data.

In many cases, the records for a selected indicator may be incomplete. Step Six involves choosing a method for the imputation of missing records. Among the most common methods are linear extrapolation and linear regression. The OECD Manual warns that too much data infilling can be "seductive and dangerous," and that no method of imputation is free from possible bias.

If too many indicators are selected from a similar area of concern, there is always the possibility that such indicators may be correlated with one another and some of them may therefore be redundant. In Step Seven, sophisticated statistical tools such as multivariate analysis or principle components analysis can be used to check for such redundant interrelationships. If any are found, the redundant indicators can be dropped from the calculation of the index. Similar techniques can also inform the search for suitable proxy indicators.

Step Eight deals with data normalization. In a multi-dimensional index with many dimensions and indicators, it is almost certain that the various data streams will involve a variety of different units of measurement. One can envisage data on debt in dollars, longevity in years, and climate change in degrees. Other indicators might be expressed as a percentage, or on a one-to-ten ordinal scale. Others might be in the form of ranked subjective descriptors. If aggregation across the dimensions or sub-dimensions is envisaged, some type of normalization scheme will be required to bring all the data onto the same page. There are several approaches. In one approach, the data for each indicator are converted into a normalized statistical distribution with mean zero and unit standard deviation. In another, all data are converted into percents, or ratios. In yet another, the data are scaled onto a zero-to-one interval, where the lower boundary is defined as the perceived minimum value for the indicator and the upper boundary as the perceived maximum. One way or another, all the data streams must be put into a compatible format suitable for aggregation.

The question of directionality in indicator data also falls under Step Eight. Some indicators (like income or wealth) have a positive impact on wellbeing as their values increase; others (like unemployment or debt) have a negative impact as they increase. Aggregation requires uni-directionality in data streams. The data for those indicators with negative directionality can be transformed into positive streams either by taking the negative of each data point (the data value multiplied by minus-one) or reciprocating each data point (the numeral one divided by the data value). While the two methods lead to somewhat different numerical results, sensitivity analysis on several indexes has suggested that the differences do not have a significant impact on overall results.

The final two steps on Table 7.3, dealing with aggregation and weighting, are sufficiently important to warrant detailed treatment in sections of their own.

The Question of Aggregation

Step Nine of Table 7.3 addresses the issue of aggregation. The eight-dimensional template put forward earlier in this chapter, each with its many sub-dimensions, and each of these requiring many indicators, represents a relatively-complete platform for the assessment of communal wellbeing, but it is a very diverse and complex playing field. Even with carefully-selected indicators and effective normalization, there are going to be significant challenges in trying to aggregate data to come up with integrated numerical measures. This will be true when aggregating across the indicators of a particular sub-dimension, or when aggregating across the sub-dimensions within a particular dimension, or when aggregating across the dimensions to reach an overall single-valued measure of wellbeing.

Once the data sets have been normalized, the simplest approach to aggregation is *additive aggregation* where the normalized indicator results are simply added and averaged. The single-valued aggregated score for a sub-dimension with four indicator scores would simply be the sum of the four scores divided by four. The problem with this approach is that it doesn't differentiate between two jurisdictions with very different patterns of scores, say one with scores {21,1,1,1} and the other with {6,6,6,6}. The aggregated score for both would be 6. An alternative approach, known as *geometric aggregation*, multiplies the four indicator scores together and then takes the fourth root. With this approach, the aggregated score for the first jurisdiction would be 2.14, and for the second, 6, suggesting that a jurisdiction with a balanced set of dimensional scores ought to be better off than one with all its strength in one dimension and great weaknesses elsewhere. Perhaps these off-kilter configurations are not that common because most indexes still use additive aggregation.

Aggregation at the sub-dimensional level, or even at the dimensional level, may seem like a reasonable proposition. It is at the overall multi-dimensional level that skepticism most often arises. Can one really expect to meaningfully integrate the effects on wellbeing of such diverse impacts as, say, access to medical care, freedom of the press, the effects of climate change, and protection of society from crime? Many wellbeing researchers question whether it is even advisable to try to integrate across the dimensions to reach a single-valued overall measure. They are dubious whether a composite index can actually achieve the desired level of congruence without sacrificing the very objectivity and transparency that is supposed to be its strength. The question has been hotly debated in the wellbeing community for many years. Table 7.5 summarizes the debate by listing the most-commonly raised advantages and disadvantages of multi-dimensional indexes that aggregate results across the dimensions to produce a single-valued outcome [20]. Perusal of Table 7.5 indicates that most of the pros and cons are paired. Simplification is good, but oversimplification is bad. A single-valued outcome makes for an effective communication tool, but the importance of internal components can get buried in the composite outcome. The results can be used to rank the wellbeing of jurisdictions against one another, but such comparisons can lead to invidious shaming of poorer societies.

While most of the researchers, public agencies, and private institutes that have addressed the overall wellbeing of society have attempted to come up with a single quantitative measure, not all assessors of societal quality-of-life have taken this route. Marc and Marque-Luisa Miringoff in their 1999 book "The Social Health of the Nation: How America Is Really Doing," argue that it is better to stick with an array of separate social indexes and not try to integrate them into a single overall measure [21]. In the *Calvert-Henderson Quality-of-Life Indicators*, the results of 12 calculations are kept as a separate array, and are not intended to be integrated into a single multi-dimensional index [22]. In 2013, the National Research Council sponsored a *Panel on Measuring Subjective Well-Being in a Policy-Relevant Framework*. In their final report the members of the panel made it known that they were "skeptical about the usefulness of any aggregate measure intended to track some average of an entire population." [23] All of these authors prefer stand-alone calculations for each dimension of wellbeing, Furthermore, they point out that a single aggregated measure is of little use for policy prescriptions, because it does not identify the particular underperforming components of wellbeing that require action.

Despite these caveats, it has always been the dream of those in the social indicators movement to develop a single multi-dimensional measure of communal

Table 7.5 Advantages and disadvantages of multi-dimensional indexes of wellbeing that aggregate results across the dimensions to produce a single-valued outcome

Advantages	• Composite indexes offer a means for presenting a simplified, holistic assessment of a complex multi-dimensional reality. • They can generally be applied at any jurisdictional scale: in the workplace, at the scale of cities or states, or at a nation-wide scale. • Most index calculations allow for tracking of component dimensions and/or individual indicators so that their specific role and importance in the overall calculation is transparent. • Regular calculations of the index can be scheduled to assess progress in jurisdictional wellbeing over time. • The single-valued numerical output and/or clear ranking among comparable jurisdictions focuses the attention of potential users, and provides an effective communication tool to reach the public, the media, politicians, policy-makers, and decision-makers. • The results of index calculations can be used to promote government accountability, and encourage policy changes that are based on measurable performance. Their publication reduces the likelihood of a public agenda that is focused on narrow interests. • A single-valued multi-dimensional index may offer an alternative to the GDP as a measure of communal wellbeing.
Disadvantages	• The structure of composite indexes may oversimplify complex issues. The importance of individual components may become buried in single-valued composite outcomes. • Lack of transparency may hinder proper interpretation of results and could lead to inappropriate policy prescriptions. • The selection of indicators, their weighting, and the methods used for aggregation across the dimensions may lead to unintended bias in the results. • There is a possibility of politically-motivated bias in the design of composite indexes in order to provide support for pre-determined policies. Results can be manipulated by agencies, political factions, politicians, and governments. • The results of the index may mirror those of the GDP without providing additional value, leading some to claim that they offer no real advantage. • Publication of rankings based on a composite index may lead to invidious comparisons between jurisdictions and shaming of those from poorer or less-developed regions. • Temporal changes within jurisdictions may move too slowly to provide meaningful indications of the need for changes in policy.

wellbeing, one that can compete with the GDP and the Dow-Jones for public attention, and prove useful in informing policy prescriptions. Certainly, a single number has the advantage of simplicity and easy comprehension. It is media-friendly and opens the possibility to widespread dissemination as a publicly-accepted measure of communal wellbeing. Newspapers and locally-focused magazines are quick to pick up on the relative rankings of cities, states, and countries that are indicated by these indexes. We have all read in local media at one time or another that our country ranks sixteenth, or that our city ranks fourth, or tenth, or sixty-ninth, in some listing of comparable countries or cities. There is little question that a single-value bottom line tends to engage the public.

The aggregation issue remains controversial, and much of the material in the next few chapters will deal specifically with how the various teams and agencies who plow these waters have addressed this core issue.

The Question of Weighting

The idea of a weighting scheme is introduced in Step Ten on Table 7.3. The idea is simple in concept but fraught with ambiguity in practice. It involves the assignment of weights to the various indicator values that are aggregated across a sub-dimension; or to the sub-dimensional values that are aggregated across a dimension; or to the dimensional values that are aggregated to produce the final single-valued output of the index. The simplest weighting scheme treats all the components equally and simply takes an arithmetic average of the component values. However, many index gurus want to weight the various components differently in order to reflect the perceived differences in their importance to the composite index as a whole. Certainly such differences exist. One could easily argue, for example, that per-capita household income has a greater impact on national wellbeing than, say, availability of fitness clubs. The weighting issue is an important one because many sensitivity studies have shown that the assignment of weights plays a crucial role in determining tradeoffs between the various indicators and dimensions, and that.large influences can be exerted on the overall results by changes in weighting.

The question is how to develop a defensible weighting scheme without introducing an unacceptable degree of subjectivity into what is claimed to be an objective exercise. If the weights are assigned subjectively by the agencies that generate the index, this becomes a step in the process that is ripe for bias. It must be recognized that most index developers, whether they are individuals, non-governmental organizations, or government agencies, have a mission, and the development of an index is part of that mission. Indexes invariably reflect the developers' value judgements about the nature of wellbeing, and setting weights is an integral part of the judgemental process. It is extremely difficult for developers not to introduce bias into weighting schemes, perhaps unintended or unrecognized, but bias nevertheless. To avoid such charges many of the agencies now convene panels of experts and stakeholders to recommend an appropriate weighting scheme for their index. Of course, the choice of experts is not itself necessarily value-free, but it is probably better than doing the weightings totally in-house.

Index developers use a variety of approaches to the setting of weights, among them equal weighting, normative weighting, and statistically-based methods. The simplest approach is to use *equal weighting*, which is viewed by some as a value-free choice, but it is nevertheless a choice in and of itself. *Normative weightings* are hardwired into the index methodology, often specified *a priori* by the index developer. Multivariate *statistical methods* such as principle components analysis are based on assessing the correlations between variables and assigning less weight to highly correlated variables. This approach avoids the possible double counting of strongly-correlated indicators or dimensions. Another approach involves relative pairwise comparisons of the *degree of importance* of the various indicator variables [24]. There are many more possibilities. A 2013 paper by researchers at the Oxford Poverty and Human Development Initiative (OSHI) lists eight different methods for setting weights in multi-dimensional wellbeing indexes. However, after presenting several of these methods in detail, they conclude that there is "no widely-accepted theoretical framework on how to set weights" in multi-dimensional indexes of wellbeing. They recommend a straightforward reliance on common sense [25].

The next two chapters introduce the reader to a variety of composite indexes. Those described in Chap. 8 are all single-dimensional. They are still *composite* in the sense that they usually involve many indicators and they aggregate results across the sub-dimensions that make up the structure of the index. Those described in Chap. 9 are all multi-dimensional, and most of them aggregate across the dimensions. Many of the single-dimensional indexes in Chap. 8 form the component building blocks of the multi-dimensional indexes of Chap. 9.

References

1. Atkinson, S. et al, Being well together: Individual subjective and community wellbeing, *Journal of Happiness Studies*, 21, 1903-1921, 2020.
2. Brundtland, G.H., *Our Common Future*, Report of the World Commission on Environment and Development, Oxford University Press, 1987.
3. [www.grossnationalhappiness.com]
4. [www.iim-edu.org/grossnationalhappiness/]
5. [www.well-beingindex.com]
6. [https://uwaterloo.ca/canadian-index-wellbeing/]
7. [www.oecdbetterlifeindex.org]
8. [www.neweconomics.org]
9. [www.economist.com/media/pdf/quality_of_life.pdf/]
10. [www.prosperity.com]
11. Stiglitz, J.E., Amartya Sen and J-P Fitoussi, *Report by the Commission on the Measurement of Economic Performance and Social Progress*, 2009.
12. Jordon, Patrick W., The Good Society Framework: Psychosocial ergonomics and quality of life, in: M. Anderson, ed., *Contemporary Ergonomics and Human Factors*, Taylor and Francis, 2012; Jordon, Patrick W., The Good Society Framework: Understanding quality of life, *Social Indicators Network News*, October, 2010.
13. Henderson, H., Lickerman, J., and P. Flynn, *Calvert-Henderson Quality of Life Indicators: A NewTool for Assessing National Trends*, The Calvert Group, 2000.
14. Herrero-Prieto, L.C. et al, Deep-rooted culture and economic development: Taking the seven deadly sins to build a well-being composite indicator, *Social Indicators Research*, 144, 601-624, 2019.
15. Brown, Lester, The eco-economic revolution, *The Futurist*, 23-32, March-April, 2002.
16. [https://composite-indicators.jrc.ec.europa.eu]
17. Van Praag, B.M.S. and A. Ferrer-i-Carbonell, *Happiness Quantified: A Satisfaction Calculus Approach*, Oxford University Press, 2004; Chakravarty, S.R., *Analyzing Multidimensional well-Being: A Quantitative Approach*, Wiley, 2017.

18. Nardo, M. et. al., *Handbook on constructing composite indicators : Methodogy and user guide*, Organization for Economic Cooperation and Development, 2008. See also : Salzman, J., *Methodological choices encountered in the construction of composite indices of economic and social well-being*, Centre for the Study of Living Standards, 2003.
19. Swain, D., *Measurement Progress: Community Indicators and the Quality of Life*, 2002; Chambers, M., *Quality Indicators for Progress: A Guide to Community Quality of Life Assessments*, 2004; *Quality of Life Progress Report*, 2006; all three reports published by the Jacksonville Community Council, Inc.
20. Nardo, 2008, op. cit.; Bandura, R., *A Survey of Composite Indices Measuring Country Performance*, United Nations Development Program, 2005 ; Booysen, F., An overview and evaluation of composite indices of development, *Social Indicators Research*, 59(2), 115-151, 2002.
21. Miringoff, M. And M-L. Miringoff, *The Social Health of Nations: How America Is Really Doing*, Oxford University Press, 1999. See also: Sharpe, Andrew, A survey of indicators of economic and social well-being, Canadian Policy Research Network, [www.cprn.org]
22. Henderson et al., op. cit.
23. Stone, A.A. and C. Mackie, eds, *Subjective Well-Being: Measuring Happiness, Suffering, and Other Dimensions of Experience*, National Academies Press, 2013.
24. Greco, S. et al, On the methodological framework of composite indices: A review of the issues of weighting, aggregation, and robustness, *Social Indicators Research*, 141, 61-94, 2019.
25. Decancq, K. and M.A. Lugo, Weights in multidimensional indices of wellbeing: An overview, *Econometric Reviews*, 32(1), 7-34, 2013.

Chapter 8
The Building Blocks of Communal Wellbeing

Single-Dimensional Indexes

The internet abounds with indexes that might be considered as having some bearing on issues of happiness and wellbeing. Studies carried out for the United Nations Development Office have identified as many as 135 of them [1]. Many of the best-known ones are multi-dimensional in nature; that is, they integrate across several of the dimensions outlined in Table 7.2 into a composite treatment that covers all the bases (or at least some subset of them). Some of these composite indexes, like the Human Development Index developed by the United Nations, the Index of Gross National Happiness from Bhutan, and the Better Life Index put out by the Organization for Economic Development and Cooperation have received mention in earlier chapters. However a detailed treatment of these indexes is postponed until Chap. 9, where the application of multi-dimensional indexes to country-by-country assessments of wellbeing is fully developed.

This chapter will zero in on *single-dimensional indexes* that focus on just one of the dimensions outlined in Table 7.2, or perhaps on only one of the sub-dimensions presented there. It is these more-focused indexes, or something very like them that often form the building blocks of the more-inclusive multi-dimensional treatments.

Table 8.1 provides a sampling of some of the better-known single-dimensional indexes that could prove useful in our travels through the world of happiness and wellbeing. They are organized under the eight-dimensional template presented in Table 7.2. The table lists not only the indexes but also the organizations that compile them and the websites where further details and results can be found.

It must be remembered that these indexes have been put together by a wide variety of organizations for a wide variety of reasons. They share only one feature in common: the desire to carry out a quantitative analysis that arrives at a single representative number that can be used to rank the performance of various jurisdictions against one another, or follow the trends over time within a single jurisdiction. Most of the indexes have been developed by organizations with their own purposes

R. A. Freeze, *The Metrics of Happiness*, Social Indicators Research Series 86,
https://doi.org/10.1007/978-3-031-10913-3_8

Table 8.1 A sampling of single-dimensional indexes that bear on issues of happiness and wellbeing

Dimension	Index	Host Organization	Website
Economy	Consumer Price Index	US Bureau of Labor Statistics	[www.bls.gov]
	Housing Affordability Index	Demographia International	[www.demographia.com]
	Global Opportunity Index	Milken Institute, Santa Monica, CA	[www.milkeninstitute.org]
	Opacity Index	Kurtzman Group for Price Waterhouse Coopers	[www.opacityindex.com]
	Index of Economic Wellbeing	Centre for Study of Living Standards, Ottawa, Canada	[www.csis.ca/iwb.asp]
Governance	Democracy Index	Economist Intelligence Unit, London, UK	[www.eiu.com]
	Global Integrity Scorecard	Global Integrity	[www.globalintegrity.org]
	Worldwide Governance Indicators	World Bank	[http://info.worldbank.org/governance]
	Worldwide Press Freedom Index	Reporters Without Borders	[www.rsf.org]
	Corruption Perception Index	Transparency International, Berlin	[www.transparency.org]
Security and Safety	Global Peace Index	Institute for Economics and Peace, Sydney, Australia	[www.economicsandpeace.org]
	Global Terrorism Index	Institute for Economics and Peace, Sydney, Australia	[www.economicsandpeace.org]
	Fragile States Index	Fund for Peace	[www.fundforpeace.org]
	Crime Severity Index	Statistics Canada	[www.statcan.gc.ca]
	National Index of Violence and Harm	Peace Studies Institute	[www.uri.edu/nivah]
Social Relationships	State of Caring Index	United Way of America	[www.unitedway.org/state of caring]
	World Giving Index	Charities Aid Foundation	[www.cafonline.org]
	Social Progress Index	Social Progress Imperative	[www.socialprogressimperative.org]
	Index of Social Health	Institute for Innovation in Social Policy, Vassar College	[www.iisp.vassar.edu]
Education		Bertelsmann-Stiftung Foundation	[www.elli.org]

(continued)

Table 8.1 (continued)

Dimension	Index	Host Organization	Website
	European Life-long Learning Indicators		
	Education For All Development Index	Global Education Monitoring Agency, UNESCO	[https://en.unesco.org/gem-report/education-all-development-index]
Health	European Health Consumer Index	Health Consumer Powerhouse, Stockholm, Sweden	[www.healthpowerhouse.com]
	Gallup-Sharecare Well-Being Index	Gallup Organization/ Sharecare	[www.well-beingindex.com]
	Child and Youth Well-Being Index	Foundation for Child Development	[www.fcd-us.org]
	Child Well-being Index	UNICEF	[www.unicef-irc.org]
	Global AgeWatch	HelpAge International	[www.helpage.org/global-agewatch]
Environment	Living Planet Index	World Wildlife Fund, Gland, Switzerland	[www.livingplanetindex.org]
	Ecological Footprint	Global Footprint Network	[www.footprintnetwork.org]
	Environmental Performance Index	Yale University Center for Environmental Law and Policy	[www.epi.yale.edu]
Infrastructure and Technology	ICT Development Index	UN International Telecommunications Union	[www.itu.int]
	Knowledge Index	World Bank Institute	[www.worldbank.org/kam]

and clientele in mind. Perhaps their results are presented to help investors, or to expose corruption, or to improve the health care system. So, while all of the listed indexes are thought to have some role to play in assessing overall quality of life, it is probably true that none of them were actually developed with that purpose in mind.

A brief description of most of the indexes listed in Table 8.1 follows. The descriptions do not provide enough detail to gain a full understanding of the methodology used to come up with the final numbers, but they will indicate the general approach that is used and the degree of complexity involved. The purpose of this exercise is to expose the highly-variable number of indicators used in the various calculations, the diversity in methodologies, and the wide-ranging nature of the data sources. As part of this overview, two of the indexes have been selected for detailed presentation; an economic index (the Index of Economic Well-being), and a social index (the Index of Social Health). In these presentations, the reader will gain a more hands-on perspective of what actually transpires in the production of these seductive and often-provocative numbers.

The sources of data that are used in the calculation of the various indexes discussed in this chapter are highlighted (or at least given passing mention) in each of the individual discussions, but the reader is reminded that a more encompassing list of sources is presented in Table A.1 in Appendix.

Economic Indexes

None of the dimensions listed in the left-hand column of Table 8.1 can compete with the Economy when it comes to the sheer number of available indicators and the wide variety of indexes based upon them. Bernard Baumohl, in his 2013 book "The Secrets of Economic Indicators," lists hundreds of them, many of which could well be seen as harbingers of communal wellbeing, at least for certain segments of the population. Among the nitty-gritty economic issues addressed in such lists are those associated with market performance, industrial production, retail sales, business cycles, money supply, currency exchange rates, foreign trade, unemployment statistics, interest rates, inflation rates, housing starts, home sales, consumer confidence, personal income, consumer spending, investor confidence, working conditions, and many other aspects of economic performance [2].

In Table 8.1, under the Economy rubric, there are just five of the many indexes that could appear there. The *Consumer Price Index* (CPI) is one of the most closely-watched national economic statistics, and one that has a direct bearing on the personal economic happiness of each of us [3]. It measures changes in the average total retail prices of a specific basket of 200 assorted consumer goods and services. These are divided into 8 groups and weighted to reflect each group's share of total consumer expenditures: housing (41%), food and beverages (15%), transportation (17%), medical care (7%), apparel (4%), recreation (6%), education and communication (7%), and other goods and services (3%). In the USA, the prices are determined by sales outlet sampling, the weights are based on the National Income and Product Accounts (NIPA), and the results are compiled and published monthly by the US Bureau of Labor Statistics (BLS). In fact, the BLS publishes two versions of the index: the CPI-W (which is thought to reflect the lifestyle of wage earners and clerical workers), and the CPI-U (which applies to all urban workers including self-employed professionals, managers, technical staff, and short-term workers).

As an indication of the ubiquitousness of economic indexes, there are at least three other popular indexes of interest to consumers, not listed in Table 8.1: the *Consumer Confidence Index* published by The Conference Board, a New York City business research group; the *Consumer Sentiment Survey* put out by the University of Michigan; and the *Consumer Comfort Index* developed by Bloomberg financial consultants. The European common market carries out similar exercises to produce the *Harmonized Index of Consumer Prices* (HICP) [4].

The second index listed in Table 8.1 under the Economy dimension is the *Housing Affordability Index*. It is produced by the St. Louis-based consulting company Demographia International and it has obvious relevance to personal wellbeing. It is discussed more fully in a later chapter with respect to the livability of cities [5]. Similar information can also be gleaned from the *Housing Market Index* put out by the National Association of Home Builders [6].

The previous indexes, while they are calculated at a communal scale, all relate to the economic wellbeing of individuals. There are also many economic indexes that serve the business community, and in the sense that a healthy business community is usually indicative of good times, these indexes can also be viewed as harbingers of communal wellbeing. The *Global Opportunity Index* (GOI), for example, is a country-by-country index designed to assist businesses and investors as they explore opportunities and strategies for overseas capital growth [7]. It provides a "data-rich framework to shed light on a nation's attractiveness to foreign investment." It was developed by the Milken Institute, an independent, non-profit, non-partisan economic think tank based in Santa Monica, CA. The institute is supported by an eclectic mix of corporate, government, and philanthropic donors, including, for example, the Bill and Melinda Gates Foundation. The GOI for a country is based on an analysis of 54 indicators grouped into 5 categories. The five categories are (1) the strength of the country's economic fundamentals, (2) the availability of financial services, (3) the costs and burdens of doing business, (4) the level of support provided by the available institutional framework, and (5) the presence or absence of international standards of practice. Many, but not all, of the GOI indicators are based on objective mining of public-access databases. For example the following seven indicators from the economic fundamentals category all come from the economic databases of the World Bank: annual GDP growth (%), GDP per capita ($US), inflation rate (%), unemployment rate (%), number of citizens of working age (% of population), number of internet users (% of population), and number of mobile phone subscribers (% of population). Once determined, each of the 54 variables is normalized into a 0–10 range, averaged *within* the categories to derive a category score, and then averaged *across* the categories to determine the GOI. Not surprisingly, the US, Canada, and the European democracies rank near the top of the GOI rankings, while most African nations rank near the bottom.

The *Opacity Index* prepared by the Kurtzman Group for PriceWaterhouseCoopers is a country-by-country measure of investment risk that emphasizes the opacity of a country's business milieu [8]. Opacity is the opposite of transparency, so that high opacity is bad. High opacity is associated with high levels of corruption, an inefficient legal system, deleterious economic policies, inadequate accounting practices, and a detrimental regulatory structure. Information on such issues as judicial independence, the status of property rights, the fairness of taxation systems, the levels of bureaucratic red tape, and the role of organized crime in daily business, are mined from such sources as the World Bank, the International Monetary Fund, Transparency International, and the International Securities Services Association.

There are also two indexes, not listed in Table 8.1, that rank the world's countries in terms of their openness to free-enterprise economic activity. The Index of Economic Freedom is generated by the Heritage Foundation in conjunction with the Wall Street Journal [9]. The Economic Freedom of the World Annual Report is published by the Fraser Institute in Vancouver, Canada [10].

Detailed Example: Index of Economic Well-Being

Our first detailed example from Table 8.1 is the Index of Economic Well-being (IEWB), produced by the Centre for Study of Living Standards (CSLS), a think tank based in Ottawa, Canada. The *raison d'être* of the Centre is to "contribute to public debate on living standards by developing and advocating specific policies through expert consensus." The Centre is funded by a mix of Canadian government agencies, business and professional organizations, labor union federations, and international agencies such as OECD and the Ford and Rockefeller Foundations.

The IEWB was developed by Lars Osberg of Dalhousie University in Halifax, Nova Scotia, and Andrew Sharpe of CSLS [11]. The index considers only the economic dimension of wellbeing, but even within that single dimension, the authors recognized the need to define four separate sub-dimensions, as outlined in Table 8.2: *Per Capita Consumption, Per Capita Wealth, Economic Equality, and Economic Security*. Each sub-dimension has several component indicators, and some of these indicators require data from more than one source. The index is usually calculated at the scale of countries. It has been applied to Canada, the USA, and to several OECD countries including the UK, Australia, Norway and Sweden. The fact that its application has been limited to developed Western nations has negated the need for indicators that reflect the economic costs of widespread extreme poverty, fragile or failed governance, ongoing internal war and conflict, and other indicators that might be required for an economic index of broader international applicability.

Looking now at some of the details in Table 8.2, let us turn first to *Per Capita Consumption*. It is calculated from four indicators. The first indicator highlighted on the top line of column 2 is *the per-capita market consumption*. In general, the higher the average per capita income of a country, the higher will be its per capita consumption. Higher values of this indicator are thus a sign of economic health. As noted in column 3, the value for this indicator is calculated from data on *average household market consumption* and the *average number of people living together per household*, both of which are usually available from publically-accessible systems of national accounts. One would think that the per-capita value would simply be equal to the household value divided by the number of householders. However, research has shown that the efficiencies of multiple-person households is better reflected if the household value is divided by the *square root* of the average number of householders (the so-called Luxemburg Income Study Equivalence Scale). This correction brings the per capita values of single-person households and multiple-family households onto an equal footing, and insures that

Table 8.2 Sixteen indicators for the Index of Economic Well-being. (Adapted from the source materials listed in [11])

Sub-dimension	Indicator	Data required	Unit
Per Capita Consumption	Per-capita market consumption adjusted for household size and life expectancy	Average household market consumption	$$
		Average number of people living together per household	
		Annual percent increase in life expectancy	
	Unpaid work per capita	Replacement wage for unpaid work	$$
	Government spending per capita	On goods and services by all levels of government	$$
	Regrettable expenditures per capita (negative)	Expenditures that do not contribute to wellbeing.	$$
Per Capita Wealth	Capital stock per capita	Average residential and non-residential capital holdings	$$
	R&D stock per capita	Share of GDP devoted to R&D	$$
	Net international investment position per capita (positive or negative)	Net foreign debt or surplus on investment monies	$$
	Natural resources stock per capita	Physical reserves of timber, minerals, and fossil fuels	$$
		Prices of these commodities	
	Human capital per capita	Accumulated public and private expenditures on education at all levels	$$
	Social cost of environmental degradation (negative)	Annual tonnes CO_2-equivelant air emissions	$$
		Social cost per tonne emitted	
Economic Equality	Income inequality	Gini coefficient	Dec Fract
	Poverty	Poverty rate	Dec Fract
		Poverty gap ratio	
Economic Security	From the risk of unemployment	Unemployment rates	Dec Fract
		Percent unemployed receiving benefits	
		Annual unemployment insurance benefits as percent of total earnings	
	From the risk of illness	Average private medical expenses as share of disposable income	Dec Fract
	From the risk of single-parent poverty	Divorce rates	Dec Fract
		Poverty rate and poverty gap ratio for single-parent families	
	From the risk of poverty in old age	Poverty rate and poverty gap ratio for elderly	Dec Fract

multiple-family consumption is not under-represented. A second correction multiplies the base value by a term that reflects the annual percent increase in life expectancy in the country under analysis. There is economic value in these extra years of life, and the consumption indicator should reflect not just the consumption per year but also the number of years an average citizen gets to consume it.

Continuing down column 2 of Table 8.2, *unpaid work* includes such endeavors as domestic work, home management, shopping and transportation, child and adult care, and volunteer activities. *Government spending* includes all outlays on goods and services by all levels of government. *Regrettable expenditures* are those that do not contribute to wellbeing, including such outlays as commuting costs, costs of divorce, household pollution abatement, and the costs of crime (including preventive security measures, and any medical or legal expenses that may arise for victims of crime). All three of these components of consumption are calculated on a per capita basis, and data for all three are usually available from the pertinent national accounts.

The next sub-dimension on the IEWB is that of *Per Capita Wealth.* There are six indicators, the first three of which are based on widely-available economic data (*per capita capital stock holdings, per capita share of GDP devoted to research and development, and per capita net foreign debt or surplus on investment monies*). The last three indicators under the wealth sub-dimension are handled by representative proxies: educational expenses to represent investment in *human capital*; air emission costs to represent *environmental degradation* (which is negative); and the value of timber, mineral and fossil-fuel reserves to represent *natural resource value*. It is recognized that a full treatment of these three areas of impact on national wealth would have to take a much broader perspective, but it is argued that the chosen proxies are suitably representative, and that the inclusion of a wider variety of similar impacts would probably not change the results much.

All of the indicators under the Consumption and Wealth sub-dimensions are measured in units of currency ($US in the USA and $CDN in Canada). Comparisons across countries use applicable currency conversion rates. Within a given country, current-year values are converted into 2002-constant-dollars using the GDP deflator or the Consumer Price Index. And finally, for the purposes of the IEWB, for each of the ten currency-based indicators, the dollar values are scaled into a %-value or decimal fraction that lies between 0 and 1, with 0 worst and 1 best.

The calculations for the six indicators under the *Economic Equality* and *Economic Security* sub-dimensions all lead to a decimal fraction directly. The *Gini coefficient* was introduced and defined back in Chap. 3. The *poverty rate* is the percent of the population whose income falls below a specific income level defined as the poverty line. The *poverty gap ratio* takes the average income of those who fall below the poverty line, subtracts it from the poverty-line income, and divides this difference by the poverty-line income.

The four Economic Security indicators reflect the probabilities of economic hardship due to *unemployment, illness, divorce, and old age*, and the investments made by governments and individuals to protect against these risks.

The 16 indicators that contribute to the IEWB (all of which are now in the form of decimal fractions), are then aggregated according to a formula that can be found in the original source materials. The formula is essentially a summation and averaging of the four sub-dimensions from Table 8.2 (Consumption, Wealth, Equality, and Security), with the value of each sub-dimension calculated as a summation and averaging of its component indicators. However the developers of the index do allow for significant weighting of the terms. For example, under the Economic Equality sub-dimension, it was the authors' opinion that poverty was a much larger drag on economic health than income inequality so they set the weights at 0.25 and 0.75 respectively. Weighting can also be applied to the four terms of the Security sub-dimension if so desired.

One of the main ideas underlying the IEWB is that individuals differ (and have the moral right to differ) over the relative weights that they assign to the various indicators. For this reason, the "app" that allows calculation of the IEWB for any desired jurisdiction now comes with an interactive weighting tool that allows the user to set any weights he or she may desire. In their reports, the authors present the results of several sensitivity analyses using various weighting schemes. In general, the results tend to show slightly different absolute values, but the time trends tend to track rather closely.

Recall that all the indicators either lead directly to decimal fractions between 0 and 1, or are scaled to do so. The annual value of the IEWB for any jurisdiction therefore also lies between 0 and 1. The final values have no meaning in an absolute sense, in that the various decimal fractions were developed from data sets with completely different units (for example, dollars for market consumption, the Gini coefficient for income equality). They have meaning only in a relative sense, for comparing one jurisdiction against another, or comparing 1 year against another within a given jurisdiction.

The data for all but two of the indicators in Table 8.2 can be gleaned from widely-available, objective, government databanks. In Canada, such databases are all supported by Statistics Canada. In the USA reference would be made to the Bureau of the Census, the Bureau of Labor Statistics, the Bureau of Economic Analysis, and perhaps other federal agencies. The two indicators that require special data mining in Table 8.2 are the natural resources stock and the social costs of environmental degradation. In both cases, the required information is available from specialized literature in these fields.

For Canada, between 1981 and 2010, the IEWB increased at a rate of 0.78% per year. Over this period, Consumption tracked strongly up, Wealth was significantly up, and Equality and Security exhibited cyclical trends that ended slightly down. During the same period, Canada's GDP increased 1.32% per year. The fact that this increase was larger than the IEWB implies that the GDP overestimated improvements in economic wellbeing (presumably because it does not take into account the economic impacts of such issues as unpaid work, regrettable expenditures, environmental degradation, income inequality, and risks to economic security).

Indexes of Governance

The presence of democratic freedoms and the absence of government corruption are among the most obvious drivers of a civil society and communal wellbeing. This is true in all countries, but has special relevance in the less-developed nations of the world.

Turning again to the list in Table 8.1, the *Democracy Index* (DI) is probably among the most straightforward of the available governance indexes. It is produced by the Intelligence Unit of the London news outlet, *The Economist*. It is based on 60 indicators in 5 categories. The categories document the presence or absence of (1) a free and fair electoral process, (2) civil liberties, (3) a functioning government system, (4) a democratic political culture, and (5) citizen political participation. The evaluation of the 60 indicators is carried out by questionnaire-based expert assessments. Some of the questions require subjective judgments, while others make reference to the results of public-opinion surveys such as the World Values Survey, the Eurobarometer, and Gallup polls. Each question has a threefold choice, worth 1, 0.5, or 0 points. An example: "Is the process of financing political parties transparent and generally accepted?" An answer of 'Yes' is scored as 1; 'Not Fully' as 0.5; and 'No' as 0. Another example: "If available from the World Values Survey, what percent of citizens have 'a great deal' or 'quite a lot' of confidence in their government?" Greater than 40% gets a score of 1; 25–40% gets 0.5; and less than 25% gets 0. The scores within each of the 5 categories are totaled and normalized into the range 0–10. The five category scores are then averaged to provide the DI. In the most recent analysis, of the 165 countries analyzed, 28 of them scored between 8 and 10 and were deemed "full democracies," 54 scored between 6 and 8 and were categorized as "flawed democracies," and the rest scored below 6 and were labeled "authoritarian," or "hybrid" (a mix of flawed-democratic and authoritarian) [12]. The question as to whether the world is becoming more or less democratic over time has recently been addressed by Jennifer Welsh, a Canadian researcher in international relations who is currently a special advisor to the Secretary-General of the United Nations. In her book "The Return of History," she decries the rise of "illiberal democracies" that promote citizen enfranchisement at election time but abuse their executive powers, particularly with respect to individual rights and freedoms, once in office [13].

Global Integrity is an NGO based in Washington, DC, that supports progress toward open and accountable governance in countries around the world. They produce the *Global Integrity Scorecard* (GIS), which was known as the *Global Integrity Index* prior to 2010. The scorecard has 6 main categories organized into 23 sub-categories. The six main categories are: (1) availability of public information and freedom of the media to report on it; (2) election integrity; (3) safeguards against government conflicts of interest; (4) transparency and fairness in public administration; (5) government oversight and controls; and (6) anti-corruption legal framework, judicial impartiality, and law enforcement professionalism. Perusal of this list shows many similarities with the Democracy Index, and indeed the two indexes cover much the same waterfront. What makes the GIS different is its clear distinction between *de jure* governance (in law) and *de facto* governance (in practice). In the questionnaire that is the basis for the scorecard, consideration of almost every indicator (over 300 of them) takes the form of paired questions. For example, under election integrity: "*In law*, do all citizens have the right to form political parties and/or run for election?" and "*In practice*, do all citizens have the right to form political parties and/or run for election?" Or another example, under anti-corruption: "*In law*, is offering a bribe to a government official illegal?" and "*In practice*, are occurrences of government bribery investigated and laws enforced?" The "in law" questions are scored as 100 for "yes" and 0 for "no." The "in practice" questions are scored as 100, 75, 50, 25 or 0, depending on the perceived degree of implementation. The GIS reports not only the answers to the questions, but also the *implementation gap,* which is the difference between the *de jure* and *de facto* scores [14]. Global Integrity also publishes a scorecard for the 50 American States. It is based on a questionnaire of 245 questions in 13 areas of state governance including such issues as campaign donation limits, open budget reporting, and registration requirements for lobbyists. In the most recent assessment, no states received an A or B grade. Three states got a C; there were 36 at D; and 11 states received an F.

The Worldwide Governance Indicators (WGI) put out by the World Bank cover some of the same ground. They use 31 internationally-respected data sources to rate 215 "countries, territories and other geographies" on 6 counts of governance (Voice and Accountability, Political Stability, Government Effectiveness, Regulatory Quality, Rule of Law, and Control of Corruption). The WGI differs from its sister indexes in that each of the six component scores is kept separately. The final result is a sixfold matrix. There is no attempt made to integrate them into a single number [15].

Freedom of the press is a fundamental right of any citizenry, the absence of which puts a strong damper on communal wellbeing. The *Worldwide Press Freedom Index* is produced by Reporters Without Borders, an organization that represents the international journalism community. The "rsf" in their web address refers to the original French name of the group, Reporters Sans Frontieres. Their index considers seven criteria: (1) *pluralism*, which is the degree to which diversity of opinion is represented in the media, (2) the *independence* of the media from the influences of government, business, or religious elites, (3) the *working environment* in which the media operates, (4) the *legislative framework* that governs journalistic activities, (5) the *transparency* of institutions and procedures, (6) the *infrastructure* that supports the production of news and information, and (7*) abuses and acts of violence* against journalists [16].

The first 6 criteria are addressed by pooling the subjective responses to an 87-question survey from selected news organizations in the country under analysis. The seventh criterion is addressed by means of a quantitative evaluation of the available statistics on abuses against journalists kept by Reporters Without Borders. The number of instances of abuse is recorded, and each instance is weighted according to its severity (harassment, assault, arrest, exile, imprisonment, or death). The scores from the first six criteria, and that for the seventh, are combined according to a formula that subjectively weights the various criteria. The scores are normalized into the range 0–100, with lower scores indicating satisfactory levels of press freedom and higher scores indicating unsatisfactory levels. In the most recent analysis, Finland, the Netherlands, and Norway led the way. Canada ranked 18th out of the 180 countries analyzed, and the USA ranked 41st with a score that puts it in the "problematic" range.

Public sector corruption is a particularly noxious drain on communal wellbeing. It can be defined as the abuse of entrusted power for private gain. Transparency International is a global organization headquartered in Berlin, with over 100 chapters worldwide, that is leading the fight against corruption. To this end, they publish the *Corruption Perception Index* (CPI) which ranks the countries of the world on such core values as transparency, accountability, integrity, solidarity, courage, and justice [17]. Among the activities that belie these values are bribery of officials, market rigging, human trafficking, police corruption, drug money laundering, cronyism, misuse of charitable donations and disaster funds, provision of counterfeit prescription drugs, and graft associated with cross-border trade. The CPI is a "once-removed" index in that it is based on a compilation of subjective assessments carried out by other institutions. The primary assessments are only accepted into the CPI calculation if they come from institutions that have been judged credible in the international marketplace. Transparency International then quantifies the subjective perceptions onto a 4-point scale, and rescales the totals into the range 0–100, where 0 is very corrupt and 100 is very clean. The Scandinavian countries ranked at the top of the 168 countries considered in the 2015 analysis. The USA ranked 16th.

Security and Safety Indexes

People are happier when they feel that they are safe and secure in their daily lives. Five of the indexes listed in Table 8.1 address these issues.

The *Global Peace Index* (GPI) is produced by the Institute for Economics and Peace, an independent, non-partisan, non-profit think tank headquartered in Sydney, Australia. The data that they use are collected and compiled by the Economist Intelligence Unit in London. The original sources include such organizations as the Stockholm International Peace Research Institute, the Uppsala University Conflict Data Program, and the UK-based International Institute for Strategic Studies (which specializes in nuclear deterrence and arms control). The index uses 22 indicators, each ranked subjectively on a 1–5 scale by an expert panel. There are two sub-indexes, one that considers *internal peace* (which is disrupted by crime and violence within the country), weighted at 60%, and one that considers *external peace* (which is brought down by militarization and participation in foreign wars), weighted at 40%. Examples of indicators that threaten internal peace include the level of violent crime, the likelihood of violent demonstrations, terrorist activity, and the annual number of homicides per 100,000 population. In 2015, according to the GPI, 81 countries became more peaceful and 78 countries became less so. Iceland and Denmark were the most peaceful; South Sudan and Iraq, the least. Canada ranked 7th; the USA 94th. With respect to the USA, it was noted that for the first time since the initiation of the GPI, gun deaths exceeded automobile-related deaths [18].

The Institute for Economics and Peace also produces a *Global Terrorism Index* (GTI). It is based on the Global Terrorism Database maintained by the National Consortium for the Study of Terrorism and Responses to Terrorism. This database currently holds records on 140,000 terrorist incidents around the world. The GTI is calculated annually on a country-by-country basis, taking into account the number of terrorist incidents, lives lost in such incidents, number of total injuries, level of property damage, and possible psychological after-effects. In Iraq in 2014, for example, there were 3370 incidents, leading to 9929 deaths and 15,137 injuries. In the USA there were 19 incidents leading to 18 deaths, most of them perpetrated by "lone wolf" attackers. In the calculation of the GTI, the number of lives lost is weighted at three times the number of incidents, and six times the number of injuries. Furthermore, the index is based on a running average of the previous 5 years, with the current year weighted at 52%, and the preceding 4 years at 26%, 13%, 6%, and 3% respectively. The index is normalized into the range 0–10, with zero being the best score and ten the worst. In 2014, the GTI for Iraq was 10, that for the USA, 4.6. Over 80% of all terrorist incidents in that year occurred in 5 countries: Iraq, Nigeria, Afghanistan, Pakistan and Syria [19].

The Fragile States Index (FSI) is another global index that focuses on the have-not countries of the world. It is calculated by the Fund for Peace, an independent NGO based in Washington, DC. It is based on 12 indicators of instability: the intervention of other states, factionalized elites, fragmented security, violation of human rights, deterioration of public services, delegitimization of the state, economic decline, uneven development, chronic emigration, group grievances, refugees and internally-displaced persons, and demographic pressures caused by overpopulation, disease, or natural disasters. The thing that makes the FSI unique is that it is calculated automatically by a proprietary software program named CAST (for Conflict Assessment System Tool). The CAST program monitors thousands of reports daily, millions of documents per year, and converts them into a numerical score. The FSI is published annually by Foreign Policy magazine [20].

The safety and security issue that hits closest to home in most Western democracies is that of crime. Police-reported crime statistics are available in most countries. Crime in the USA is reported in the Uniform Crime Reports put out by the Federal Bureau of Investigation, and in the National Crime Victimization Surveys published by the Bureau of Justice Statistics. Differentiation is made between *violent crime* (which includes murder, manslaughter, rape, robbery, and aggravated assault), and *property crime* (which includes burglary, larceny, motor vehicle theft, and arson). Based on the historical data, both types of crime peaked in the USA in the early 1990s and have been declining ever since. The difficulty with the raw crime reports is that they don't provide enough differentiation between the various crimes in terms of how such crimes impact the public at large. In Canada, researchers at Statistics Canada have tried to address this problem with their *Crime Severity Index* (CSI) [21]. In this approach, the various categories of crime are weighted according to their "seriousness." The weights are based on sentencing data available from criminal court records. They are calculated as the incarceration rate for that crime times the average length of prison sentence (in days). Using this formula, murder has a weight of 7042; manslaughter 1822; robbery 583; vehicle theft 84; and marijuana possession 7. The CSI is calculated by multiplying the number of incidents of a particular type of crime in a given jurisdiction by the weight for that offense; adding the totals together for all offenses; and standardizing the result by setting its base value to 100 for the year 2006. The CSI can be generated for any level of jurisdiction desired: national, provincial, or metropolitan. As with the raw crime rates, the CSI also indicates a reduction in crime in recent years. The most recent calculation of the CSI for the city of Toronto, for example, was 65.

The *National Index of Violence and Harm* was originally developed by the Peace Studies Institute at Manchester University in Indiana. It has recently been taken over by researchers at the University of Rhode Island. It uses 19 variables to define 2 sub-indexes for the USA, 1 that reflects levels of personal violence and 1 that reflects societal violence [22].

Another security-based index not listed in Table 8.1 is the *World Risk Index* which ranks the level of risk in 173 countries using 4 sub-dimensions and 28 indicators [23].

Social Indexes

Social indexes are designed to measure the role of social relationships in generating happiness and wellbeing. They reflect the strength of marital and family bonds, the role of friendships and participation in group activities, the pleasure gleaned from cultural and spiritual activities, and the feelings of satisfaction that arise from helping others.

The first two indexes listed in Table 8.1 under the Social dimension relate to the joy of helping others. The United Way of America (UWA) promotes their *State of Caring Index* (SCI) as a measure of the level of caring and compassion of the nation [24]. It is based on the UWA comprehensive community assessments, which are themselves based on a questionnaire that is presented to citizens and stakeholders in telephone and face-to-face interviews. Among the stakeholders consulted are community leaders, social service providers, and citizen advisory committees. The questionnaire focuses on 36 indicators in 7 areas. Among the key indicators are the percentage of the population living below the poverty level, the percentage of families headed by a single parent, the teenage birth rate, the incidence rate of elder abuse and neglect, the availability of prenatal care, the percent of income given to charity, and the per-capita charitable amounts raised by UWA. The index is calculated on a state-by-state basis, and on a county-by-county basis within states.

The *World Giving Index* (WGI) treads similar ground to the SCI but on a worldwide basis. It is produced by the Charities Aid Foundation, a UK-based NGO that provides advice and service to philanthropic organizations. Their *raison d'être* is to "motivate society to give more." The WGI is touted as "the world's leading study of generosity." [25]. It is based on the results of the Gallup World Poll which reaches 150,000 people in 140 countries annually. The three key questions on the Gallup questionnaire that inform the WGI are: (1) Have you helped a stranger recently? (2) Have you donated money to charity this year? And (3) Do you currently volunteer to a charitable organization? The responses from a given country are tabulated, and the countries ranked. Surprisingly, the highest-ranked country in the 2016 assessment was not one of the usual Western democracies but rather the Asian state of Myanmar. Perhaps the people of Myanmar were celebrating their return to the roster of democratic countries after the elections of 2015 which ended 25 years of autocratic military rule.

The final two indexes listed under the Social Relationships dimension in Table 8.1 reflect a broader mandate. The *Social Progress Index* (SPI) measures "the extent to which countries provide for the social needs of their citizens." It is produced by the Social Progress Imperative, a Washington-based NGO chaired by Michael Porter, an economist with the Harvard Business School. "Social progress" is defined as the "capacity of a society to meet the basic human needs of its citizens, establish the building blocks that allow citizens and communities to enhance and sustain the quality of their lives, and create the conditions for all individuals to reach their full potential." [26]. The concepts that underlie the SPI are based on the "capabilities approach" pioneered by Amartya Sen, discussed back in Chap. 3. The SPI has 3 sub-dimensions, 4 components for each sub-dimension, and 3-to-5 indicators for each component, a total of 53 in all. The indicators cover such issues of social wellbeing as shelter, health, sanitation, nutrition, equality, inclusion, sustainability, personal freedom, and safety. Their contributions to the SPI are all based on objective data from publically-available databases. The SPI differs from many other indexes of wellbeing on two counts. First of all, despite the leadership of a Harvard economist, the SPI contains no economic variables. It covers only the non-economic dimensions of social performance, and is therefore completely independent of the GDP. Secondly, its indicators measure outcomes, not inputs. Its health indicators, for example, are based on citizen wellbeing, not on the amount of public funding given to healthcare. The data for each indicator is transformed onto a 0–100 scale by defining worst-case (0) and best-case (100) scenarios. The indicator data are weighted and aggregated to produce a component score, averaged across the components to get a sub-dimensional score, and averaged across the sub-dimensions to get the SPI. The five highest-ranked countries in the 2016 analysis were Norway, Sweden, Switzerland, Iceland and New Zealand. Canada ranked 6th and the USA 16th.

Lack of equality in opportunity between the genders is a source of unhappiness for many women in the world. There are several indexes not listed in Table 8.1 that deal with gender equity issues. The World Economic Forum puts out the *Global Gender Gap Index* (14 indicators) [27]. The United Nations Development Program has its *Gender Inequality Index* (5 indicators) [28]. The organization Social Watch publishes the *Gender Equity Index* (11 indicators) [29].

Four further social indexes of interest not listed in Table 8.1 are the *Index of Social Development* (6 sub-dimensions, 200 indicators, 193 countries) published by the International Institute of Social Studies at Erasmus University in Rotterdam, Netherlands [30], Social Watch's *Basic Capabilities Index* (3 sub-dimensions, 5 indicators, 167 countries) [31], the *Social Inclusion Index* (2 sub-dimensions, 21 indicators, 16 countries) put out by Americas Quarterly [32], and the *Multiculturism Index* (3 sub-dimensions, 8 indicators, 21 OECD countries) published by Queens University in Kingston, Ontario [33].

Detailed Example: Index of Social Health

One of the earliest attempts to measure social welfare in something other than purely economic terms took place in the late 1980s at Fordham University where the husband-wife team of Marc and Marque-Luisa Miringoff created the Institute for Innovation in Social Policy. Since the death of Marc Miringoff in 2004, the Institute has been housed in the Department of Sociology at Vassar College in Poughkeepsie, NY, under the direction of Marque-Luisa Miringoff. The *raison d'être* of the Institute is the "investigation of social indicators as a way to improve the reporting and understanding of social conditions" in America. The *Index of Social Health* (ISH) is the centerpiece of the Institute's work. The results are reported at irregular intervals (every 3 years or so), and have led to the publication of two books that summarize the social health of the nation or as the authors put it in the subtitle of one of the books: "How America is really doing." [34].

The ISH is applied on a state-by-state basis leading to a ranking of the 50 states from best to worst. It uses 16 indicators, 4 of which (unemployment rate, weekly wages, affordable housing, and income inequality) are economic in nature, and the rest unavowedly social. Most of the indicators are negative rather than positive; that is, they measure the extent of problems that detract from social health, rather than the conditions that make direct positive contributions toward it. A positive outcome for a state comes from that state having a low incidence of the detracting problems. All of the indicators have objective sources of data available. All but two of them come from credible federal government databases. The two exceptions come from equally-credible non-governmental sources (a national database on teenage drug use housed at the University of Michigan, and the results of a widely-accepted index on housing affordability). There are no subjective components in the calculation of the ISH.

Table 8.3 lists the 16 indicators and their sources. They are ordered by stage of life. Three indicators apply to childhood social health (infant mortality, child abuse, and child poverty), three to youth issues (teenage suicide, teenage drug abuse, and high school completion rates), three to adult concerns (unemployment rates, weekly wages, and health insurance coverage), two to the elderly (poverty, and healthcare costs), and five that apply to all ages (homicides, alcohol-related traffic fatalities, food insecurity, affordable housing, and income inequality). The exact definitions of some of the indicators have changed slightly over the years, as have a couple of the

Table 8.3 Sixteen indicators for the Index of Social Health. (Adapted from the source materials listed in [34])

Age	Issue	Indicator	Source
Childhood	Infant mortality	Number of deaths in the first year of life per 1000 live births	National Center for Health Statistics
	Child abuse	Number of children under 18 involved in reports of abuse per 1000 population	Department Health and Human Services
	Child poverty	Percentage of children under 18 living in poverty	Bureau of the Census
Youth	Teenage suicide	Deaths by suicide, ages 15–24, per 100,000 population	National Center for Health Statistics
	Teenage drug abuse	Percentage of 12th-graders who have used illicit drugs in the past year	University of Michigan: Monitoring the Future Program
	High school completion	Percentage of 18–24 year-old who are not enrolled in school and who have not completed high school	Bureau of the Census
Adulthood	Unemployment	Unemployed as a percent of civilian labor force	Bureau of Labor Statistics
	Weekly wages	Average weekly earnings, workers in private industry	Economic Report to the President
	Health insurance coverage	Percentage of total population without health insurance	Bureau of the Census
Old Age	Poverty among elderly	Percentage of population over 65 living in poverty	Bureau of the Census
	Healthcare costs for the elderly	Out-of-pocket healthcare costs, age 65 and over	Bureau of Labor Statistics
All Ages	Homicides	Murders and non-negligent manslaughters per 100,000 population	FBI Uniform Crime Reports
	Alcohol-related traffic fatalities	Traffic deaths involving alcohol as a percentage of all traffic deaths	National Highway Traffic Safety Administration
	Food insecurity	Percentage of households that do not have access to enough food for an active, healthy life for all household members	Department of Agriculture, Economic Research Service
	Affordable housing	Percentage of home owners spending 30% or more of monthly household income on mortgage payments	Housing Affordability Index
	Income inequality	Gini coefficient	Bureau of the Census

data sources. The second indicator under "Old Age" has had several incarnations (life expectancy at age 65, elderly suicide rates, and the healthcare costs that are on the current roster). It is also worth noting that one of the indicators (affordable housing) is actually based on another index, our first example of something that is quite common in the measurement of wellbeing: the output from one index providing the input to another.

The methodology that is used to arrive at the ISH for each state is actually quite simple. For each of the 16 indicators, the 50 states are put in rank order from 1 to 50 (1 being best and 50 worst), based on the data gleaned from the appropriate database. These 16 numbers are then averaged for each state, and this average is subtracted from 50 (i.e. if the averaged rank equals 10, then 50 minus 10 equals 40). This latter value is then expressed as a percentage of 50 (i.e. 40/50 equals 80%). Dropping the % gives that state's ISH (in the example, ISH equals 80). The range of possible values is 1–100. A value above 80 is considered excellent, 60–79 above average, 40–59 average, 20–39 below average, and less than 20 poor. In the most recent assessment, Minnesota led the way with a score of 75.0, closely followed by Iowa, New Hampshire, Nebraska and Vermont. New Mexico was at the bottom with a score of 26.8, just ahead of Mississippi and Arizona.

The ISH can also be calculated for the nation as a whole. The same 16 indicators are used, but on a national rather than a state scale. The value for a given indicator for a given year is taken from the appropriate database, and then converted into a percentage of the maximum value ever recorded for that indicator over the years. The % is dropped and the 16 scores are arithmetically averaged to produce the nationwide ISH. Like the state values, the national value lies between 0 and 100, with 0 the worst possible score and 100 the best. In the most recent assessment the national ISH was 50.2. Since 1970 it has varied between 45 and 65, with the best scores being recorded in 1973 and 2000, and the worst in 1982 and 1993.

Looking at the indicators in more detail, the authors of the ISH found that seven of them improved in the period 1970–2011 while nine of them declined. The seven that improved were infant mortality, teenage drug abuse, high school completion rates, poverty among the elderly, homicide rates, alcohol-related traffic fatalities, and affordable housing. Interestingly, the three indicators that showed the greatest correlations with the overall trends of the ISH were child poverty, high school completion rates, and health insurance coverage.

Educational Indexes

In 1996, UNESCO sponsored an International Commission on 'Education for the Twenty-First Century.' The chairman was the prominent French economist Jacques Delors who also served three terms as the President of the European Commission (the executive arm of the European Union). In their final report, the commission highlighted the "four pillars of learning:" *Learning to Know*, *Learning to Do*, *Learning to Live Together*, and *Learning to Be*. The first pillar involves the acquisition of knowledge via the formal educational route (learning in the classroom); the second refers to vocational and work-related training (learning on the job); the third focuses on such learned traits as tolerance, openness, and trust (learning in the community); and the fourth reflects the learning opportunities provided by cultural activities, sports participation, and social media (learning at home) [35]. In 2006, the Canadian Council on Learning used the UNESCO framework to develop a *Composite Learning Index* (CLI) for Canada that was used to assess the links between learning conditions and social outcomes in 4500 Canadian communities [36]. Unfortunately, the federal-government funding that sustained the program was cut off in 2010 and only one reckoning of the CLI was ever published.

The four pillars still live, however, in the first educational index listed in Table 8.1, the *European Lifelong Learning Indicators* (ELLI), which were developed by an international team of experts using the UNESCO framework and following the Canadian model [37]. The ELLI program is administered by the private charitable foundation, Bertelsmann Stiftung, which is based in Gutersloh, Germany, but also maintains offices in Barcelona, Brussels and Berlin. The goals of Bertelsmann Stiftung are "inspiring people, shaping the future, and participating in a globalized world." The ELLI provide a comprehensive review of learning conditions in 27 European Union countries using 36 indicators grouped under the 4 UNESCO pillars. As an example, consider the seven indicators under the 'Learning to Know' pillar: (1) total public expenditures on education as a percent of gross national income, (2) percentage of children 4–6 in formal pre-school education, (3) performance of 15-year-olds on the PISA reading scale, (4) performance of 15-year-olds on the PISA math scale, (5) performance of 15-year-olds on the PISA science scale, (6) percentage of people 25–64 who have participated in some kind of formal education or vocational training in the past 12 months, and (7) percentage of the workforce 30–34 with post-secondary education of some kind. The PISA scales are produced by the Program for International Student Assessment of the Organization for Economic Cooperation and Development (OECD). The other data comes from the European Union Statistics on Income and Living Conditions. Each of the indicator scores are standardized onto a 0–100 scale, then weighted and averaged in a statistically-sophisticated way (using factor analysis and least-squares regression), to produce the four ELLI scores, one for each pillar. When applied on a country-by-country basis, the ELLI scores were found to be highly correlated with a suite of desirable social outcomes such as high mean net income, high GDP per capita, low unemployment rates, favorable Gini coefficient, positive self-reported health status, level of life satisfaction, and solid ratings on the Environmental Performance Index. The top-ranked countries in this European exercise were Denmark, Sweden and the Netherlands; the lowest were Greece, Bulgaria and Romania.

The second educational index listed in Table 8.1, the *Education for All Development Index* (EDI), also has a UNESCO connection, in that it is prepared by an agency that is closely associated with UNESCO, and which relies heavily on data that is archived at the UNESCO Institute for Statistics in Montreal, Canada [38]. The index is actually put together by the same team that publishes the annual Global Education Monitoring (GEM) Report, and the calculation of the index is an integral part of that effort. The index is determined on a country by country basis and values are available for a suite of over 120 countries around the world. The index features four sub-dimensions (called domains by GEM) with just one proxy indicator per domain. The four domains are Primary Education, Adult Literacy, Quality of

Education, and Gender Equity. The proxy for the first domain is the *percent of eligible children engaged in primary education*, and that for the second is simply the *adult literacy rate*. Several proxies were considered to represent the third domain, the quality of education in a country, including student-teacher ratios, and others. However, studies showed that the proxy most highly correlated with learning outcomes was *the survival rate to Grade 5*, and it was this indicator that was incorporated in the calculation. The proxy for gender equity is taken as an equal weighting of three terms, all based on *male-to-female participation ratios, the first in primary education enrolment, the second in secondary education enrolment, and the third in adult literacy rates*. In the 2010 reckoning, the top four spots in the EDI rankings were held by Japan, Sweden, Norway, and the UK. The USA ranked 25th.

There are several other educational indexes calculated at the national level that are not included in Table 8.1. The most widely quoted is probably the *United Nations Education Index* (UNEI), which is actually one of the three components of the broader UN Human Development Index. It uses only two indicators: the expected years of schooling in a country's educational system, and the mean years of schooling actually received by its youth. In the UNEI, Australia, Denmark and New Zealand top the list. The USA is ranked 8th and Canada 12th [39].

There is also a *Right to Education Index* (RTEI) published by an anti-poverty advocacy group, the RESULTS Educational Fund, which addresses "the right to education being respected, protected and fulfilled" in a country. Special attention is paid to the educational opportunities of girls, children with disabilities, indigenous and minority groups, and rural communities [40].

Lastly, one can draw attention to three indexes that measure the educational milieu from the student perspective. The first is the *Multi-Dimensional Student's Life Satisfaction Scale* (MSLSS) developed by Scott Heubner, an educational psychologist at the University of South Carolina. It features 5 domains (Family Life, Friends, School, Living Environment, and Self), and is determined on the basis of responses to a 40-item questionnaire [41]. Robert Cummins of Deakin University in Melbourne, Australia, whose Personal Wellbeing Index was featured in Chap. 6, also puts out a specialized version for students, the *Personal Wellbeing Index – School Children* (PWI-SC) [42]. And Joseph Sirgy of Virginia Polytechnic University has published widely on the quality of life of students at the college level [43].

Health Indexes

Health is one of the most important drivers of human happiness and wellbeing. Most jurisdictions have two types of index to measure the healthcare systems in their arena. The first type reflects the level of satisfaction with healthcare provision from a consumer standpoint. The second focuses on the actual medical health of the citizenry.

The first index listed under the Health dimension in Table 8.1, the *European Health Consumer Index* (EHCI), is a good example of the first type [44]. It is put out by the Health Consumer Powerhouse, a Swedish health-policy think-tank that specializes in comparing European healthcare systems. The ECHI uses 48 indicators in 6 areas: (1) patient rights, (2) access to care, (3) treatment outcomes, (4) range and reach of services, (5) prevention, and (6) use of pharmaceuticals. The results are based on the responses to an annual questionnaire sent to over 1000 patient organizations in 36 countries. Each of the questions on the questionnaire bears a one-to-one correspondence with one of the 48 indicators. Under the 'access to care' heading, for example, there are six questions: (1) Can you expect same-day access to your family doctor? (2) Can you gain direct access to a specialist? (3) Is major elective surgery delivered within 90 days of diagnosis? (4) Is cancer therapy started within 21 days of treatment selection? (5) Can a CT scan be obtained within 7 days? (6) Is the waiting time in hospital between arrival and attention less than 1 h? The scoring system is quite unique. Each responder has three options, scored on a 3–2–1 scale. For the listed 'access-to-care' questions, a 3 means "almost always," 2 means "more than 50% of the time," and 1 means "less than 50% of the time." For many of the indicators in the other five areas, 3 means "good," 2 means "fair," and 1 means "poor." The scores are summed within each area and then converted into a decimal fraction of the maximum available for that area (which may be different for each of the six areas due to the differing number of indicators for each area). For the six-question access-to-care example introduced above, the minimum score available is 6 (all 1s) and the maximum is 18 (all 3s). The range of possible decimal fractions is therefore 0.33–1.00 (and this will be true for each area no matter the number of questions). The decimal fraction is then multiplied by 1000 leading to a range of scores for each area from 333 to 1000. The final index is an average of the six area scores so it too has a range 333–1000. The leading countries in the most-recent EHCI listing were The Netherlands, Switzerland and Norway. However, a further input-output analysis that compared medical outcomes with healthcare spending produced a "bang-for-the-buck" ranking led by Macedonia, Estonia and the Czech Republic.

In the USA, feedback from health system users is used to calculate the *Consumer Assessment of Healthcare Providers and Systems* (not listed in Table 8.1). The system is hosted by the Agency for Healthcare Research and Quality, a branch of the US Department of Health and Human Services. Results are disseminated to health plan providers, state agencies, purchaser groups, Medicare and Medicaid agencies, and children's health insurance programs [45]. At the global level, the World Health Organization publishes an *Index of Overall Health System Performance.*

The final four listings under the Health dimension in Table 8.1 are all examples of the second type of health index, those that focus directly on the health status of the citizenry. First, let us consider the *Gallup-Sharecare Well-Being Index* (GSWBI). The Gallup Organization's polling activities in the United States reach over 300,000 individuals over 18 years of age every year through live telephone surveys. The questions and responses cover a wide range of topics, and subsets of the polling results are used as data in many varied applications. Answers to the health-based questions on the Gallup poll are analyzed with the collaboration of *Sharecare,* a web-based "health and wellness engagement platform," founded by Jeff Arnold of

WebMD fame and TV's Dr. Mehmet Oz. It zeroes in on the influence of health on overall wellbeing. The index covers 6 health domains and uses 42 specific indicators. The six domains are Physical Health, Emotional Health, Healthy Behaviors, Workplace Environment, Satisfaction of Basic Necessities, and Overall Life Evaluation. Among the specific issues covered on the questionnaire are the incidence of colds and flu, the number of sick days taken per month, the levels of stress and depression reported by responders, the use of exercise regimes, the practice of good nutrition, the regularity of visits to doctor and dentist, and the degree of access to health insurance. The scores for each of the six domains are normalized into a 0–100 range and then aggregated into a single composite index. The index can be computed at the scale of communities, cities, regions or states, both for comparative purposes across jurisdictions and for time series analysis within jurisdictions [46].

The next two indexes listed in Table 8.1 address the hugely important issue of the wellbeing of children. Family and communal happiness is probably impossible in countries, or specific regions of countries, or for particular groups within countries, where the wellbeing of children is problematical. This is especially the case for the children of war-torn countries uprooted by violence and conflict within or across their borders. A 2015 UNICEF report on *The Growing Crisis for Refugee and Migrant Children* suggests that there may be as many as 17 million internally-displaced children in the world, and over 11 million child refugees and asylum seekers. Over 50% of them come from just 5 countries: Syria, Afghanistan, Somalia, Sudan, and the Democratic Republic of Congo [47].

No soulless calculation could do justice to the tragedies that accompany these chronicles of lost innocence in war-torn countries. The two indexes listed in Table 8.1 treat the more tractable issue of childhood wellbeing in the industrialized western democracies. The *Child and Youth Well-Being Index* (CWI) is an American effort funded by the New-York-City-based Foundation for Child Development. It was originally developed by the Federal Interagency Forum on Child and Family Statistics, but is now hosted in the Department of Sociology at Duke University [48]. The index is calculated for the United States as a whole. It utilizes 28 indicators defined over seven domains. The domains are Family Economic Well-Being, Safe/Risky Behavior, Social Relationships, Emotional/Spiritual Well-Being, Community Engagement, Educational Attainment, and Health. Among the specific indicators are median family income, child poverty rates, percentage of families with secure parental employment, teenage birth rates, high-school and college graduation rates, reading and math test score statistics, and measures of the rate of adolescent violent crime (both as victims and offenders). The numerical value of the index showed a long steady decline in the first 20 years after it was introduced in 1975, followed by a 10-year period of steady recovery. Since 2003 there have been some short-term volatility in some of the domains, but overall, very little change has been recorded. Although the level of wellbeing of children and youth in America is much higher than that in many other countries, it is apparent that the problems that do exist are somewhat resistant to solution.

The similarly-named *Index of Child Well-being* (ICW) is an international index that covers similar ground. It is produced by UNICEF at their Innocenti Office of

Research in Florence, Italy. It uses 26 indicators in 5 sub-dimensions to rank child wellbeing in 29 industrialized countries. The five sub-dimensions are: Material Wellbeing, Health and Safety, Education, Behavior and Risks, and Housing and Environment. Among the indicators are child poverty rates, birthweights, immunization rates, participation rates in early childhood education, the availability of healthy breakfasts, regular exercise, and the prevalence of teenage smoking, cannabis use, or alcohol abuse. The "child deprivation rate" for a country is defined as the percentage of children who lack 2 or more of the following 14 items: 3 meals a day, 1 meal per week of meat/poultry/fish, fresh fruits and vegetables every day, books in the home, outdoor leisure equipment, regular leisure activities, educational toys in the home, money for school events, homework desk, internet connection, some new clothes, 2 pairs of properly fitting shoes, friends allowed to visit, and special occasions like birthdays celebrated [49].

An even broader coverage is provided by the *Child Development Index* (not listed in Table 8.1) put out by the Save the Children Foundation, a worldwide NGO based in London, England. It uses just 3 domains (Education, Health, and Nutrition) but has been calculated for 141 countries [50].

The study of the wellbeing of children is a well-developed sub-discipline within the happiness movement. UNICEF has been producing reports on the *State of the World's Children* since 1979. The US Federal Interagency Forum on Child and Youth Statistics has published a set of *Key National Indicators of Wellbeing for America's Children* since 1997. An *International Society for Child Indicators* was established in 2006, and the journal *Child Indicators Research* in 2008 [51].

There are health indexes designed for the other end of life as well. The *Global AgeWatch Index* put out by HelpAge International compares countries on their treatment of seniors. It features 4 sub-dimensions and 13 indicators, and has been calculated for 91 countries [52]. The four sub-dimensions are Income Security, Health Status, Employment and Education, and Enabling Environment. Among the 13 country-wide indicators are pension income coverage, poverty rate in old age, GDP per capita, life expectancy at 60, access to public transportation, availability of social connections for seniors, and conditions of physical safety. Data are mined from data bases at the World Bank, the World Health Organization (WHO), the Organization for Economic Co-operation and Development (OECD), and the Gallup Polls.

Environmental Indexes

Environmental issues can play an important role in the determination of personal happiness and communal wellbeing, but there are significant problems in developing a meaningful index for a given country or jurisdiction under analysis. The primary problem lies with the incredibly wide range of topics that fall under the environmental umbrella. Developers of an environmental index might be expected to consider such diverse issues as air quality, water quality, greenhouse gas emissions, ozone depletion, climate change, soil erosion, desertification, acidification, eutrophication, deforestation, biodiversity, animal habitat protection, wetland management, resource depletion, disaster protection, noise pollution, energy production, and waste management. Water quality issues alone may involve several aqueous media: streams, lakes, groundwater, and oceans. Air quality issues may be outdoor, involving toxic chemicals, particulates, smog, and odor; or they may be indoor, involving radon, lead or asbestos. Habitat issues may relate to wildlife, fish, or avian species. Expertise in these various issues comes from widely disparate fields including hydrology, meteorology, oceanography, agriculture, forestry, fisheries, engineering, resource economics, risk analysis, and many branches of health sciences, including toxicology, epidemiology, and immunology. The scales of interest may range from global, to national, to regional, to local. An index may be developed for a variety of different purposes, including advocacy, education, strategy development, policy development, or adaptive management.

In short, it is a complex business, the result of which is that there are hundreds of environmental indexes that have been developed for one purpose or another. The International Institute for Sustainable Development in Winnipeg, Canada, has identified 838 initiatives around the world that tend in this direction [53]. Some are being carried out by international agencies like the United Nations Environmental Program (UNEP), the World Bank, and the Organization for Economic Cooperation and Development (OECD); others by national government agencies like the US Environmental Protection Agency (EPA), and Environment Canada (EC); still others by environmental advocacy groups like Worldwatch, the Environmental Defense Fund, and the World Resources Institute. A 2019 paper by an Australian environmentalist reviews 12 indexes of sustainable progress and critiques their ability to bond human wellbeing to the health of the environment [54].

Our coverage here, as outlined in Table 8.1, is limited to a brief description of one of the more-focused environmental indexes, the Living Planet Index; a somewhat more detailed description of the premiere composite index, the Environmental Performance Index; and a reminder to look back in Chap. 4 at the description there of the Ecological Footprint.

The *Living Planet Index* (LPI) was developed by the Zoological Society of London together with the Swiss-based World Wildlife Fund (WWF). It treats only one issue of environmental concern, that of biodiversity. The LPI is a "measure of the world's biological diversity, based on population trends of vertebrate species from terrestrial, freshwater, and marine habitats." [55]. The time series of population data are weighted "to give more weight to more species-rich systems, realms and groups," and aggregated into a single value that lies between 0 and 1 (or at least it has done since the LPI was standardized to a value of 1.0 for the year 1970). During the period from 1970 to the present, worldwide biodiversity has declined by 38% for terrestrial systems, 36% for marine systems, and 75% for freshwater systems. The LPI is now below 0.

The most widely-quoted environmental index for application on a country-by-country basis is the *Environmental Performance Index* (EPI) based at the Yale University Center for Environmental Law and Policy, in collaboration with the

Center for International Earth Science Information Network at Columbia University, and the World Economic Forum. The Yale Center for Environmental Law and Policy is a joint research institute between the Yale School of Forestry and Environmental Studies, and the Yale Law School, with support from the Yale Data-Driven Environmental Solutions Group. The Center tries "to incorporate fresh thinking, ethical awareness, and analytically-rigorous decision-making tools into environmental law and policy." Development and application of the EPI is aided by a roster of 74 "expert contributors" from universities, international agencies, government programs, and private institutes around the world.

The EPI has been published every second year since 2006. It is a country-by-country analysis that transforms raw data sets into numerical indicator scores that are aggregated into a single index score for each country. Over the years there have been many changes in the indicators used and in the sources of information on which they are based. The most recent version, put out in 2016, uses 19 indicators, addressing 9 environmental issues, grouped into 2 sub-dimensions [56]. The *Environmental Health* sub-dimension covers human environmental impacts. The *Ecosystem Vitality* sub-dimension covers ecosystem impacts.

The first thing to note is that not all possible environmental issues are included in the index. There is no direct reference to groundwater contamination by industrial chemicals, for example, or population growth, or natural disasters, although there are indicators that may peripherally impinge on some of these missing issues. Moreover, even for those issues that are addressed, many of them are treated by just one proxy indicator out of the many that could possibly have been chosen: nitrogen efficiency as a proxy for all agricultural impacts, for example, or wastewater treatment statistics as a proxy for all water-related ecosystem impacts. These limitations are not highlighted here as a criticism of the index. They represent the unavoidable tradeoffs that have to be made, given the unbroachable number and complexity of environmental concerns. There is much information in the EPI reports on how these issues and proxies were selected, and one is left with an impression of much thoughtful deliberation.

The Environmental Health sub-dimension covers three issues: *Health Impacts*, *Air Quality*, and *Water and Sanitation* (which are assigned weights of 33% each). The Health Impacts indicator is taken directly from the Global Burden of Diseases, Injuries and Risk Factors (GBD) published by the Institute for Health Metrics and Evaluation (IHME). The GBD measures the annual burden on society of 79 health-risk factors in terms of deaths, years of life lost, and disability-adjusted life years. The EPI uses the data from just 5 of the 79 risk factors (unsafe water, unsafe sanitation, outdoor air pollution, household air pollution, and ozone pollution), which are the ones most appropriate to the environmental-health focus.

The Air Quality issue involves four indicators that cover exposures to particulate matter, nitrogen dioxide, and the contaminants released by burning solid fuel (coal, charcoal, wood, dung, or crop residues), all of which are implicated in the occurrence of respiratory diseases and lung cancer. Data on exposure to particulate matter comes from a satellite program based at Dalhousie University in Canada and the Global/Urban Mapping Program. Data on exposure to nitrogen dioxide comes from the

Tropospheric Emissions Monitoring Internet Service. Calculation of the household air quality indicator is carried out using data that treat both the percentage of the population burning solid fuel and the health risk so engendered. Data on usage comes from the World Health Organization Global Health Observatory Data Repository. Data on health risk comes from the IHME's GBD.

The Water and Sanitation issue is addressed using two indicators, one for sanitation and one for water supply. Each of these indicators has two components, one that addresses access and one that addresses health risk. In both cases, the access data comes from a joint monitoring program of the World Health Organization and UNICEF; while the health risk data comes again from the IHME's GBD.

The Ecosystem Vitality sub-dimension covers six issues: *Water Resources* (with a weight of 25%), *Biodiversity and Habitat* (25%), *Agriculture* (10%), *Forests* (10%), *Fisheries* (5%), and *Climate and Energy* (25%). The 12 proxy indicators that are used to define these issues vary widely in nature and in the sources of the data. Consider as examples: Percentage of domestic terrestrial biome area that is protected (determined in part from the United Nations World Database on Protected Areas); Annual loss in tree cover between 2000 and 2014 in areas with greater than 39% tree cover divided by 2000 forest extent (from Global Forest Watch); and Change on CO_2 Emissions per unit GDP, 2002–2012 (from World Resources Institute Climate Analysis).

The EPI is calculated on a different basis than any of the other indexes examined thus far. For each of the 19 indicators, the final values are based on a "proximity-to-target" approach that assesses how close each country is to an identified policy target. For every indicator, two benchmarks are identified: a *High-Performance Benchmark* (HPBM) and a *Low-Performance Benchmark* (LPBM). For indicators that are defined in terms of percentages, the LPBM and HPBM values may simply be 0 and 100. Or, depending on how the indicator is defined, the two may be inverted. In some cases, the HPBM is based on expert opinion. In many cases where there is no particularly obvious choice, the HPBM and LPBM are set as the 1st percentile, or the 99th percentile, or some other percentile, of the available global data.

Once the LPBM and the HPBM have been set for every indicator, they are all converted onto a 0–100 range, and each of the 19 indicator variables are linearly interpolated between their 2 defined bounds. The values are then aggregated according to the percentage weights noted above for each of the 2 sub-dimensions, and the 2 sub-dimensions are averaged (i.e. given 50% weight each) to produce the final EPI score for the country under analysis.

In the 2016 EPI report, the five most environmentally friendly countries were Finland, Iceland, Sweden, Denmark and Slovenia. The bottom five were Afghanistan, Niger, Madagascar, Eritrea and Somalia. Canada ranked 25th, the USA 26th out of 180 countries.

Two other environmental indices not listed in Table 8.1 are the *Environmental Vulnerability Index* (3 sub-dimensions, 50 indicators, 235 countries and territories) put out by the United Nations Environmental Program [57] and the *Sustainable Society Index* (3 sub-dimensions, 21 indicators, 151 countries) published by the Sustainable Society Foundation [58].

There is also a new index of interest, just announced in 2019, and not yet in wide use, but interesting in concept. The *Inclusive Sustainable Transformation Index* (with 8 sub-dimensions and 27 indicators) attempts to "capture the extent to which a country has developed a modern industry- or service-based economy that at the same time protects the environment and is gender-inclusive." It is based in part on meeting the United Nations Sustainable Development Goals (SDGs). The development team includes representatives of both China and the USA. The results do not upset expectations. In the list of 200 ranked countries: European, North-American, and Southeast-Asian countries score well; South-American countries are below average; and African countries are near the bottom [59].

Indexes of Infrastructure and Technology

The level of technological advancement in a country seems to be highly correlated with the happiness and wellbeing of its citizens. There are many indexes that track this facet of society. Table 8.1 lists two of them.

As a first example, consider the *Information and Communication Technology (ICT) Development Index* published annually by the International Telecommunications Union, a UN agency based in Geneva, Switzerland. The ICT index is carried out on a country-by-country basis. It can be applied in a comparative sense, to chart the differences between countries with respect to ICT development, or in a time-series sense within one country to determine the extent to which that country has the potential to enhance growth and development of ICT technology [60]. The index uses 11 indicators to arrive at one benchmark measure for each country. The indicators are spread among 3 sub-dimensions: *Access* (which accounts for 40% of the overall score), *Use* (40%), and *Skills* (20%). Among the indicators that fall under the first of these three headings are: percentage of households with a home computer, percentage of households with internet access, and international internet bandwidth per internet user; under the second heading: fixed and mobile broadband subscriptions per 100 inhabitants; and under the third: mean years of schooling, and secondary and tertiary school enrollments as a percentage of the eligible population. The indicators are equally weighted within each of the three sub-indexes, and then aggregated according to the percentages noted above to produce the final index value.

The second example is the *Knowledge Index* produced by the World Bank Institute. It uses 3 sub-dimensions and 9 indicators, and has been calculated for 146 countries [61]. It is designed to measure a country's "potential and ability to generate, adopt, and diffuse knowledge." The three sub-dimensions are Education and Human Resources, Innovation System, and Information and Community Technology. Indicators for the first sub-dimension include years of schooling, and secondary and tertiary education enrolment rates. The second sub-dimension tracks the number of patents granted, the number of scientific papers published, and the value of royalty payments paid out. The third sub-dimension utilizes data on telephone hookups, computer stats, and internet usage.

There are three other tech indexes not listed in Table 8.1 that bear mention. The World Economic Forum publishes the *Networked Readiness Index* (4 sub-dimensions, 54 indicators, 144 countries) [62]. The United Nations Development Program produces the *Technology Achievement Index* (4 sub-dimensions, 8 indicators, 72 countries) [63]. And Cornell University sponsors the *Global Innovation Index* (2 sub-dimensions, 84 indicators, 142 countries) [64].

Weaknesses and Annoyances

If one were to dig out the detailed reports associated with each of the indexes highlighted in this chapter, it is likely that not one of them would come without a lengthy discussion of problems, weaknesses, and cautions. The developers of indexes of happiness and wellbeing are well aware that their creations are far from perfect. The subject is just too multilayered for anyone to feel that they have got their hands around it, fully and completely. There are nitty-gritty technical issues that dog the practical application of most indexes, and there are broader cultural and social concerns that can bring the entire scope and design of an index into question.

Among the most ubiquitous technical issues are those associated with data. There can be problems with the uniformity of data, and of data-collection methodologies, across countries, or even within them. There can be data-lag issues that delay the availability of data from some sources, necessitating the use of older, possibly out-of-date data for some components of the index, or for some jurisdictions under consideration, and leading to analyses that are based on out-of-synch data sets. Most common of all are data gaps that require some method of fill-in. For missing data points within a time series, linear interpolation is the most common approach. For data points before or after the available time series, most indexes use extrapolation forward or backward on the trend. All of the makeshift accommodations that are used to address these issues have the potential to introduce unintended biases and uncertainties into the results.

There can also be technical issues within the calculation procedures. The potential problems associated with directionality, normalization, aggregation, and weighting have already been discussed in Chap. 7. The final value of an index can be very sensitive to each of these procedures.

Perhaps more important than the technical issues are the broader issues associated with the basic underlying design of an index. How were the indicators selected? Does the selection reflect any unconscious cultural bias? Does it perhaps reflect the conscious ideological bias of an advocacy group? Does it have relevance to both higher-income jurisdictions and lower-income jurisdictions? Is the calculation procedure too complex, with extraneous dimensions or indicators that may be cross-correlated, and/or have data requirements that are in excess of what is available? Or, on the contrary, is the calculation procedure too simplistic, with too few indicators to fully reflect the intricacies of happiness and wellbeing? All of these issues will impact on the public perceptions of the index, the level of confidence it engenders in the political realm, and the effectiveness and influence it brings to policy deliberations.

A Summary of Results for the USA and Canada

To bring some closure to this chapter, Table 8.4 displays the percentile scores and country rankings for the USA and Canada for the 15 single-dimension indexes from Table 8.1 that produce global cross-country calculations. For those indexes that have ranges of 0–100 or 0–1, the percentiles are taken directly from the published scores. For those indexes with open-ended ranges, the percentiles are linearly interpolated between the highest and lowest scores in the lists of published results. For those indexes with reverse scales, the percentiles have been reciprocated, so that for all the indexes in Table 8.4, the higher the percentile, the better the performance.

Table 8.4 Summary of results for the USA and Canada for a set of selected single-dimensional indexes

Index	Number of countries	USA percentile (%)	USA ranking	Canada percentile (%)	Canada
Global Opportunity Index	136	71	19	77	6
Index of Economic Well-being	14	48	13	58	8
Democracy Index	167	80	21	92	6
Worldwide Press Freedom Index	180	78	41	85	18
Corruption Perception Index	175	74	17	81	10
Global Peace Index	163	64	103	93	8
Global Terrorism Index	130	49	36	25	66
Fragile States Index	178	66	20	76	10
World Giving Index	140	99	2	96	6
Social Progress Index	159	85	19	89	2
Child Well-Being Index	29	15	26	45	17
Global AgeWatch	96	79	9	84	5
Environmental Performance Index	180	85	26	85	25
ICT Development Index	175	81	15	76	25
Knowledge Index	146	91	9	91	6

Both the USA and Canada rank very highly on most of the indexes, although Canada outperforms the USA overall. The two areas where both countries score poorly are with respect to global terrorism and child wellbeing. The global terrorism scores have declined rather precipitously for many countries in recent years due to the increased incidence of home-grown terrorist incidents. As for the child well being scores, it must be noted that this index only covers 29 Western nations, and that these include several Scandinavian and other European nations which have much more highly-developed social programs than the United States, certainly, and even Canada, as well. To end on a positive note, both countries rank near the top in charitable giving as reflected in the World Giving Index.

References

1. Bandura, R., *A Survey of Composite Indices Measuring Country Performance,* United Nations Development Program, 2005; Yang, Lin, *An Inventory of Composite Measures of Human Progress*, United Nations Development Program, 2014. [hdr.undp.org/sites/default/files/inventory_report_working_paper.pdf]
2. Baumohl, Bernard, *The Secrets of Economic Indicators*, 3rd ed., Financial Times Press, 2013.
3. Boskin, M.J., Consumer Price Indexes, in David R. Henderson, ed., *Concise Encyclopedia of Economics* (2nd ed.), Library of Economics and Liberty, 2008.
4. [www.investopedia.com]
5. [www.demographia.com]
6. [www.nahb.org]
7. [www.milkeninstitute.org]
8. [www.opacityindex.com]
9. [www.heritage.org]
10. [www.fraserinstitute.org]
11. Osberg, Lars and Andrew Sharpe, *The Index of Economic Well-Being*, Centre for Study of Living Standards, Ottawa, Canada, 2001; Osberg, Lars and Andrew Sharpe, How should we measure the economic aspects of well-being? *Review of Income and Wealth*, 51(2), 311-336, 2005; Osberg, Lars and Andrew Sharpe, *Beyond GDP: Measuring Economic Well-Being in Canada and the Provinces,1981-2010*, Centre for Study of Living Standards, Ottawa, Canada, Research Report 2011-12, 2011. [www.csls.ca]
12. [www.eiu.com]
13. Welsh, Jennifer, *The Return of History*, House of Anansi Press, 2016.
14. [www.globalintegrity.org]
15. [http://info.worldbank.org/governance/wgi/index.aspx]
16. [www.rsf.org]
17. [www.transparency.org]
18. [www.economicsandpeace.org]
19. [www.economicsandpeace.org]
20. Messner, J. and Nate Halen, *Fragile States Index*, Fund for Peace, 2016. [www.fundforpeace.org]
21. [www.statcan.gc.ca]
22. [www.uri.edu/nivah]
23. [www.worldriskreport.org]
24. [www.unitedway.org/stateofcaring]
25. [www.cafonline.org]

26. Stern, Scott, Amy Wares and Tamar Hellman, *Social Progress Index, Methodological Report*, Social Progress Imperative, 2016. [www.socialprogressimperative.org]
27. [www.weforum.org/issues/global-gender-gap]
28. [http://hdr.undp.org/en/data]
29. [www.socialwatch.org]
30. [www.indsocdev.org]
31. [www.socialwatch.org]
32. [http://americasquarterly.org]
33. [www.queensu.ca/mcp/index.html]
34. Miringoff, Marc and Marque-Luisa Miringoff, *The Social Health of the Nation: How America Is Really Doing*, Oxford University Press, 1999; Opdyke, Sandra and M.L. Miringoff, *The Social Health of the States*, Institute for Innovation in Social Policy, Vassar College, 2008. [www.iisp.vassar.edu]
35. Delors, Jacques, et. al., *Learning: The Treasure Within*, Report of the International Commission on Education for the Twenty-First Century, UNESCO, 1996.
36. Cartwright,F., J. Mussio, and C. Boughton, *Developing the Composite Learning Index: A Framework*, Canadian Council on Learning, 2006.
37. Saisana, Michaela, ELLI Index: *A Sound Measure for Lifelong Learning in the European Union*, Joint Research Centre, Institute for the Protection and Security of the Citizen, European Union, 2010; *ELLI Index Europe, Indicators in Depth*, Bertelsmann Stiftung, 2010. [www.elli.org]
38. [https://en.unesco.org/gem-report/education-all-development-index]
39. [hdr.undp.org/en/content/education-index]
40. [www.rtei.org]
41. Heubner, E.S. et al, Further validation of the multi-dimensional students life-satisfaction scale, *Jour. Psychoeducational Assessment*, 16(2), 118-134, 1998; Heubner, E.S. et al, *Manual for the MSLSS*, University of South Carolina, Dept. Psychology, 2001.
42. Cummins, R.A and A.L.D. Lau, *Manual: Personal Wellbeing Index – School Children (PWI-SC)*, School of Psychology, Deakin University, Melbourne, Australia, 2005.
43. Sirgy, M.J., S. Grzekowink and D. Rahtz, Quality of college life of students: Developing and validating a measure of well-being, *Social Indicators Research*, 80(2), 343-360, 2007.
44. Bjornberg, Arne, *European Health Consumer Index Report*, Health Consumer Powerhouse, 2016. [www.healthpowerhouse.com]
45. [www.ahrq.gov]
46. [www.well-beingindex.com]
47. Garin, Emily, *Uprooted: The Growing Crisis for Refugee and Migrant Children*, UNICEF, 2015.
48. Land, K.C., ed, *The Well-Being of America's Children: Developing and Improving the Child and Youth Well-Being Index*, Springer, 2012.
49. UNICEF, *Child Well-Being in Rich Countries: A Comparative Overview*, UNICEF Office of Reseaech – Innocenti, Report Card 13, 2016. [www.unicef-irc.org]
50. [www.savethechildren.org.uk]
51. Lamb, V.L. and K.C. Land, Worldwide view of child well-being, Chapter 19, *Global Handbook of Quality of Life: Exploration of Well-Being of Nations and Continents,* edited by W. Galatzer, et. al., Springer, 2015; Ben-Arieh, A., The child indicators movement: Past, present and future, *Child Indicators Research*, 1, 3-16, 2008.
52. [www.helpage.org]
53. [www.iisd.org]
54. Patrick, R. et al, Human wellbeing and the health of the environment: Local indicators that balance the scales, *Social Indicators Research*, 146,651-667, 2019.
55. McRae, L., R. Freeman and V. Marconi, *The Living Planet Index*, in "The Living Planet Report," N.Oerlemans, ed., World Wildlife Fund International, Gland, Switzerland, 2016. [www.livingplanetindex.org]

56. Environmental Performance Index, *Global Metrics for the Environment, 2016 Report,* Yale Center for Environmental Law and Policy, 2016. [www.epi.yale.edu]
57. [www.vulnerabilityindex.net]
58. [www.sustainabilitysocietyindex.com]; Van de Klerk, G. and A. Manuel, A comprehensive index for a sustainable society: The SSI – the Sustainable Society Index, *Ecological Economics*, 66, 228-242, 2008.
59. Lin, J.Y., C. Monga and S. Standaert, The Inclusive Sustainable Transformation Index, *Social Indicators Research*, 143, 47-80, 2019.
60. International Telecommunications Union, *Measuring the Information Society Report*, 2016. [www.itu.int]
61. [www.worldbank.org/kam]
62. [networked readinessindex.org]
63. [http://hdr.undp.org]
64. [www.globalinnovationindex.org]

Chapter 9
The Wellbeing of Nations

Multi-dimensional Composite Indexes of Nationwide Communal Wellbeing

In this chapter our attention turns to the multi-dimensional composite indexes of wellbeing that have been applied at the national or international level. These indexes represent our first detailed look at the types of socially-relevant and all-encompassing measures that have been the long-time dream of the social indicators movement since its inception. These are the indexes that are seen as possible candidates to replace the GDP with a more suitable measure of human wellbeing. These are the constructs that attempt to integrate the impacts of social relationships, the environment, health, education, security, governance, and technological advancement, onto the purely economic framework that infuses GDP-based assessments.

Table 9.1 provides a listing of several such indexes that have been at the forefront in the calculation of nationwide communal wellbeing. The criteria for inclusion on the table are that these indexes have been widely used over some years, and that they are still in use today. Many of them were originally developed by individuals or small teams of wellbeing researchers working in relative obscurity. Most are now administered by well-known non-governmental organizations or institutes. The table lists the name of each index, its acronym, the developer or sponsoring agency, the year of first launch, the number of dimensions included in its multi-dimensional schema, the total number of individual indicators used in its overall calculation, and a website where more detail can be found.

All of the indices listed in Table 9.1 are *multi-dimensional* in that they include consideration of more than one dimension of wellbeing, sometimes as few as 3 or 4, more often as many as 8 or 9, and in one case, 11. They are *composite* in that all of them integrate across the various dimensions to produce a single-valued numeric result. They are *communal* in that their calculations are carried out on a societal rather than an individual basis. And they are *nationwide* in that they are usually

R. A. Freeze, *The Metrics of Happiness*, Social Indicators Research Series 86,
https://doi.org/10.1007/978-3-031-10913-3_9

Table 9.1 Multi-dimensional composite indexes of nationwide wellbeing

Name		Developer	Launch	Dims	Inds	
Human Development Index	HDI	United Nations Development Programme	1990	3	4	[http://hdr.undp.org]
World Happiness Report	WHR	United Nations Sustainable Development Solutions Network	2012	6*	6	[http://unsdsn.org/happiness]
Quality of Life Index	QLI	Economist Intelligence Unit	2005	9*	9	[www.economist.com/theworldin/2005]
Happy Life Years	HLY	Ruut Veenhoven, World Database of Happiness	1996	2	2	[www2.eur.nl/fsw/research/veenhoven]
Happy Planet Index	HPI	New Economics Foundation, London UK	2006	3	3	[www.happyplanetindex.org]
Genuine Progress Indicator**	GPI	Redefining Progress	1995	3	26	[http://rprogress.org]
Canadian Index of Wellbeing	CIW	Canadian Institute of Wellbeing	2011	8	64	[https://uwaterloo.ca/canadian-index-wellbeing/]
Weighted Index of Social Progress	WISP	Richard J. Estes, University of Pennsylvania	1984	10	40	[www.miqols.org/toolbox/isp.html]
Gross National Happiness Index–A	GNH-A	International Institute of Management, Las Vegas NV	2005	7	30+?	[www.iim-edu.org/grossnationalhappiness/index.htm]
Gross National Happiness Index-B	GNH-B	GNH Center, Bhutan	2010	9	33	[www.grossnationalhappiness.com]
Better Life Index	BLI	Organization for Economic Cooperation and Development	2011	11	24	[www.oecdbetterlifeindex.org]
Prosperity Index	LPI	Legatum Institute, London, UK	2007	9	104	[www.prosperity.com]
Best Countries Ranking		US News and World Report	2016	9	65	[www.usnews.com/news/bestcountries]
Wellbeing Index	WI	Robert Prescott-Allen	2001	10	57	[www.iied.org]
Good Country Index	GCI	Simon Anholt, Anholt-Gfk-Roper	2014	7	35	[www.goodcountryindex.org]

*See text

**Based on earlier Measure of Economic Welfare (MEW) - 1972; and Index of Sustainable Economic Welfare (ISEW) - 1989

applied on a country-by-country basis, either to compare and rank countries at a given point in time, or to track the performance of a single country over time.

The types of dimensions that make up the multi-dimensional fabric of these composite indexes were originally listed back in Chap. 7 in Table 7.1. The scope of each of these dimensions was further clarified in Table 7.2. Detailed descriptions of many of the single-dimensional components that constitute the building blocks of the multi-dimensional calculations, and across which the composite indexes are integrated, were described in Chap. 8. A summary of data sources for these indexes, and for the ones discussed in this chapter, can be found in Table A.1 in Appendix.

The indexes included in Table 9.1 are listed in the order in which they are discussed in this chapter, rather than in the order in which they were launched. To place this evolution into better context, the reader should refer to Table 9.2 which provides an historical timeline that puts these nationwide models of wellbeing in order of their launch date, together with many of the other seminal events that have taken place in the history of wellbeing studies, all of which have already received coverage in earlier chapters. The historical timeline provided in Table 9.2 is weighted toward those ideas and indexes that have been developed with a strong motivation to provide alternatives to the GDP as a measure of national wellbeing.

The Forerunners

Chapter 3 described the revolution in economics that gave birth to the social indicators movement in the late 1960s and early 1970s. Economists began to see the limitations of the GDP as a measure of human wellbeing, and began searching for measures that would be more broadly-based. In the USA, suggestions as to what aspects of life might be included in such a measure came from Raymond Bauer's 1966 treatise on *Social Indicators*, Frank Andrews and Stephen Withey's 1976 book on *Social Indicators of Well-Being*, and the series of reports put out by the US Bureau of the Census in 1973, 1977 and 1980 under the title *Social Indicators: Selected Data on Social Conditions and Trends* [1]. As further prods to the movement, it was in 1972 that the King of Bhutan began talking about Gross National Happiness, and in 1974 that the first issue of the journal *Social Indicators Research* appeared.

There is no question that these ideas resonated strongly with the various agencies of the United Nations, but it would be well over a decade before the United Nations Development Programme actually produced a working index designed to replace the GDP. The UN's Human Development Index (HDI) was launched in 1990 and its history and methodology is fully described in the section that follows this one. The HDI is the initial listing in Table 9.1 because it was the first multi-dimensional index to be widely used by those other than its developers, and it is still in wide use today. However, it was certainly not the first composite index to be put forward. At least three academically-based economics research teams took up the challenge years

Table 9.2 Timeline of ideas and indexes developed to provide alternatives to the GDP as a measure of national wellbeing

1934	Simon Kuznets of the U.S. National Bureau of Economic Research develops the National Income and Product Accounts that are eventually used as the basis for the calculation of the USA's Gross Domestic Product (GDP)
1944	At a UN conference held at Bretton Woods, New Hampshire, 44 Allied nations agree that the GDP will be the standard measure for assessing and comparing the economies of each member state.
1972	The king of Bhutan introduces the philosophy of Gross National Happiness (GNH) as a more meaningful measure of national wellbeing than the GDP.
1972	William Nordhaus and James Tobin of Yale University introduce the Measure of Economic Welfare (MEW).
1973	British economist E.F. Schumacher publishes "Small Is Beautiful: Economics As If People Mattered," and a US-based team under the Club of Rome publishes "The Limits to Growth," both of which are critical of GDP-based traditional economic theory.
1974	The journal "Social Indicators Research" begins publication.
1976	Frank M. Andrews and Stephen B. Withey of the University of Michigan publish their report on "Social Indicators of Well-Being" in the US.
1979	Morris David Morris of Brown University develops the Physical Quality of Life Index (PQLI) for the U.S. Overseas Development Council.
1984	Richard J. Estes of the University of Pennsylvania publishes the Weighted Index of Social Progress (WISP).
1985	Economist Amartya Sen publishes his book on "Commodities and Capabilities" in which he enumerates the flaws of the GDP as a measure of human wellbeing.
1987	The UN World Commission on Environment and Development chaired by Bro Harlem Brundtland issues its report on "Our Common Future," which argues for a global economy based on sustainable development.
1988	Feminist economist Marilyn Waring argues in her book "If Women Counted" that the GDP grossly undervalues the economic value of women's work to society.
1989	Herman Daly and John Cobb launch the Index of Sustainable Economic Welfare (ISEW).
1990	The UN Development Program launches the Human Development Index (HDI).
1995	The US-based Redefining Progress launches the Genuine Progress Indicator (GPI).
1996	Ruut Veenhoven introduces the concept of Happy Life Expectancy (HLE) based on data from his World Database of Happiness. Repackaged as Happy Life Years (HLY) in 2004.
2000	The Calvert-Henderson Quality-of-Life Indicators are published.
2005	The US-based International Institute of Management launches the GNH Index (GNH-A).
2006	The UK-based New Economics Foundation launches the Happy Planet Index (HPI).
2007	An international conference on "Beyond GDP" is held in Brussels, Belgium.
2007	The State of the USA Program is founded to develop a Key National Indicator System.
2007	The UK-based Legatum Institute launches the Prosperity Index (LPI).
2009	The Sarkozy Commission report is published on the "Measurement of Economic Performance and Social Progress."
2009	The Gallup Poll launches its happiness survey in the US.
2010	The Center for Bhutan Studies launches the Bhutan GNH Index (GNH-B).
2011	OECD launches the Better Life Index (BLI), and publishes its first "How's Life?" report.
2011	The Canadian Index of Wellbeing (CIW) is launched.
2012	The UN publishes its first edition of the "World Happiness Report."
2012	A UN Resolution decrees March 20 as the annual International Day of Happiness.

before the UN. They are the true forerunners of the many multi-dimensional indexes that form the backbone of this Chapter.

The first of these was the Measure of Economic Welfare (MEW), developed in 1972 by two economists from Yale University working under the auspices of the National Bureau of Economic Research. William Nordhaus and James Tobin considered their progeny as "a primitive experimental measure" designed to address "the more obvious discrepancies between the GDP and true economic welfare." These perceived flaws in the GDP, at least with respect to its use as a measure of communal wellbeing, were discussed in Chap. 3. They include its failure to properly value leisure time, its failure to value unpaid household work, its avoidance of the negative externalities associated with environmental degradation, and its inclusion of so-called "defensive" government expenditures which have no direct effect on household economic welfare (like those associated with military defense, police protection, public health, and disaster response). MEW calculations start with the per-capita GDP, then add value for the first two of these "discrepancies," and subtract value for the second two. The MEW is an American construct and it has never been applied to other countries for comparative purposes. It makes use of data that are largely available in the National Income and Products Accounts (the so-called NIPA accounts). In their original report, Nordhaus and Tobin applied the MEW retroactively to the period 1929–1965. They found that the MEW calculations indicated a growth in wellbeing over this period in the United States, but that the rate of growth of the MEW index was significantly less than that of the GDP [2]. In 2018, William Nordhaus was awarded the Nobel Prize in Economics, at least in part for his role in developing the Measure of Economic Welfare.

While the MEW itself is no longer in use, and therefore does not appear in Table 9.1, it was the direct progenitor of the *Index of Sustainable Welfare* (ISEW), produced by Herman Daly and John B. Cobb in 1989, and the ISEW was itself the direct precursor of the *Genuine Progress Indicator* (GPI), which *is* still in wide use, and *does* appear in Table 9.1. A more detailed treatment of this genealogic trail is included in the section on the GPI later in this chapter.

The second forerunner of note was the Physical Quality of Life Index (PQLI), developed in the late 1970s by a social scientist at Brown University with the pleasingly palindromic name of Morris David Morris [3]. He did so on-assignment from the U.S. Overseas Development Council, an independent, international, policy-research institute based in Washington DC, which was looking for an alternative measure to the GDP to judge the social advancement of the poorer countries in the world. Morris was the first to use objective data from publically-available, international databases, and to apply his index to a wide suite of the world's countries. The PQLI had just three indicators: basic literacy rate, infant mortality, and life expectancy at age 1. Critics found fault with the complete absence of any economic component, and pointed out that the two childhood-health indicators were far too closely correlated to be used as independent measures. Perhaps because of these caveats, or perhaps because it was simply ahead of its time, the PQLI never took off. It is no longer in use, and for this reason does not appear in Table 9.1, but despite its faded importance, modern researchers owe a debt of gratitude to Morris and the

USODC for this pioneering precursor of later composite indexes of nationwide communal wellbeing.

The first full-blown multi-dimensional index of national wellbeing was produced by Richard J. Estes of the School of Social Policy and Practice at the University of Pennsylvania. He first conceptualized his ideas in a 1976 paper, and then fully developed them in a book published in 1984 [4]. He called his original creation the Index of Social Progress (ISP), but it was soon replaced by the more-sophisticated Weighted Index of Social Progress (WISP). The WISP has been in continued use since its inception, but primarily as a research tool by Estes and his colleagues. It nevertheless qualifies for inclusion in Table 9.1, and a more complete description of its structure and use appears in a separate section later in this chapter.

These early contributions by Nordhaus and Tobin on MEW, Morris on PQLI, Estes on WISP, and Daly and Cobb on ISEW, deserve the many accolades they have received over the years. They led the way toward the explosion of ideas that burst forth in the new millennium on how to move "beyond GDP."

The Human Development Index

The earliest composite index to receive wide international usage is the *Human Development Index* (HDI), first introduced by the United Nations Development Program (UNDP) in 1990. The results of the HDI rankings have appeared at regular intervals ever since, and although there are now many composite indexes of greater complexity, the HDI remains at the forefront. It is the most-widely disseminated and most-widely quoted of the nationwide indexes, and is considered the strongest candidate to replace the GDP as the measurement of choice in the assessment of human happiness and wellbeing.

The birth of the HDI can be credited to four world-renowned economists, all of whom came from the Indian subcontinent. The original push came from within the UNDP, led by the Pakistani economist Mahbub ul Haq who wanted to "shift the focus of development economics from national income accounting to people-centred policies." [5]. He saw the need for a measure that would better reflect a nation's human achievement than the then-current emphasis on GDP and economic growth. In this, he was strongly influenced by the work of the Cambridge-based economist, Amartya Sen, who had espoused similar ideas in his 1985 book *Commodities and Capabilities* [6]. Sen argued that the wellbeing of a country should be measured by what its citizens can "be and do" not by what they "have." He saw human development as an effort to advance political, economic and social freedoms, so that citizens would have ample opportunity to fully develop their inborn capabilities. In 1989, ul Haq put together an advisory committee that included Sen, the Oxford-based economist Sudhir Anand, and the British Labour politician Megnhad Desai. The HDI saw first light in the 1990 Human Development Report of the UNDP. Many of the methodological treatises that followed were authored by Anand and Sen. In his autobiographical speech at the 1998 ceremony where he was awarded the Nobel

Prize in Economics [7], Sen spoke nostalgically of his contributions to the birth of the HDI, stating that his involvement brought him "great delight." As for ul Haq, the UN now sponsors an annual award in his name for "lifetime service to human development."

The HDI was founded on six basic principles: (1) It must reflect the fundamental purpose of human development, which is to enlarge people's choices. (2) It must use a limited number of indicators in order to keep the index simple and manageable. (3) It must be a single composite index, not a plethora of separate indexes. (4) It must cover both social and economic choices. (5) It must be sufficiently flexible in both coverage and methodology to allow gradual refinements as better alternatives become available. And (6) it's development must not be inhibited by the apparent lack of reliable or up-to-date data series [8].

With these principles in hand, the founders decided on a three-dimensional structure to reflect what they saw as the three primary drivers of human wellbeing: Health, Knowledge, and Living Standard (or in our terminology from Chap. 7: Health, Education, and Economy). It was their initial desire to have just one proxy indicator for each dimension, and in this they initially succeeded. Their indicator for the Health dimension was taken as life expectancy at birth (in years); for Knowledge, the adult literacy rate (in percent); and for Living Standard, the country's per-capita GDP (in Purchasing Parity Power dollars, $PPP). The reader may recall from Chap. 3 that $PPP are widely used in international monetary comparisons, with one $PPP having the same purchasing power in the domestic economy of the country under analysis as one $US has in the US economy. The $PPP conversion rates for almost all of the countries in the world are available from the International Comparison Programme published by the World Bank [9].

The specific indicators in the HDI structure have changed somewhat over the years. The indicators that are currently in use were introduced at the time of the most recent revisions in 2010. Life expectancy at birth remains unchanged as the Health indicator. The Living Standard indicator has undergone the minor transformation from GDP per capita to GNI per capita (where GNI is the Gross National Income of a country as defined back in Chap. 3, a value that is not significantly different from the GDP for most countries). Adult literacy has been entirely removed from the calculation and replaced by two new indicators for the Knowledge dimension: expected years of schooling (EYS), and mean years of schooling (MYS), where EYS is defined as the number of years of schooling that a child of school entrance age can expect to receive if prevailing patterns of age-specific enrolment rates persist through the child's life, and MYS is defined as the average number of years of schooling that have actually been received by people aged 25 and older. With the 2010 revisions in place, the HDI remains a three-dimensional construct, but the number of specific indicators has increased to four [10].

Life expectancy data (LE) for the HDI is taken from a database maintained by the UN Department of Economic and Social Affairs. Data on per capita GNI comes from the World Bank, the International Monetary Fund, and the UN Statistical Division. Data on EYS and MYS comes from a variety of sources: the UNESCO Institute for Statistics, UNICEF Multiple Indicator Cluster Surveys, OECD's Education-at-a-

Glance Indicators, the Demographic and Health Survey data from the global consulting firm ICF, and the Dataset of Educational Attainment maintained by Harvard economist Robert Barro and his Korean colleague Jong-Wha Lee [11].

The methodology for calculating the HDI for a given country from the raw data is relatively straightforward [12]. The first step is to normalize each of the four indicator values into a decimal fraction. This is done by setting a minimum and a maximum value for each indicator, based on the range of values observed around the world. The developers of the HDI consider the minimums as "natural zeros" and the maximums as "aspirational targets." For LE, the selected range is [20,85] years; for EYS, [0,18] years; for MYS, [0,15] years; and for per-capita GNI, [100,75,000] $PPP. For the first three indicators, normalization onto a [0,1] range is carried out using a simple linear relationship. Because of the huge observed range in per capita GNI, and the perceived non-linear relationship between GNI and HDI, the raw data for per capita GNI is transformed by taking the natural logarithm (the ln function) of the actual value (and of the minimum and maximum values) before normalizing it onto the [0,1] range. (Note that the ln of 100 is 4.61 while that of 75,000 is 11.22). The logarithmic transformation emphasizes the diminishing marginal utility of higher incomes on human happiness and wellbeing.

In the second step, the two Knowledge indicators, EYS and MYS, are reduced to a single decimal fraction by taking their arithmetic mean (which implies an equal weighting of these two components).

In the final step, the three decimal fractions representing the three dimensions are aggregated into a single result by taking the geometric mean, that is, by multiplying them together and then taking the third root of the resulting number. In the original 1990 formulation the aggregation was carried out using the arithmetic mean; the switch to the geometric mean took place as part of the 2010 revisions. The appropriateness of this approach to aggregation across the dimensions was discussed in Chap. 7. Either approach implies equal weighting of the three component dimensions. Given that the three terms of the HDI are all decimal fractions, so too is the HDI. The HDI for any given country will always be a decimal fraction lying between 0.000 and 1.000.

As an example of an HDI calculation, take the 2018 values for the USA: LE = 79.5 years (normalized to 0.915); EYS = 16.5 years (normalized to 0.917); MYS = 13.4 years (normalized to 0.893); and per capita GNI = 54,941 PPP$ (ln value = 10.91; normalized to 0.953). The arithmetic mean of the EYS AND MYS is 0.905. The geometric mean of [0.915, 0.905, 0.953] is 0.924, which is therefore the HDI for the USA for 2018.

The most recent calculations of the HDI were carried out for 189 countries in 2018 [13]. The highest value was 0.953 (for Norway) and the lowest was 0.354 (for Niger). The top five countries were Norway, Switzerland, Australia, Ireland, and Germany. The lowest five were Burundi, Chad, South Sudan, Central African Republic, and Niger. Canada ranked 12th and the USA 13th. A total of 59 countries were judged as high-HDI (greater than 0.80), 92 as moderate-HDI (0.55–0.80), and 38 as low-HDI (less than 0.55). The global average HDI was 0.728. This represents a significant improvement over the initial 1990 value of 0.598. The authors acknowledge the "considerable progress," but also note the many "persistent deprivations and disparities."

Where data permits, the HDI calculations allow the disaggregation of the results to clarify disparities between rich and poor, male and female, urban and rural, and between various ethnic groups or regions. In this mode, the HDI provides clearer direction to policy makers as to what is needed for the improvement of nationwide communal wellbeing.

The HDI is certainly not accepted by all. There have been many studies that have critiqued the HDI and found it wanting in one or more of its aspects. Most have suggested potential improvements, additions, or replacements. A report published by the UNDP in 2011 provides an objective and relatively complete summary of these studies, and also provides full references to a large suite of them [14]. The various criticisms can be grouped into a set of relatively-few general premises: (1) Many critics hold that the three-dimensional structure is too sparse. They are supportive of more-inclusive composite indexes that include consideration of environmental sustainability, governance, national security, and technological advancement. (2) Others find fault with the choice of proxy indicators, which they find oversimplified. (3) Some critics draw attention to the somewhat arbitrary methods of aggregation and weighting across the dimensions and the apparent sensitivity of the results to the selected weighting schemes. (4) Others are opposed to aggregation at all. They find single-valued indexes to be of dubious value, exhibiting instead a preference for multi-dimensional dashboards. (5) There is also concern that basing calculations on mean values of the four indicators may be evading the implications of distributional inequalities. And lastly, (6) there is much discussion in the literature about the apparent close correlation between the HDI and GNI per capita, and whether the HDI actually reveals anything about a country's status that is not already clear from the GNI or GDP alone.

The first four items in this list are really just matters of opinion, and all of them relate to the obvious trade-off between the desire for a simple, transparent, and media-friendly index, and the added rigor that might be achieved with a more-complex representation of national well being.

The desire for indexes with more dimensions and more indicators has of course spawned many multi-dimensional national indexes, the most noteworthy of which are described in the rest of this chapter. Of interest here is the response of the UN Development Programme itself. Despite ul Haq and Sen's original desire to avoid a "plethora of separate indexes," the UNDP in their 2010 revisions to the program embarked on exactly that route. They now publish four additional indexes (*Inequality-Adjusted HDI, Gender Development Index, Gender Inequality Index, and Multidimensional Poverty Index*), and five statistical dashboards (*Quality of Human Development, Life-Course Gender Gaps, Women's Empowerment, Environmental Sustainability, and Socioeconomic Sustainability*). Furthermore, there is also a *Human Sustainable Development Index* (HSDI) that was also launched in 2010, not by the UNDP, but by the International Geosphere Biosphere Program (IGBP) [15]. It is calculated in identical fashion to the HDI but with the addition of one additional dimension to represent a country's environmental impacts. Addition of this dimension leads to one additional proxy indicator in the form of per-capita carbon emissions (in CO_2 equivalents). The addition of an environmental dimension does not lead to large changes in the ranking of most countries relative to the HDI, although some highly-developed countries do show some slippage. In the 2010 listings, the Scandinavian countries remain near the top; Canada slides from 8th to 23rd; and the USA from 4th to 24th. The biggest effects are on the oil-producing nations of the Middle East like Qatar, Kuwait, and United Arab Emirates, all of which lose more than 50 places relative to the HDI. The 2010 HSDI may turn out to be a one-off as the IGBP completed its mission in 2015 and presumably the HSDI died with it.

Returning to the list of potential HDI shortcomings, it can be seen that the fifth item raises the issue of whether it is appropriate to base calculations on the mean values of the four indicators, or whether consideration of the *distribution* of these variables within a given country might influence rankings. A country with wide disparities in its internal distribution of longevity, educational attainment, or income, could exhibit a very different level of national wellbeing than one with more equitable distributions, even though calculations based on the means might not show it. This same point was made back in Chap. 3 with respect to the per-capita GDP in the discussion of the Gini coefficient. Two of the new UN-sponsored indexes noted above, the *Inequality-Adjusted HDI*, and the *Multidimensional Poverty Index*, are designed to address the issue of distributional inequities, albeit in quite different ways.

In the *Inequality-Adjusted HDI* (or IHDI), the inequality measure is taken as the ratio of the geometric mean to the arithmetic mean of the distributions for each indicator variable, where the arithmetic mean is defined as the sum of a set of n numbers divided by n, and the geometric mean is the nth root of the product of n numbers. The ratio of geometric to arithmetic means is applied as a multiplicative correction factor to the unadjusted, normalized values of each of the four indicator variables. Because the geometric mean is always smaller than the arithmetic mean, the correction always produces a lower value. The IHDI thus discounts the HDI according to the extent of inequality in a country. The greater the inequality, the lower is the IHDI relative to the HDI.

In-country distributional data on income are available from the World Bank International Income Distribution Database, the UN World Income Inequality Database, the European Union Study of Income and Living Conditions, and the Luxembourg Income Study. Those for longevity and educational attainment can be mined from the same databases used to calculate the HDI.

The 2018 IHDI calculations show reductions relative to the HDI for every country considered. The least reduction was 3.6%, for Japan, and the greatest was 45.3%, for the African island nation of Comoros. On average, the global loss was roughly 20%. By and large, the ranked order of countries is quite similar for the IHDI and HDI. Canada's ranking is the same in both listings; the USA loses 11 places in the IHDI.

Another distributional aspect of the HDI that has caught some critics' attention is the fact that gains in one dimension could offset losses in the other two. Perhaps most inappropriately, increases in the welfare of the best-off individuals in a country could offset decreases in the welfare of the worst-off. To obviate this criticism, the UNDP introduced the *Multidimensional Poverty Index* (MPI) in 2010. The MPI is a *deprivational* index which does not allow HDI-style offsets. It is designed for use in developing nations; it is not applied to high-HDI countries. There are still three dimensions, but now ten indicators, and all the indicators are defined in a negative sense. For example, the years-of-schooling indicator under the Education dimension is now stated in the negative as "no household member has completed 5 years of schooling." If true, that household is judged as "deprived." The percentage of deprived households in a country is aggregated for each indicator over all the households in the country from available surveys and estimates. Among the other deprivational indicators are: "no electricity," "no access to safe drinking water," "shared or unimproved sanitation facilities," "evidence of nutritional malnourishment," "a child lost to illness or accident," and "does not own a car or truck." The MPI is administered for the UNDP by the Oxford Poverty and Human development Initiative (OPHI) at Oxford University [16]. The 2018 dataset provides MPI values for 104 developing nations.

A recent paper has drawn attention to yet another distributional issue. Many countries differ in the proportions of older and younger people in their demographic makeup, and it is held that these differences could have a significant impact on the HDI. To address this issue, a demographically-adjusted HDI is proposed, in which the GNI per capita term is replaced by GNI per adult, and the LE-at-birth term is replaced by the LE of the current population [17].

The final item in the critics list, about the added value of the HDI as a measurement tool relative to using the GNI or GDP alone, is certainly worthy of consideration. According to the UNDP's own calculations, the correlation coefficient between the ranking of countries based on the HDI and one based on the GNI is 0.87, which indicates a high degree of correlation. In the 2018 calculations, only 30 of the 189 countries exhibited rankings that differed by more than 20 places between the two approaches. Only a very few countries would see a change in their status as high, moderate, or low-HDI, if a change were made from one approach to the other. These findings will receive further attention in a separate section near the end of this chapter.

As counterpoint to these criticisms, let us re-examine the societal role of the HDI, and its various spinoffs, in terms of the three primary goals outlined for the social indicators movement back in Chap. 3. These were: (1) to monitor changes over time in a broad range of social phenomena that extend beyond traditional economic indicators, and include indicators of wellbeing and quality of life; (2) to contribute to public enlightenment through social reporting both to the general public and policy makers; and (3) to provide information for monitoring and evaluation of public policy, searching for the common good, and deciding on how to reach it. It can be argued that the HDI has played a positive role on all three fronts [18].

World Happiness Report

The United Nations is closely associated with another set of world rankings that are in no way related to the Human Development Index. These rankings appear in the World Happiness Report (WHR) which is published annually by the Sustainable Development Solutions Network (SDSN), a program that operates under the auspices of the UN. The *raison d'etre* of the SDSN is to "mobilize global scientific and technological expertise to promote practical solutions for sustainable development, including implementation of the UN Sustainable Development Goals and the Paris Climate Agreement." The SDSN tries to meet its goals through compacts with member institutions which include "universities, research institutes, civil society organizations, and other knowledge centers." The World Happiness Report is designed to "survey the science of measuring and understanding subjective wellbeing." Emphasis is on the *subjective* approach to measurement. The editors apparently feel that national rankings ought to be based on the levels of happiness reported by individual citizens of a country in general population surveys, rather than on objective contributing factors like educational attainment or GDP per capita, as are used in the Human Development Index. At the very least, they see the WHR rankings as a counterpoint to those produced by the HDI. In fact, despite the differences in their source material, it has been shown that the correlation between the HDI and the central dependent variable used in the WHR rankings is very high [19]. To the extent that the two sets of rankings mirror one another, as they tend to do, each provides some confirmation for the other, and the two rankings taken together can be viewed as providing a stronger case than either taken alone.

The WHR is edited by three of the world's leading researchers in the science of wellbeing: John Helliwell, Richard Layard, and Jeffrey Sachs. Helliwell is a Canadian economist, a professor emeritus at the University of British Columbia, and the co-director of the Social Interactions, Identity and Wellbeing Programme at the Canadian Institute for Advanced Research. Layard is a British labour economist, a lifetime peer in the British House of Lords, and the founder of the Centre for Economic Performance at the London School of Economics. Sachs holds dual appointments in the School of International and Public Affairs, and the School of Public Health, at Columbia University. He is also director of the Earth Institute, an interdisciplinary network of professionals whose mission is to address the complex issues facing the Earth. He is an anti-poverty crusader who has written 15 books, 3 of them New York Times bestsellers.

The format of the WHR is that of a collection of chapters each authored by an invited expert on one or another aspect of a central theme. There have been seven editions, the first appearing in 2012 and the most recent in 2019. Among the themes that have been addressed are the social foundations of happiness, the role of parenthood, the importance of ethical behavior, the negative influence of mental illness, the effect of migration between countries, and the implications of all these issues for public policy. More to the point for our purposes, each edition includes a ranking of the world's countries with respect to their communal wellbeing, and an analysis of the main life factors that contribute to each country's place on the world listing.

The ranking of a country on the WHR list is based solely on the mean value of the responses from that country to the Cantril ladder-of-life question on the Gallup World Poll (GWP). The reader may recall from Chap. 6 that this question takes the following form: "Please imagine a ladder, with steps numbered from zero at the bottom to ten at the top. The top of the ladder represents the best possible life for you and the bottom of the ladder represents the worst possible life for you. On which step of the ladder would you say you personally feel you stand at this time." Each responder picks one of the steps, by number, and the GWP provides the statistics for all the responses from a given country. The mean value for each country will be a number between 0 and 10.

The most recent rankings in 2019, are actually based on the pooled results from the 3-year period 2016–2018. There are 156 countries with sufficient data to be included in the analysis. The five top-ranked countries are Finland, Denmark, Norway, Iceland, and the Netherlands. The five bottom countries are Rwanda, Tanzania, Afghanistan, Central African Republic, and South Sudan. Finland's score was 7.77, South Sudan's 2.85. Canada ranks 9th with a score of 7.28. The USA ranks 19th at 6.89. The distribution of worldwide happiness shows a mean value of 5.41 [20].

There is a lot of consistency in the year-to-year rankings, with the same few countries filling the top ten and bottom ten slots. They sometimes appear in slightly different order, but the good life experienced by northern Europeans, and the misery of many parts of Africa, which first appeared in the objective rankings of the Human Development Index, show up again here in the subjective rankings of the World Happiness Report.

The feature that makes the World Happiness Report unique is not the rankings themselves but a further analysis that is carried out to decompose each country's life evaluation score into component percentages that reflect the estimated contributions to the overall score of six possible determinants of happiness and wellbeing. The six possible determinants selected by the WHR team are: (1) natural log of GDP per capita, (2) healthy life expectancy, (3) social support, (4) freedom to make life choices, (5) generosity, and (6) perceptions of corruption. The methodology is designed to determine "how much each of these variables is estimated to contribute to explaining international differences in life evaluation scores."

The first step in the calculations is to define a representative value for each of the six variables for every country. The GDP-per-capita value comes from the World Development Indicator database maintained by the World Bank (in $PPP, adjusted to constant 2011 dollars). The healthy life expectancy value is taken from the World Health Organization's Global Health Observatory Data Repository. Values for the other four variables are all defined as the mean national values from the responses to specific yes/no questions on the Gallup World Poll. For social support, the question is: "If you were in trouble do you have relatives or friends you can count on to help you whenever you need them?" For social freedom: "Are you satisfied with your freedom to choose what you do with your life?" For generosity: "Have you donated money to a charity in the past month?" For corruption: "Is your perception that corruption is widespread throughout government and/or business?"

In step 2, six scatterplots are produced with the overall life evaluation score for every country plotted against that country's value for each of the six variables. A least-squares regression analysis is carried out on each of the six plots to determine the regression coefficients that define the average worldwide relationship between each of the variables and the life scores. On each scatterplot, some countries will lie above the regression line and some below. It is also possible to record the lowest observed value for each given variable (i.e. the value for the country that ranked 156th out of 156 for that variable).

In step 3, for each variable for each country, the pertinent regression coefficient is multiplied by the difference between that country's value for that variable and the lowest observed value for that variable. The final result is a percentage influence for each of the key variables for each country in the analysis. In the report, the results are presented as a bar graph, with the length of the bar for each country equal to its life-evaluation value, and each bar color-coded into six segments, the length of each one being proportional to the percentage influence estimated to be exerted on that country by the six possible determinants. It is felt that this type of breakdown could be of direct use to policy makers in each country, with the necessary steps to improve wellbeing implicitly related to the particular mix of underlying determinants in that country. For what it is worth, the percentage influence of the six variables, averaged over the world's countries came out to be: social support (34%), GDP per capita (26%), healthy life expectancy (21%), freedom to make life choices (11%), generosity (5%), and perceptions of corruption (3%).

The World Happiness Report is not to be confused with the similarly-named World Database of Happiness which figured prominently in Chap. 6, but which is not in any way associated with this UN programme.

The Quality of Life Index

The ranking exercise in the World Happiness Report (WHR) actually has a precursor, albeit one that has appeared only irregularly and under several different names. The sponsoring agency is the Economist Intelligence Unit (EIU), which is the information-gathering and research arm of The Economist newspaper in London, England. Like the WHR, their Quality-of-Life Index (QLI) uses average country-by-country scores from life satisfaction surveys as a starting point. Like the WHR, these values are then regressed against a set of objective indicators representing various possible contributing factors, taken from publically-available international datasets. In the WHR, the regression coefficients are used only in an explanatory sense; in the QLI, they are used as weights in the final tally of the index.

In the 2005 assessment, which is the only one that is widely quoted, nine contributing factors (or dimensions, if you will) were found to be significant. Each dimension was defined with just a single indicator. *Material Wellbeing* was represented by GDP per capita; *Health* by life expectancy at birth; *Job Security* by the unemployment rate; *Family Life* by the divorce rate; *Community Life* by the level of membership in community organizations; *Climate and Geography* by the country's average latitude; *Political Freedom* by a dataset put out by Freedom House; *Political Stability* by a set of internal EIU ratings; and *Gender Equality* by the ratio of male to female earnings [21].

Another assessment was carried out by the EIU in 2013, clearly using the same model, but now called the Where-to-be-Born Index. This new name is apparently a serious reincarnation of the name used for a tongue-in-cheek analysis published by the EIU in 1988. In that earlier version, countries were rated not only on the usual dimensions of economy, health, freedom, and so on, but also on a "philistine factor" that highlighted a perceived lack of cultural sophistication, and a "yawn factor" that was applied to countries that the EIU ranking team found boring.

It is unclear whether the Quality-of-Life Index (or the Where-to-be-Born Index) is to be resurrected on any kind of regular or irregular schedule. It appears that the EIU is now putting all its ranking efforts into the Global Livability Index (GLI) which ranks cities rather than countries. The GLI will receive its due attention in Chap. 10.

Happy Life Years

We have already met the Dutch happiness researcher Ruut Veenhoven back in Chap. 6 where he was highlighted as the founder and webmaster of the online World Database of Happiness, and a founding editor of the Journal of Happiness Studies. He is also responsible for a national happiness ranking system based on the concept of Happy Life Expectancy (HLE), as it was called when first presented in 1996, or Happy Life Years (HLY), as it has become known since Veenhoven repackaged the idea in 2004 [22].

Veenhoven shares the opinion of the editors of the World Happiness Report that national rankings ought to be based on the subjective levels of happiness reported by individual citizens of a country in general population surveys, rather than on databases for objective contributing factors as are used in the calculation of the Human Development Index. In this, he makes use of his own World Database of Happiness (WDH), which includes the results of every happiness poll that has ever been published for every country in which such polling has been carried out. It includes the findings of the World Values Surveys (since 1981) and the Gallup World Poll (since 2005), as well as countless other national and international polls.

Almost all of these polls and surveys ask responders at some point to evaluate their overall level of happiness or life satisfaction by answering a single standard question of the form: "Taking all things together, how satisfied or dissatisfied are you currently with your life as a whole?" Respondents are usually asked to rate their life satisfaction on a 10-point scale. Sometimes the question is posed using the 11-point Cantril ladder of life. Occasionally, 3-, 5-, or 7-point scales are used. In the WDH all responses are linearly converted onto a [0–10] range. For each survey on record in a given country, the WDH then averages all the individual scores, in order to provide a nation-wide satisfaction-with-life score for that survey. Veenhoven further recommends averaging these survey-by-survey scores over a 10-year period, in order to smooth out any anomalies, and to make the numbers more comparable across nations.

These nation-wide life-satisfaction scores can, on their own, be used as a basis for comparative rankings, as is done in the UN's World Happiness Report (albeit with a smaller subset of polling results than are included in the WDH). In 2004, the more-detailed available data in the WDH allowed such enhanced calculations to be made for 67 countries. By 2014, the date of the most recent calculations, a total of 158 countries were included. Of these, six countries (Costa Rica, Mexico, Iceland, Norway, Switzerland, and Canada) produced average self-reported life-satisfaction scores greater than 8.0 on the [0–10] scale.

However, Veenhoven felt, as did the developers of the HDI, that longevity records in a given country represent a sufficiently-important harbinger of national wellbeing that they cannot be ignored. In order to include a lifespan term, he proposed the concept of Happy Life Years (HLY), where the HLY score for a country is defined as the average 10-year satisfaction-with-life score for the country (on a scale of 0–10), multiplied by the average life expectancy in the country (in years), divided by 10. For example, a country with an average life satisfaction score of 8.0 and an average life expectancy of 80 years, would produce an HLY score of 64.0. The HLY is always a number between 0 and 100, and it has units of years.

The life expectancy data comes from the usual sources. The satisfaction-with-life data comes directly from the World Database of Happiness. For the 10-year period 2005–2014 covered in the most recent rankings [23], Cost Rica was the highest-ranked nation in the world with an HLY of 67.9 years. It was closely followed by Iceland, Denmark, Switzerland, and Canada. The bottom five countries were Benin, Sierra Leone, Burundi, Tanzania, and Togo. The lowest value, for Togo, was a shocking 14.8 years.

The USA ranked 24th with an HLY of 57.5 years. In the period 1973–2014, the USA picked up 6.1 years. However, satisfaction-with-life scores remained relatively flat during this period, and almost all of the increase can be attributed to gains in longevity.

As with the HDI, critics of Veenhoven's HLY methods also find fault with his use of only mean values of national life-satisfaction data in his calculations. They feel that such an approach could bury the impacts of distributional inequalities. As with the founders of the HDI, he has responded with a companion index, in this case called the Inequality-Adjusted Happiness of Nations (IAH) index [24]. Recall that in the Inequality-Adjusted HDI (or IHDI) discussed earlier, the inequality correction is taken as the ratio of the geometric mean to the arithmetic mean of the data. In the IAH, Veenhoven takes a different route. His inequality correction depends on mining the data in the World Database of Happiness for both means and standard deviations of the life-satisfaction data, and using their ratio to come up with inequality-corrected input data. Life expectancies are not corrected. As with the

IHDI relative to the HDI, the IAH scores are always lower than the HLYs. As with the HLYs, IAH scores are measured in years, with a theoretical range of [0,100] and a practical range of, say [10, 65]. Low scores are bad; high scores are good. Intermediate scores imply either that average happiness is high but that there is a sizeable inequality in the level of happiness, or that average happiness is medium but equally so across the populace. At the time of its introduction in 2005, Denmark had the highest IAH (based on a mean life satisfaction of 8.2, and a standard deviation of 1.8), while Tanzania had the lowest (based on a mean of 3.2, and a standard deviation of 3.6).

The Happy Planet Index

The *Happy Planet Index* (HPI) is the brainchild of Nic Marks, a British statistician who founded the Centre for Wellbeing at the New Economics Foundation (NEF) in London England. The NEF describes itself as an independent "think-and-do tank" that "inspires and demonstrates real wellbeing." The Happy Planet Index was launched in 2006 and has been updated triennially ever since. Its creators are quick to point out that the HPI is not measure of happiness, per se. Its country-by-country rankings do not identify the most livable countries, or the most-developed, in any traditional sense. Rather, it is a measure that captures the degree to which long and happy lives can be achieved while leaving the smallest possible environmentally-damaging footprint. It is "a measure of the ecological efficiency of supporting wellbeing." It is another way to introduce an environmental dimension into the calculations, an alternative if you will, to the Sustainable HDI (the HSDI) introduced in the earlier section on the UN's Human Development Index.

In the simplest light, the HPI is defined as [Life Satisfaction times Life Expectancy] divided by Ecological Footprint [25]. The alert reader will note that the numerator of this expression is equivalent to the Happy Life Years (HLYs) defined in the previous section, so that the HPI can be more compactly defined as [Happy Life Years divided by Ecological Footprint]. The alert reader will also note that the HPI does not include any term that reflects the economic dimension. There is no consideration of a country's GDP or any other measure of income or material wealth. Presumably, economic health contributes to the Life Satisfaction term but it is not a direct part of the calculation.

As for the Ecological Footprint (EF), it was described back in Chap. 4. It is best understood as a measure of the level of consumption in a country, and the world-wide impact of such consumption on the environment. It is defined as the amount of land area that is required to sustain a given population at current levels of consumption, technological development, and resource efficiency. It has units of hectares per capita. It turns out that for the current world population, there are 1.73 ha available for each person living on earth. If all the countries in the world had an EF of 1.73 ha per capita, it would imply that the world's resources were being developed sustainably, and that they were being shared equally among the world's population. Of course, that is not the case. Most countries have scores well above the sustainable level, and only a few have scores below. Low EF scores for a given country imply good environmental stewardship. High EF scores imply that a country's consumption levels are outstripping the ability of the world's ecosystems to support them. Because the EF term appears in the denominator of the HPI expression, lower EF values lead to higher HPI scores for that country. Higher HPI values are good, lower values are bad.

The value of the Life Satisfaction (LS) term in the HPI calculation for a given country is initially taken as the mean value of the distribution of responses from the Cantril ladder-of-life question on the Gallup World Poll. The Life Expectancy (LE) value (in years) is initially taken as the mean value of the longevity distribution as found in the country-by-country mortality tables held by the UN Department of Economic and Social Affairs. For almost all of the countries included in the analysis, scores for a country's Ecological Footprint (in hectares per capita) can be gleaned from the Global Footprint Network. In those few countries where data in the GFN are not complete, missing values of EF are imputed from multiple linear regression against other factors known to influence EF like per-capita CO_2 emissions, population density, and the latitude of the countries' major cities.

Calculation of the HPI for a country from the raw data on LS, LE, and EF, is actually somewhat more complicated than the bare-bones description given above. The basic data are actually massaged in three ways during the calculation: (1) to adjust for distributional inequities, (2) to correct for undue influence of one or other of the indicator variables on the overall result, and (3) to scale the results so that the final HPI values are bounded by the range [0,100].

In the first step of this threefold adjustment, the distributional inequities in life satisfaction and life expectancy are handled in exactly the same way as was done for the four indicator variables in the Inequality-Adjusted Human Development Index (IHDI) discussed in an earlier section of this chapter. That is, the original datasets are mined for both their arithmetic means and their geometric means. The original unadjusted values for LS and LE are then multiplied by the ratio of the geometric to arithmetic means to produce the inequality-adjusted LS and LE values. The EF value, being a singular deterministic calculation, is not adjusted.

In the second step, the original data distributions for LS and LE are mined not only for their arithmetic and geometric means, but also for their standard deviations, and the coefficient of variance (defined as the ratio of the standard deviation to the arithmetic mean) is calculated for each of these indicator variables. In order to insure that neither component dominates the overall HPI score, the inequality-adjusted LS and LE values in the numerator of the HPI expression are scaled in such a way that their coefficients of variance are equal to one another. And finally, a scaling adjustment is made to the EF value so that the HPI is equally sensitive to changes in the denominator of the HPI expression as it is to changes in the numerator.

In the third step, the upper bound of the HPI is set to 100 using a scaling correction that is designed to produce an HPI = 100 for the utopian country where all of its citizens have a Life Expectancy of 85 years, all of them rate their Life

Satisfaction as 10 out of 10, and the country's Ecological Footprint is equal to or below 1.73 ha per person.

Taken together, the second and third steps result in the addition of four scaling constants to the simple HPI expression introduced earlier. Further details on the three-step procedure that leads to these constants and their use in the final calculation of the HPI for a given country can be gleaned from the Methods section on the HPI website [26].

The most recent HPI calculations were reported in 2016. However due to the apparently unavoidable delays that occur between data collection and publication, the 2016 analysis was based largely on data from 2012. The report includes consideration of 178 countries, and while the upper bound for the HPI has been carefully scaled to be 100, the sad fact is that there is no country in the world that produced an HPI score greater than 50. Furthermore, perusal of the detailed rankings indicates a world order that is very different from that produced by indexes that emphasize economic success and material wealth. The particular influence of the Ecological Footprint, and the absence of positive credit for economic health, leads to an entirely different suite of countries at the top of the pack. The top ten HPI countries in the 2016 ranking were Costa Rica, Mexico, Columbia, Vanuatu, Vietnam, Panama, Nicaragua, Bangladesh, Thailand and Ecuador. Those western European and North American countries that often lead international ranking exercises performed universally poorly: Germany 81st, Japan 95th, UK 108th, Canada 111th, France 129th, and USA 150th.

The Genuine Progress Indicator

In the unstated but undeniable competition to see which one of the various constructs might prove most popular as the favored alternative to the GDP as a measure of human wellbeing, there are two clear front-runners. The first is the United Nations' Human Development Index (HDI) discussed earlier in this chapter. The second is the Genuine Progress Indicator (GPI) to be discussed now. (The careful reader might note that if everyone were on the same page, the GPI would be an "Index" and its contributing components "Indicators." However the founders of the GPI, being early in the game and before terms had solidified, chose to call their progeny an "Indicator" and its components "Factors.")

The GPI is a direct descendant of The Measure of Economic Welfare (MEW), the pioneering forerunner developed in 1972 by William Nordhaus and James Tobin, and the Index of Sustainable Economic Welfare (ISEW) developed in 1989 by sustainability guru Herman Daly and further expounded in his 1994 book with the environmental philosopher John Cobb: "For the Common Good." [27]. The GPI was launched in 1995 by the Bay Area think tank, Redefining Progress, under the leadership of John Cobb's son, Clifford Cobb, and a team of research associates committed to the further development of a "green GDP." [28]. The launch was accompanied by an article in Atlantic Monthly entitled: "If the GDP is up, why is

America down?" [29]. It was also buttressed by a joint public statement of support from 400 economists, statesmen, and business leaders, including several Nobel laureates. The most detailed description of the methodology appeared in 2006, and that report has remained as the GPI bible ever since [30].

As it turns out, by 2008, Redefining Progress had closed its doors. However the GPI lives on. One summary assessment that appeared on the internet identified 94 studies carried out with either the GPI or ISEW methodology between 1989 and 2019. The great majority of these studies were set at a nationwide scale, but many others were applied at the scale of states, provinces, cities, or regions.

All three of the constructs (MEW, ISEW, and GPI) in this family of indexes are designed to determine whether or not a country's economic growth, in the form of increased production of goods and expanding services, actually leads to an improvement in wellbeing for the citizens of the country. They all rest on the hypothesis that most free-market activities have costs as well as benefits and that these costs must be properly taken into account in any meaningful measure of social progress [31]. Unlike most of the other indexes described in this chapter the MEW/ISEW/GPI methodology does not step outside the GDP blueprint to produce a completely independent construct. Rather, all three start with a measure of nationwide personal consumption expenditures taken from a country's national accounts (the NIPA accounts in the USA), just like the GDP does. There are then three further steps. In Step 1, the personal consumption value is adjusted to take into account the inequalities in the distribution of income. In Step 2, additions are made to the adjusted consumption value to account for non-market contributions to wellbeing such as volunteer time, parenting, and homemaking. In Step 3, deductions are made for purely defensive expenditures like the costs of crime prevention or pollution cleanup, and for the undesirable side-effects of economic progress like the degradation and depletion of natural capital.

The three indexes differ only in the number of adjustments that are made. The MEW started with just a few; the ISEW added a few more; and the GPI carries the idea through to the point where 26 different factors are included in the calculation. Every one of the factors has units of dollars, just as the GDP does, so the GPI can be seen very clearly as a direct alternative to the GDP.

There are at least two different ways one might view the organization of the GPI, one in which each factor is classified into one of the three dimensions that are usually ascribed to the GPI: Economic, Social, and Environmental; and one which differentiates between two blocks of factors, one that measures a nation's current level of economic welfare, and one that indicates the sustainability of its economic development. Table 9.3 outlines the GPI factors according to the second scheme. The right-hand column clarifies the various factors that are addressed, and identifies which ones add value to the GPI and which ones deduct value from it.

Comparison of the GPI and the GDP for the USA over the past 25 years indicates a widening gap between the two measures. Both show improvement, but the increase in wellbeing as measured by the GPI is much smaller than the increase in economic activity indicated by the GDP. It is apparent, as ecological economists have argued for many years, that much of the benefit of economic growth is often countered by

Table 9.3 Calculation methodology for the Genuine Progress Indicator. (Adapted from the source material listed in [30])

Current economic welfare	Consumer spending	• Fundamental building block of GPI is consumer expenditures on goods and services from National Accounts.
		• Actual consumer expenditures on durable goods replaced by value of services derived from the stock of durable goods (rate of depreciation on goods, rate of interest on income invested in goods).
		• Adjusted for inequality of distribution of personal income.
		• Less cost of commuting.
		• Less costs of auto accidents.
		• Less costs of household pollution abatement.
		• Less costs of crime (medical expenses, legal expenses, property damage, costs of crime prevention).
		• Less costs of family breakdown (divorce costs, separate residences, legal fees, harm to children).
	Government spending	• Added value of roads and highways.
		• All other government expenditures (military defense, scientific research, policing, weather prediction, etc.) are considered defensive and are not included in GPI.
	Non-market production and leisure	• Added value of household work.
		• Added value of parenting time.
		• Added value of volunteer work.
		• Less value of lost leisure time.
	External factors	• Less costs of underemployment (unemployed, involuntary part-time, effects of work-life restraints, etc.).
		• Less costs of air pollution (human health, acid rain damage, loss in property value, agricultural damage, loss of aesthetics, etc.).
		• Less costs of water pollution (human health, ecological damage, loss of recreation value, aesthetics, etc.).
		• Less costs of noise pollution.
Sustainable economic development	Depletion of natural resources	• Less cost of depletion of non-renewable natural resources, especially oil and gas (calculated as replacement value of alternative energy to future generations).
		• Less value of lost farmland (to urbanization, and to loss in soil quality).
	Net capital investment	• Annual change in net foreign investment position (plus or minus).
		• Annual change in domestic capital investment (plus or minus).

(continued)

Table 9.3 (continued)

	Long-term ecological damage	• Less cost of global warming from CO_2 emissions.
		• Less cost of ozone depletion from CFC emissions.
		• Less value of lost wetlands.
		• Less value of lost forests.

the social costs that are engendered, leading to little societal gain from a welfare perspective [32].

The original GPI methodology is now very long in the tooth, and the proliferation of GPI studies around the world has led to much customization, and much divergence in the approach used by various users. In recent years there have been many calls for the development of a GPI 2.0 that would update the GPI accounting protocols to provide the necessary flexibility while maintaining some level of international and scale-independent consistency [33].

The Canadian Index of Wellbeing

The six multi-dimensional indexes presented thus far have all been based on a very limited number of dimensions. Let us now turn to the remainder of the composite indexes listed in Table 9.1, all of which consider a much larger suite of dimensions and indicators. Rather than emphasizing either subjective self-reported data, or externally-available objective data, as most of these simpler indexes do, most of the more-complex constructs find a place for both types of data in their makeup.

First up is the *Canadian Index of Wellbeing* (CIW) [34]. As a starting point, this choice could be viewed as somewhat odd, because the CIW is one of the latest entries in Table 9.2. Furthermore, it differs from most other nationwide composite models in that it is designed for application only in its home country, not for multi-country international comparisons. However, the choice makes sense in another context. Not only does the CIW feature one of the largest sets of indicator variables, but it also boasts one of the most symmetric and transparent structures, and one of the simplest and most straightforward methodologies for the calculation of its single-number result. The reader will get a soft introduction to the scope of these multi-dimensional constructs without getting bogged down in excessive detail.

Tables 9.4 and 9.5 lists the dimensions and indicators for the CIW. There are eight dimensions, and eight indicators per dimension (for a total of 64). The eight dimensions are: (1) Community Vitality, (2) Democratic Engagement, (3) Education, (4) Environment, (5) Healthy Populations, (6) Leisure and Culture, (7) Living Standards, and (8) Time Use. Perusal of the table clarifies the types of issues that the developers of the CIW thought were germane to Canadian wellbeing. Thirty-five of the indicators are defined as percentages of the Canadian population that can be identified in some specific way (sometimes the entire population, sometimes selected subsets of the entire population like the labour force, or those in a particular age

Table 9.4 Indicators for the Canadian Index of Wellbeing (first four dimensions). (Adapted from the source materials listed in [34, 35])

Community Vitality	Percentage of population reporting unpaid participation in any activities on behalf of a group or organization in past year (formal volunteering)
	Percentage of population with 5 or more close friends
	Crime Severity Index
	Percentage of population who have experienced discrimination in past 5 years based on ethno-cultural characteristics
	Percentage of population who feel safe walking alone after dark
	Percentage of population who believe that most or many people can be trusted
	Percentage of population who provide unpaid help to others on their own
	Percentage of population reporting a somewhat or very strong sense of belonging to community
Democratic Engagement	Percentage of voter turnout at federal elections
	Percentage who volunteer for a law, advocacy, or political group
	Gap in percentage turnout between older and younger voters
	Percentage reporting they are very or fairly satisfied with the way democracy works in Canada
	Percentage with a great deal or quite a lot of confidence in federal parliament
	Ratio of registered to eligible voters
	Percentage of women in Parliament
	Percentage of Members of Parliament who send communications to constituents
Education	Percentage of children aged 0–5 years for whom there is a regulated centre-based child care space
	Amount of time spent in talk-based activities with children aged 0–14 years
	Ratio of students to educators in public schools
	Average expenditure per public school student ($2013)
	Percentage of population aged 25 years and older participating in education-related activities
	Average annual undergraduate tuition fees ($2015)
	Percentage of Canadians 20–24 year of age completing high school
	Percentage of 25–64 year old in population with a university degree
Environment	Ground level ozone (population weighted in parts per billion)
	Absolute greenhouse gas emissions (megatonnes of CO_2 per year)
	Primary energy production (petajoules)
	Residential energy use
	Total farm land (hectares)
	Viable Metal Reserves Index
	Ecological Footprint
	Annual water yield in Southern Canada (km^3)

Table 9.5 Indicators for the Canadian Index of Wellbeing (last four dimensions). (Adapted from the source materials listed in [34, 35])

Healthy Populations	Percentage self-rated health as excellent or very good
	Percentage self-rated mental health as excellent or very good
	Percentage with self-reported diabetes
	Life expectancy at birth, years
	Percentage of daily or occasional smokers among teens aged 12–19 years
	Percentage of Canadians with a regular medical doctor
	Percentage of population getting influenza immunization
	Percentage of population with absence of health limitations
Leisure and Culture	Average percentage of time spent on the previous day in social leisure activities
	Average percentage of time spent on the previous day in arts and culture activities
	Average number of hours in the past year volunteering for culture and recreation organizations
	Average monthly frequency of participation in physical activity lasting over 15 min
	Average attendance per performance in past year all performing arts performances
	Average visitation per site in past year to all National Parks and National Historic Sites
	Average number of nights away per trip in the past year on vacation trips to destinations over 80 km from home
	Expenditures in past year on all aspects of culture and recreation as a percentage of total household expenditures
Living Standards	Gini coefficient
	After tax median income of economic families ($2013)
	Percentage of persons in low income
	Percentage of households that are moderately or severely food insecure
	Percentage labour force with long-term unemployment
	Percentage of labour force employed
	Canadian Imperial Bank of Commerce Index of Employment Quality
	Housing affordability based on Shelter Consumption Affordability Ratio
Time Use	Percentage of Canadians 25–64 years of age working over 50 h per week at main job
	Percentage of 15–64 year old reporting high levels of time pressure
	Average daily amount of time with friends
	Percentage of labour force working under 30 h per week, not by choice
	Percentage of Canadians who report 7–9 h of good quality essential sleep
	Mean workday commute time for individuals working for pay
	Percentage of individuals working for pay with flexible work hours
	Percentage of labour force with regular weekday work hours

group). Four of the indicators are defined as percentages of something else, like time spent in various activities. Four are economic entities measured in dollars.

The sources of the raw data for the 64 indicators represent a melding of both subjective and objective databases. Some of the indicators are based on self-reported data from national questionnaires (e.g. *self-rated mental health status, daily amount of time spent with friends, percentage time spent in arts and culture activities*), some are based on objective public datasets (e.g. *percentage voter turnout at federal elections, average annual undergraduate tuition fees, after-tax median income, greenhouse gas emissions*), and some involve direct integration of available single-dimensional indexes which themselves have been calculated on the basis of their own suite of indicators (*Crime Severity Index, Index of Employment Quality, Viable Metal Reserves Index, Ecological Footprint*). Two of these indexes, the Crime Severity Index, and the Ecological Footprint, have been presented and discussed in some detail in earlier chapters.

Most of the necessary datasets are archived by Statistics Canada. These include the Canadian General Social Survey, the Canadian Community Health Survey, the Labour Force Survey, the Survey of Household Spending, the Canadian Income Survey, the Elementary/Secondary Education Survey, the Ethnic Diversity Survey, the Canadian Survey of Giving, the Tuition and Living Accommodation Costs Survey, and the Canadian Residents Travel Survey. Among the objective databases that are accessed by the CIW are those of Environment Canada, Parks Canada, Childcare Canada, Elections Canada, and the Canada Census.

The CIW also differs from many of the other national indexes in that it deals only with percentage changes to each indicator, not with their absolute values [35]. The raw data for the year 1994 are used as the base value for all of the indicators, each of which is set to a dimensionless value of 100 for that year. The datum for a specific indicator from a later year is divided by the 1994 datum and then multiplied by 100. Take *life expectancy at birth*, for example. The raw datum for 1994 was 78.2 years, whereas by 2014 it had risen to 82.1 years. The ratio of the two is 1.0498, leading to a dimensionless value of 104.98, indicating a percentage improvement in that indicator of 4.98% over the period 1994–2014.

If one examines the 64 indicators in Tables 9.4 and 9.5 in detail it can be seen that some of them, like *life expectancy at birth*, are defined such that a positive percentage increase in the dimensionless indicator value represents an improvement in wellbeing. Others, like *absolute greenhouse gas emissions*, are defined such that a positive increase implies a decline in wellbeing. In fact, 16 of the 64 CIW indicators are so defined. For these negatively-defined indicators, the percentage changes are adjusted by multiplying them by -1. As a result, for all the indicators, no matter how they are defined or adjusted, a positive value represents an improvement in wellbeing, a negative one a decline.

Once all the indicator values have been calculated (in terms of their percent improvement or decline), they are equally weighted and arithmetically averaged within each dimension. Then all of the dimensions are equally weighted and arithmetically averaged to produce the final output.

The CIW is intended primarily to track the trends in Canadian wellbeing over time. To this end, even though the index was only launched in 2011, calculations have been made for all years back to 1994. The most recent report, published in 2016

[36], provides results for the period 1994–2014. During this period the CIW increased by 9.9%, indicating an improvement in the wellbeing of Canadians.

Data are also available for each of the dimensions for the same period. Most of them increased along with the overall CIW: Education (+32%), Healthy Populations (+16%), Community Vitality (+14%), Democratic Engagement (+13%), Living Standards (+11%), and Time Use (+3%). Two of the dimensions registered a decline: Environment (−3%), and Leisure and Culture (−9%). The developers of the CIW feel that this type of breakdown should be of direct use to policy makers. They call the CIW the "ultimate policy tool" for Canadians.

The results published in 2016 also shed light on the question of whether composite models have anything to offer over and above the information provided by the GDP. It is noted that the GDP increased by 38.0% during the 1994–2014 study period while the CIW increased by only 9.9%. So, even though the CIW and GDP are correlated (in that they both increased in lock step), the increase in the GDP greatly over-predicts the true gains in citizen wellbeing. Policies that lead to increased GDP undoubtedly help those at the upper end of the income spectrum, but they are less beneficial to ordinary Canadians. The developers of the CIW conclude that it does provide additional intelligence over and above that provided by the GDP in helping identify the wellbeing needs of Canadians.

The history of development of the CIW bears telling, in that it too, like the index itself, followed a relatively-seamless and efficient path. Although the CIW has had the ongoing support of Canada's federal government, the CIW was not developed under government auspices. The idea for a national wellbeing index was first broached within the Atkinson Charitable Foundation, an activist philanthropic organization founded by Joseph Atkinson, long-time publisher of the Toronto Star newspaper, and a fierce advocate for social justice and the rights of working people. During the period 1999–2010 the Foundation laid the groundwork for the CIW, making use of Canadian wellbeing experts like Alex Michalos, John Helliwell, Mark Anielski and Ronald Colman, hosting meetings of interested stakeholders, funding research in the wellbeing community on indexing issues, supporting the development of background papers for each of the selected dimensions, promoting public discussion groups, and establishing a CIW Advisory Board. To chair the Advisory Board, the Foundation selected Roy Romanow, a former premier of the province of Saskatchewan, and an ardent supporter of the CIW. Romanow has become the public face of the CIW, giving speeches to all and sundry, writing articles in popular magazines, and keeping the CIW front and center in the Canadian media. In 2010 the Atkinson Foundation ceded leadership of the CIW to the Faculty of Applied Health Sciences at the University of Waterloo in Waterloo, Ontario, which is now the host agency for the index and the home of the CIW data repository. The first iteration of the CIW itself was launched in 2011. Its stated mission is "to help policy makers and decision makers to understand the consequences of their actions for Canadian wellbeing," and "to measure national progress toward (or away from) a vision that constitutes sustainable wellbeing." The catchwords on the masthead of all CIW documents are "Measuring what matters/Making measures matter."

The Weighted Index of Social Progress

The Index of Social Progress (ISP) and its successor the Weighted Index of Social Progress (WISP) have been highlighted earlier in this chapter as being among the earliest multi-dimensional indexes of national wellbeing. They were developed in the late 1970s and early 1980s by Richard J. Estes of the University of Pennsylvania. The structure and methodology of WISP has remained remarkably constant, with only minor changes in the 35 years from its original format to its current version. Application of WISP has been largely limited to Estes and his coworkers, who have used it as a methodological centerpiece for a prodigious stream of academic studies on a wide variety of topics that are all loosely connected to the theme of national wellbeing.

A description of the current version of WISP can be found in two articles in the journal *Social Indicators Research* [37]. The index has ten dimensions, with between one and six indicators for each dimension, for a total of 40. The dimensions are: (1) economic, (2) education, (3) health, (4) demography, (5) environment, (6) welfare effort, (7) status of women, (8) social chaos, (9) defense effort, and (10) cultural cohesion. All of the specific indicators under the various dimensions are objective, based on data gleaned from publically-available databases produced by such agencies as the United Nations, World Bank, OECD, International Monetary Fund, Red Cross, and the like. They include such widely-used variables as per capita GDP, unemployment rate, GINI score, adult literacy rate, school completion rates, life expectancy at birth, infant mortality rate, and many other well-defined objective indicators that allow calculation of the sub-indexes for each of the ten dimensions.

Twenty-three of the indicators (like per-capita GDP, and school completion rates) are defined such that higher numbers have a positive influence on the index; 17 (like the unemployment rate, and infant mortality rate) are defined such that higher numbers have a negative influence. These latter indicators are appropriately converted in the calculations of each sub-index.

The final three dimensions in the above list may deserve comment. The "social chaos" dimension covers the same areas of concern as are treated in more recent indexes under the rubric of "safety, security, and governance." The indicators that are defined for this dimension cover such issues as political rights, civil liberties, crime, corruption, and violence.

The dimension entitled "defense effort" has just one indicator: military expenditures as a percent of GDP. In WISP, these expenditures are viewed as a form of military preparedness and are treated as a positive, whereas in many of the more recently-developed indexes, military involvement in foreign or civil wars counts as a negative.

Perhaps the most controversial of Estes' dimensions is that of "social cohesion." Homogeneity in ethnicity, religion, and language (in terms of the percentage of the population sharing same) is viewed as a positive. This would appear to fly in the face of the more liberal view that preaches the value of diversity. This issue is sufficiently important to warrant a separate discussion later in this chapter.

Unlike the Canadian Index of Wellbeing and many other national indexes which weight each indicator and each dimension equally to come up with a composite score, the WISP index is true to its name, weighting the indicators within each dimensional calculation, and weighting the dimensions to come up with a composite score. The weightings in WISP are not set on the subjective whims of the developers. They are the result of a sophisticated multivariate statistical analysis. To quote Estes: "Weights were derived through a two-stage principle-component and varimax factor-analysis in which indicator and sub-index scores were analysed separately for their relative contribution toward explaining the variance associated with changes in social progress over time. Standardized indicator scores were multiplied by their respective factor loadings, averaged within their sub-index, and the average sub-index scores were in turn subjected to a second statistical weighting. The resulting values for the two-stage statistical weighting process formed the basis for computing the composite WISP score." [38].

The WISP index has been calculated somewhat irregularly over the years to rank the nations of the world. The most recent exercise, for 2018, has been picked up by the International Society for Quality of Life Studies (ISQOLS) and appears on their website [39]. The top five countries in the ranking are Denmark, Germany, Austria, Japan and Sweden. The bottom five are Somalia, Yemen, Sierra Leone, Chad, and the Central African Republic. Canada ranks 25th, and the USA 39th.

Gross National Happiness Index: American Version

Of course, the granddaddy of all this alt-GDP thinking is the concept of Gross National Happiness (GNH), first popularized in the early 1970s in the kingdom of Bhutan. In its earliest manifestations, it was not so much a quantitative calculation as it was a set of goals for government policy, designed to include social and environmental targets as well as purely economic ones. The Bhutanese government did not get around to creating The Centre for Bhutan Studies and GNH Research until 1999, and did not produce a GNH Index until 2010. In the meantime they were partially scooped by the International Institute of Management (IIM), a Las-Vegas-based think tank, who came out with a GNH Index based on the Bhutanese concepts in 2005. In Table 9.1 these two indexes are identified as GNH-A (for American version) and GNH-B (for Bhutanese version). As another way to differentiate between them, the American IIM index is sometimes called the Gross National Wellness Index (GNW).

We say "partially scooped" because, although there is no doubt that the IIM developed such an index, they have never released the full details in the public domain. The IIM is a private entity that offers licensing to use their index on a for-fee basis. An outline of the index can be accessed from materials posted on the IIM website [40]. The website also exhibits considerable sensitivity to the respective roles of IIM and the Centre for Bhutan Studies in developing the ideas of a GNH Index, and many pleas for recognition of IIM's priority. There is even reference to an academic paper that accuses Bhutan of inventing a tradition that doesn't really exist, and a favorable quotation of the anti-Bhutan slogan that GNH really stands for Gross National Hypocrisy because of Bhutan's alleged unfair treatment of its Hindu Nepalese minority [41].

It is clear from the outline that there are seven dimensions in the structure of the GNH-A Index and the score for each dimension is determined by a combination of subjective results from a specially-designed life-satisfaction survey and objective statistical data for a number of indicator variables. Among the indicator variables that receive mention in the white paper are consumer debt, consumer price index, income distribution, disposable income, antidepressant usage, numbers of psychotherapy patients, rate of occurrence of chronic illnesses, obesity levels, purchasing power, number of labor lawsuits, divorce rates, crime rates, levels of air and water pollution, and involvement in domestic or foreign conflicts.

Presumably the GNH-A index has been applied to various American jurisdictions, probably including the USA as a whole, and perhaps to other countries as well, but if so, the results have not been widely disseminated.

Gross National Happiness Index: Bhutanese Version

Now to the Bhutanese version of their own index, the GNH-B Index in Table 9.1. It was launched by the Centre for Bhutan Studies (CBS) in 2010, and is fully detailed in a 2012 report [42]. The index is designed for use in Bhutan itself and has not been used to assess or rank other countries. It is based on core Buddhist principles that value "serving others, living in harmony with nature, and realizing one's own innate wisdom." The revised Bhutanese constitution of 2008 directs government "to promote those conditions that will enable the pursuit of Gross National Happiness."

The Bhutanese GNH Index has 9 dimensions and 33 indicators, many of which have multiple sub-indicators, leading to a grand total of 124 variables that come under consideration. The dimensions are: (1) Psychological Wellbeing, (2) Health, (3) Education, (4) Culture, (5) Time Use, (6) Good Governance, (7) Community Vitality, (8) Ecological Diversity and Resilience, and (9) Living Standards. Table 9.6 lists the 33 indicators, and specifies the number of variables used with each indicator.

The approach is completely subjective, in that the data on which the computations are based come solely from a questionnaire designed by the CBS and circulated to carefully-chosen subsets of the Bhutanese citizenry. The questionnaire includes a number of items designed to identify the demographic status of the responder (age, gender, education, occupation, etc.), and then a long set of questions organized under the 9 dimensional domains, the 33 indicator areas, and bearing a one-to-one correspondence to the 124 variables.

The GNH-B Index is a highly-original construct. Its uniqueness lies in its specification of a "threshold sufficiency level" for each indicator (or in some cases

Table 9.6 Dimensions, indicators, number of variables, number of sufficiency thresholds, and weights for the Bhutanese Gross National Happiness Index, GNH-B. (Adapted from the source materials listed in [42])

Dimensions	Indicators	Number of variables[a]	Number of sufficiency thresholds	Weights (%)
Psychological wellbeing	Life satisfaction	5	1	33
	Positive emotions	5	1	17
	Negative emotions	5	1	17
	Spirituality	4	1	33
Health	Self-reported health	1	1	10
	Healthy days per month	1	1	30
	Long-term disability	1	1	30
	Mental health	10	1	30
Education	Literacy	1	1	30
	Schooling	1	1	30
	Knowledge	5	1	20
	Value	5	1	20
Culture	Language	1	1	20
	Artisan skills	13	1	30
	Cultural participation	1	1	30
	The way to harmony	2	2	20
Time Use	Work	1	1	50
	Sleep	1	1	50
Good Governance	Political participation	2	2	40
	Political freedom	7	1	10
	Service delivery	4	4	40
	Government performance	7	1	10
Community Vitality	Social support	2	2	30
	Community relationships	2	2	20
	Family	6	1	20
	Safety	1	1	30
Ecological Diversity and Resilience	Pollution	7	1	10
	Environmental responsibility	1	1	10
	Wildlife damage to crops	2	1	40
	Urban issues	4	1	40

(continued)

Table 9.6 (continued)

Dimensions	Indicators	Number of variables[a]	Number of sufficiency thresholds	Weights (%)
Living Standards	Per-capita household income	1	1	33
	Assets	3	3	33
	Housing quality	3	3	33

[a] Not including those used solely for demographic identification

for each variable). Take the first indicator in Table 9.6, for example. An individual's Life Satisfaction score is determined on the basis of five questions on the CBS questionnaire. The responder is asked to rate his or her level of contentment with respect to health, occupation, family, standard of living, and work/life balance. For each of these variables the responder is offered a 1–5 Likert scale. The lowest possible total for the five variables is 5, the highest 25. The threshold sufficiency level is set at 19. If an individual's self-reported total score for these 5 variables is equal to or greater than 19, then that individual is judged to have attained sufficiency with respect to the Life Satisfaction indicator. If he or she scores less than 19, then that individual has identified an insufficiency in that aspect of his or her Gross National Happiness.

Most of the indicators, including the one just given, are designed so that there is just one sufficiency threshold for each indicator. Some, however, have more than one threshold. Note, for example, in Table 9.6, that the Service Delivery indicator under the Good Governance dimension has four variables and four thresholds, with one threshold defined for each variable. The four proxy variables for government service delivery are: (1) distance to nearest health care centre, (2) waste disposal service, (3) access to electricity, and (4) water supply and quality. The respective sufficiency thresholds are: (1) less than a 1-h walk, (2) proper disposal, (3) full access, and (4) an "improved" supply of good quality. In all cases with more than one threshold per indicator, some type of averaging is done to come up with a single threshold at the indicator level. In the Service Delivery example, overall indicator sufficiency requires sufficiency in all four of the variables.

Among some of the other sufficiencies required by the various indicators or variables are the ability to read and write (Literacy), the number of days spent in cultural pursuits in the past year (Cultural Participation), average number of hours of sleep (Time Use), percent of income donated to charity (Social Support), percent of time engaged in meditation (Spirituality), perceived intensity of seven environmental threats (Pollution), and per-capita household income (Living Standards). Some of the thresholds have been set on the basis of international standards (work laws, UN recommendations, environmental standards, etc.); others are normative judgements made by the CBS based on consultations with experts and focus-group discussions. For any individual responder to the CBS questionnaire there are only two outcomes for each indicator: either the sufficiency threshold is met or it is not.

The first step in calculating the GNH-B Index is to weight the sufficiencies or insufficiencies according to the percentage weights indicated in the right-hand column of Table 9.6. The second step is to determine the percentage of weighted sufficiencies met on each responder's questionnaire (0–100%). On the basis of studies of the Bhutanese citizenry, the CBS has decided that those who satisfy 66% or more of the weighted sufficiency thresholds can be considered "Happy" whereas those below 66% are "Not-Yet-Happy." The third step of the calculation therefore involves a statistical assessment of all the questionnaires from a particular survey to determine what percent of the Bhutanese population are happy (H_{hap}) and what percent are not-yet-happy (H_{nyh}). The final step is to assess only the not-yet-happy cohort to see what is the average number of weighted sufficiency thresholds not met (A_{stnm}) by this segment of the population. The GNH-B Index is then given by:

$$\text{GNH} - \text{B} = H_{hap} + \left(H_{nyh} \times A_{stnm}\right)$$

In the data presented for the 2012 report, 40.8% of Bhutanese are happy ($H_{hap} = 0.408$), 59.2% are not-yet-happy ($H_{nyh} = 0.592$), and the not-yet-happy cohort averages 56.6% of weighted sufficiency thresholds not met ($A_{stnm} = 0.566$). The GNH-B Index for Bhutan for 2010 is therefore 0.743. The possible range is [0, 1] and higher values indicate greater Gross National Happiness.

The Bhutanese GNH Index is by far the most elegant wellbeing index in terms of its ability to identify and direct needed policy changes. By gathering statistics on which thresholds are least-often met, the CBS provides the government of Bhutan with data that can be seen as a direct screening tool for government policies and programmes. Moreover, the results can be "unpacked" using the demographic data provided on the questionnaires to determine where the greatest insufficiencies abound: by district, by age, by gender, by educational level, and by occupation. For the data reported for Bhutan in the 2012 report, rural districts had more insufficiencies than urban, females more than male, the elderly more than the young, and the least-educated more than the better-educated. As for occupation, civil servants and monks were the happiest, farmers and housewives the least happy. Contributions to unhappiness were roughly equal across the dimensions, but the greatest effects were from lack of education and insecurity in living standards. A policy assessment by the CBS suggested that increases in GNH would require sustained and coordinated efforts on the part of individuals, communities, and government.

The Better Life Index

One of the more-widely-quoted national indexes is the Better Life Index put out by the Organization for Economic Cooperation and Development (OECD) [43]. It provides country-wide rankings, but only for the 35 OECD countries (and 3 key partner countries), all of which are among the more-developed countries in the world. The top five in the 2017 report are Norway, Australia, Iceland, Canada, and Denmark. The USA is 10th.

The Better Life Index has a traditional structure, similar to many of the other indexes treated in this chapter. It has 11 dimensions, with between 1 and 4 indicators per dimension, for a total of 24 in all. The dimensions are: (1) Housing, (2) Income, (3) Jobs, (4) Community, (5) Education, (6) Environment, (7) Civic Engagement, (8) Health, (9) Life Satisfaction, (10) Safety, and (11) Work-Life Balance. As examples of the 24 indicators, consider 4 of the dimensions, each of which has 2 indicators: Income (household net adjusted disposable income, and household net wealth), Civic Engagement (voter turnout rate, and stakeholder engagement in developing regulations), Health (life expectancy, and self-reported health), and Safety (homicide rate, and feeling safe walking home alone). As this sample suggests, some of the indicators are subjective and come from national surveys like the Gallup World Poll, others are objective and come from national accounts or international databases like those available from the UN and the OECD itself. All the indicators can be seen as well-chosen proxies for the broad suite of issues encompassed by each dimension.

The aggregation of indicator scores also follows the usual path. For each indicator a minimum value (worst possible outcome) and a maximum value (best possible outcome) are defined, and scores are then normalized onto a [0, 1] range. Indicators that are defined negatively are inverted. In default mode, the indicator scores are averaged within each dimension, and then averaged across the dimensions, giving rise to equal weighting of all indicators. One unique feature of the Better Life Index is an option for the user to assign any weights he or she desires to any or all of the indicators, thus creating a customized index that can be tailor-made to meet the predilections of any user (for good or for ill).

The Prosperity Index

The Prosperity Index is published by the Legatum Institute in London, England. The Institute is the educational and philanthropic arm of the Dubai-based private investment firm, the Legatum Group. The Institute was founded in 2007, and its current leader is Baroness Philippa Stroud, a Conservative member of the British House of Lords who is well-known as an anti-poverty crusader and fighter for social justice. The *modus operandi* of the Institute is to "promote policies that create pathways from poverty to prosperity." In the eyes of the Legatum Group, such policies will have twofold goals: to accumulate material wealth, and to enhance wellbeing. There will be economic drivers and social drivers, and they will "work together in a relationship where each benefits and enhances the other."

The Legatum Prosperity Index (LPI) [44] is designed to rank the countries of the world on the grounds of the Legatum worldview. It has nine dimensions (called pillars), two of which define the needs of an "open economy" (Economic Quality, and Business Environment), four of which identify an "inclusive society" (Governance, Personal Freedom, Social Capital, and Safety and Security), and three of which characterize an "empowered people" (Education, Health, and Natural Environment). Each pillar has between 9 and 13 indicators (called variables) for a total of 104 in all.

The selection criterion that was used to select each of the 104 indicators is known as the five-A approach. Indicators must be Applicable (resonant, and relevant to policy), Actionable (targetable, and responsive in the short-to-medium-term), Agnostic (internationally comparable and consistent), Adaptable (have scope for improvement over time), and Accessible (logical and statistically robust).

The LPI uses both objective sources (about 2/3 of the indicators) and subjective sources (about 1/3). Objective sources include international organizations (United Nations, World Bank, International Monetary Fund, World Health Organization, and others), non-governmental organizations (Freedom House, Amnesty International, and Transparency International), and academically-archived databases. Subjective data come from the Gallup World Poll and the Executive Opinion Survey of the World Economic Forum (WEF).

The LPI uses both input and output indicators. The first priority is given to output variables that are direct measures of outcomes that are components of a prosperous life (like life expectancy at birth, or percentage of citizens with safe water delivery). An auxiliary role is given to input variables that cultivate or safeguard conditions for prosperity but do not measure them directly (like tolerance for ethnic minorities, or trust in local police).

Each indicator is assigned a weight of 0.5, 1.0, 1.5, or 2.0. The weights are assigned by the LPI team on the basis of: (1) relevance and significance of the indicator "as informed by the academic literature," (2) expert opinions from advisors, and (3) degree of compatibility with Legatum Institute's views of prosperity.

As an example of the LPI indicators, consider the following 8 variables (out of 12) selected from the Business Environment pillar. For each indicator, the source, the weighting, and the possible range of values are indicated. The sources are: E = WEF Executive Opinion Survey, W = World Bank Development Indicators, and G = Gallup World Poll.

- Affordability of financial services (E, 1.0, 1–7)
- Hiring and firing practices (E, 0.5, 1–7)
- Intellectual property protection (E, 1.5, 1–7)
- Ease of getting credit (W, 2.0, 0–100)
- Ease of resolving insolvency (W, 1.0, 0–100)
- Ease of starting a business (W, 1.0, 0–100)

- Perception of starting a new business (G, 1.0, 0–1)
- Perception of working hard and getting ahead (G, 1.5, 0–1)

As further less-detailed examples, consider 4 (of 12) indicators from the Health pillar (immunization rates against measles, improved sanitation facilities, obesity prevalence, and satisfaction with healthcare), 4 (of 12) from the Personal Freedom pillar (death penalty, conscription, governmental religious restrictions, and LGBT tolerance), and 4 (of 10) from the Social Capital pillar (opportunity to make friends, voter turnout, availability of help when in trouble, trust in local police).

As has been seen with other national indexes, some indicators are logged, some capped, and some inverted. In the LPI all indicator scores are then normalized onto a [0, 100] range. Each indicator's normalized score is multiplied by its weight; the indicator scores are summed across the pillar; and the nine pillars are averaged to get the LPI.

In the most recent calculation in 2018, the LPI was calculated for 149 countries. The top five were Norway, New Zealand, Finland, Switzerland, and Denmark. Canada ranked 8th, the USA 17th. The bottom five countries were Sudan, Chad, Yemen, Central African Republic, and Afghanistan. The global mean LPI was 58.8 (on a scale of 0–100). Since its inception in 2007, the global LPI has risen from 56.8 to 58.8. The LPI is highly correlated with GDP per capita, life satisfaction scores from the Gallup World Poll, and the UN's Human Development Index.

US News and World Report Best Country Rankings

The newest country ranking on the block was first published in 2016 by the American newsmagazine US News and World Report [45]. Their 2019 Best Country Rankings are based on a global survey of over 20,000 people in 36 countries from 4 regions (the Americas, Asia, Europe and the Middle East, and Africa). To qualify for inclusion, a country has to satisfy all four of the following criteria: (1) be one of the top 100 countries in terms of GDP, (2) be one of the top 100 countries in terms of foreign investment inflows, (3) be one of the top 100 countries in terms of international tourism receipts, and (4) be one of the top 150 countries in the 2016 calculation of the UN Human Development Index. In all, 80 countries so qualified, representing 80% of the world's population, and 95% of the global GDP. However, many of the world's poorer countries, especially those in Africa, are not included, so while the US News rankings may be comparable with other rankings at the top, they are not comparable at the bottom.

The methodology for the Best Country Rankings was developed by David J. Reibstein, a professor of marketing at the Wharton School at the University of Pennsylvania, together with input from the BAV Group, a subsidiary of the global marketing agency, VMLY&R. The US News rankings are much more inclined toward material wealth and business opportunity than are most of the ranking systems discussed earlier in this chapter. Proof of this leaning comes from the methodology, wherein each of the nine dimensions that make up the structure of the ranking system is weighted on the basis of a country-by-country global correlation between the dimensional data and the countries' per capita GDP. Dimensions that demonstrated a stronger relationship with the wealth metric were weighted more heavily.

The nine dimensions and their weightings are as follows: (1) Adventure—2.00%, (2) Citizenship—15.88%, (3) Cultural Influence—12.96%, (4) Entrepreneurship—17.87%, (5) Heritage—1.13%, (6) Movers—14.36%, (7) Open for Business—11.08%, (8) Power—7.95%, and (9) Quality of Life—16.77%. The highest weighted dimension is Entrepreneurship; the lowest is Heritage.

The survey that is used to determine the rankings provides the responder with a set of 65 attributes (spread over the nine dimensions) and asks how closely the responder thinks each attribute applies to each country. Consider for example the five attributes under the Adventure dimension (friendly, fun, pleasant climate, scenic, and sexy), the six attributes under the Cultural Influence dimension (culturally significant, fashionable, happy, modern, prestigious, and trendy), the ten attributes under the Entrepreneurship dimension (connected to the world, educated population, entrepreneurial, innovative, easy access to capital, skilled labor force, high level of technical expertise, transparent business practices, well-developed infrastructure, and a strong legal framework), or the nine attributes under the Quality of Life dimension (good job market, affordable, economically stable, family friendly, income equality, politically stable, safe, well-developed education system, and a well-developed public health system). The Movers dimension is a version of the BAV Group's Brand Asset Valuator which is held to be predictive of a country's future economic growth. The attributes under this dimension value originality (different, distinctive, dynamic, and unique).

The attribute scores for each country are corrected for outliers; negative attribute scores are inverted; and all scores are normalized onto a universal [0, 100] scale. The normalized attribute scores are averaged within each dimension, and then the dimensional scores are totalled using the weighting scheme discussed above.

The top ten countries in the 2019 calculation were Switzerland, Japan, Canada, Germany, UK, Sweden, Australia, USA, Norway and France. The results are also used to produce subsidiary lists of the Best Countries for Women, for Study Abroad, for Comfortable Retirement, for Solo Travel, to Start a Career, to Start a Business, to Raise Kids, and more.

The Wellbeing Index

Robert Prescott-Allen is a consultant on sustainable development based in Victoria, British Columbia. In 2001 he published a book entitled: "The Wellbeing of Nations: A Country-by-Country Index of Quality of Life and the Environment." In the book he outlined a Wellbeing Assessment methodology and carried it out for 180 countries around the world. He described his book as "the ultimate travel guide for a sustainable future" and his methodology as providing "a real metric for measuring sustainability and wellbeing." [46].

Prescott-Allen's Wellbeing Assessment differs from many of the other exercises described in this chapter in that it gives equal weight to human wellbeing and ecosystem wellbeing. It does so by defining two separate indexes, a Human Wellbeing Index (HWI) and an Ecosystem Wellbeing Index (EWI), for each country under analysis. The average of the two indexes is a country's overall Wellbeing Index (WI). All three indexes are developed so that their final scores lie in the range [0, 100].

In addition to the WI, a country's wellbeing status is also represented graphically on a Barometer of Sustainability, which is a two-dimensional plot of HWI versus EWI. On this plot, every country is represented by a single point. Those countries (mostly-first-world) that have achieved a high HWI, but at the expense of serious environmental degradation (low EWI), are identified as "ecosystem-deficit" countries. Those countries (mostly in Africa) that have a low HWI, but have made little demand on the environment (and hence have a high EWI), are identified as "human-deficit" countries. In the 2001 analysis, 32 countries showed an ecosystem deficit, while 27 exhibited a human-deficit. The remainder of the 180 countries were "double-deficit." No countries were identified as high-functioning on both counts. The highest reported WI (for Sweden) was 64.0.

The HWI and EWI are constructed using five dimensions each, so that the full WI has a total of ten. The HWI uses 26 indicators and the EWI uses 31, for a total of 57. The dimensions of the HWI are: (1) Health and Population, (2) Wealth, (3) Knowledge and Culture, (4) Community, and (5) Equity. The dimensions of the EWI are: (6) Land, (7) Water, (8) Air, (9) Species and Genes, and (10) Resource Use. Most of the dimensions cover more than one element of wellbeing and use multiple indicators to do so. For example, the Wealth dimension includes indicators of both *household* wealth (average family income, percentage of population with insufficient food, percentage of population with access to safe water and basic sanitation), and *national* wealth (GDP per capita, inflation rate, unemployment rate, debt service costs as a percentage of GDP). The Equity dimension covers both *household* equity (ratio of the average income of the richest 20% of the population to that of the poorest 20%), and *gender* equity (ratio of male to female income, ratio of male to female school enrolment rates, and percentage of women in parliament). On the EWI side, the Air dimension covers both *global* atmospheric conditions (per capita greenhouse gas emissions, per capita use of ozone-depleting substances), and *local* air quality (average concentrations in representative cities of concentrations in air of SO_2, NO_2, CO, ozone, lead, and particulates). The Species and Genes dimension covers both *wild* diversity (threatened wild plant species as a percentage of total wild plant species, threatened wild animal species as a percentage of total wild animal species), and *domesticated* diversity (number of not-at-risk breeds per million head of domesticated animal species, ratio of threatened breeds to not-at-risk breeds of domesticated animal species). The wild plant species that are taken into account include flowering plants, conifers, and ferns. The wild animal species include mammals, birds, amphibians, and reptiles. The domesticated animal species include most common livestock.

Consideration of the indicators highlighted above make it clear that many of the 57 indicators are quite detailed in and of themselves. Among some of the other indicators included under the various HWI or EWI dimensions are such items as military expenditures as a percentage of GDP, homicide rates, number of internet users as a percentage of population, average energy consumption per hectare, average energy consumption per person, food produced per harvested hectare, fertilizer use per harvested hectare, annual percentage change in native forest cover, and degraded land as a percentage of cultivated or modified land area, weighted according to the severity of degradation.

Despite the apparent complexity of many of the indicator definitions, indicators were chosen in large part on the basis of availability. Data for all the indicators are available from 31 public-access sources (from international agencies like WHO, IMF, OECD, UNESCO, and FAO, or from NGOs like Freedom House, World Energy Council, World Wildlife Fund, UN Children's Fund, Transparency International, and the International Institute for Strategic Studies).

The raw data for the various indicators, which of course come in a wide variety of units, are all normalized onto a [0, 100] scale. Unlike all the other normalizations that have been seen for other indexes, the Prescott-Allen normalization is not necessarily linear. Rather than just defining a minimum and maximum raw score, a set of breakpoints are defined (usually five) and the normalization is piecewise linear between the breakpoints. In any case, the final result is a set of indicator scores between 0 and 100 for every indicator for every country.

Every dimension has several indicators, and the way the indicators are integrated to get the final dimensional score is quite complex. Sometimes two or more of the indicator scores are combined by taking their average. Sometimes it is done by taking the lowest value. Sometimes a weighted average is used. All of the weights and combinatorial specifications are hardwired into the methodology.

As an example of weighting, consider the Species and Genes dimension described above. In calculating the overall dimensional score, the average value of the two normalized wild-diversity indicator scores is weighted twice as heavily as the average value of the two normalized domesticated-diversity indicator scores. As a further example, one can look at the Community dimension. It has nine normalized indicator scores: (A) political rights rating, (B) civil liberties rating, (C) press freedom rating, (D) corruption perception rating, (E) military expenditures as a percentage of GDP, (F) homicide rate, (G) rape rate, (H) robbery rate, and (J) assault rate. First (A), (B), (C), and (D) are averaged to produce (K). Second, (G), (H), and (J) are averaged to produce (L). Third, (F) and (L) are averaged to produce (M). Fourth, (E) and (M) are averaged to produce (N). And lastly, the overall dimensional score is taken as the lower of (K) and (N). Most other dimensions have calculation procedures of similar complexity.

The five human-wellbeing dimensional scores are averaged to get the HWI, and the five ecosystem-wellbeing dimensional scores are averaged to get the EWI. The WI for a country is the average of the HWI and the EWI. In the 2001 analysis presented in Prescott-Allen's book (based on data from the late 90s), the top five WI scores are for Sweden, Finland, Norway, Iceland, and Austria. Canada ranked 7th and the USA 27th. The bottom scores came from Saudi Arabia, Uganda, Afghanistan, Syria and Iraq.

Looking separately at the two component indexes of the WI, it can be seen that the HWI rankings are rather similar to the overall ranking lists for other indexes, with high scores exhibited by the Scandinavian countries and other countries from the western bloc. The EWI rankings, on the other hand, are quite revealing. The top twenty spots include many African countries. Most oil-producing countries like Saudi Arabia and Iran sink very close to the bottom. On the EWI list, Canada ranks 110th and the USA 147th.

The Good Country Index

In his presidential inaugural address, John F. Kennedy challenged Americans to "ask not what your country can do for you," but to "ask what you can do for your country." In founding the Good Country movement, the British internationalist Simon Anholt made a different challenge: Ask not what your country can do for you, he urged, ask what your country can do for humanity.

The *Good Country Index* (GCI) differs from all preceding nationwide composite indexes discussed in this chapter in that it makes no attempt to assess the internal level of communal wellbeing in any country. Rather it attempts to measure the external global impact of a country's policies and behaviours on the world as a whole. It measures "not how *well* each country is doing but how *much* it is doing." It identifies how countries balance their duties to their own citizens with their responsibilities to the wider world. The stated goal of the GCI is to determine how much each country contributes to humanity, and how much it takes away [47].

Simon Anholt is an independent policy advisor, an honorary professor at East Anglia University, and an advocate for international cooperation and engagement between countries. He is best known for his innovative ideas on how nations can improve their national identities and reputations [48]. He has acted as a policy advisor to many countries including the Netherlands, South Korea, Sweden, Germany, New Zealand, and Switzerland, as well as to such international agencies as the United Nations, the World Bank, and the World Economic Forum. He is the founder and publisher of the Anholt-Gfk-Roper Nation Brands Index which ranks the countries of the world on the state of their national identity. In some ways, the Good Country movement is an outgrowth of Anholt's nation branding work, and the two enterprises are still quite closely connected, in that his managing partner for the Good Country Index is Robert Govers who is also a leading figure in the nation-branding community and the founding chairman of the International Place Branding Association.

The GCI is calculated using 7 dimensions, with 5 indicators per dimension, for a total of 35 indicators in all. The seven dimensions are: (1) Science, Technology and

Knowledge, (2) Culture, (3) International Peace and Security, (4) World Order, (5) Planet and Climate, (6) Prosperity and Equality, and (7) Health and Wellbeing. While these dimensions may look very similar to those used in other composite models of wellbeing, the emphasis here is totally different. The individual indicators do not reflect what countries do at home, only how they meet their responsibilities to a wider world. Compare, for example, five indicators that are commonly found under the Health and Wellbeing heading in traditional composite indexes, with those found in the GCI.

For the traditional models, one encounters measures of internal health and wellbeing like:

- Life expectancy at birth.
- Percentage of citizens with a regular medical doctor.
- Percentage of population getting influenza immunization.
- Occurrence of child and adult obesity.
- Availability of affordable, accessible health care.

For the Good Country Index, the measures reflect external global impact on health and wellbeing:

- Amount of food aid shipped to other countries.
- Exports of pharmaceuticals.
- Voluntary excess contributions to the World Health Organization.
- Humanitarian aid contributions.
- Prevention of drug trafficking through drug seizures.

The indicators under the other dimensions are equally appropriate to the objectives of the index. They include such measures as: exports of creative goods and services, number of peacekeeping troops sent overseas, number of treaties signed under peaceful conflict resolution, foreign investment outflow, international cooperative patent applications, and percentage of population that contributes to international charities. Twelve of the 35 indicators are defined negatively, but their data are then inverted in the usual way to ensure compatibility. Among the negatively-defined indicators are: exports of weapons and ammunition, exports of hazardous waste, CO_2 emissions, and UNESCO dues in arrears as a percent of overall contribution.

For many of the GCI indicators (25 of the 35, in fact), the raw data are divided by the country's GDP, in order to define a measure that is relative to the size of a country's economy. By defining such measures as, say, humanitarian aid, or international patent generation, relative to a country's GDP, the developers of the index avoid penalizing smaller or poorer countries for their smaller economies.

Sources of raw data for the 35 indicators lie with many of the usual international agencies including the United Nations, the World Bank, Reporters Without Borders, and the Global Footprint Network, but also with some more specialized sources like the Charities Aid Foundation World Giving Index, Henley and Partners Visa Restriction Index, the World Food Information System of the World Food Programme, Fairtrade International, the Basel Convention Hazwaste Fact Sheets, the International Trade Centre of the World Trade Organization, the Armed Conflict

Dataset maintained by the University of Uppsala and the Oslo Peace Research Institute, and the Global Cyber Security Index put out by the cybercrime prevention organization HostExploit.

The methodology of calculation of the GCI is relatively straightforward. For every country under analysis, for each of the 35 indicators, the raw datum is divided by the GDP, when appropriate, and negative indicators are adjusted for compatibility. The values are then normalized into a decimal fraction in the range [0, 1] with 0 being best and 1 worst. The value for each dimension is the average of the five indicator scores for that dimension. All the countries are then put in ranked order for each dimension. The Overall GCI ranking is the average of the seven dimensional rankings.

The most recent calculation of the GCI was carried out in 2017 (but using data from 2014 due to the time lapse that occurs in bringing databases up to date). It included consideration of 163 countries. The top ten ranked countries, in order from the top, were the Netherlands, Switzerland, Denmark, Finland, Germany, Sweden, Ireland, United Kingdom, Austria, and Norway. The bottom five ranked countries, in order from the bottom, were Afghanistan, Libya, Iraq, Yemen, and Chad. Canada ranked 14th and the USA 25th. Among other countries with large economies, Japan was 21st, Russia 65th, and China 76th. Top-ranked countries can be seen as "doing a lot for the common good, relative to the size of their economies." Bottom-ranked countries are "hindering the common good, or at least can be seen as free-riders." Any country with a ranking greater than 82nd can be seen as contributing to humanity, any country below 82nd as taking away.

The developers of the GCI note that the biggest challenges facing mankind are global and borderless, things like climate change, drug trafficking, terrorism, pandemics, and poverty. Solutions require international cooperation and coordinated action. They see the publication of the GCI as a tool in the fight to change the culture of governance worldwide.

They recognize that the GCI tells only half the story, and that citizens are justly interested in the effect of their government's policies on a country's internal happiness and wellbeing. They encourage people to consider GCI rankings alongside reputable and reliable measures of domestic performance in order to see both halves of the story.

Summary of Country Rankings

Table 9.7 provides a summary of the top ten and bottom ten countries from eight of the multi-dimensional composite indexes of nationwide communal wellbeing that have been covered in this chapter. Seven of them look very much alike, with the top ten nations highlighted by the Scandinavian countries, other western European nations, Australia, New Zealand, and Canada. This is true even for the Good Country Index which measures quite a different thing than the others. The outlier is the Happy Planet Index, whose top ten includes several South American nations. Readers may

Table 9.7 Summary of country rankings from multi-dimensional composite indexes of nationwide communal wellbeing

Index	Human Development Index	World Happiness Report	Happy Life Years	Happy Planet Index	Weighted Index Social Progress	Legatum Prosperity Index	Wellbeing Index	Good Country Index
Acronym	HDI	WHR	HLY	HPI	WISP	LPI	WI	GCI
Countries	189	156	158	140	162	149	180	163
Top Ten	Norway	Finland	Costa Rica	Costa Rica	Denmark	Norway	Sweden	Netherlands
	Switzerland	Norway	Iceland	Mexico	Germany	New Zealand	Finland	Switzerland
	Australia	Denmark	Denmark	Columbia	Austria	Finland	Norway	Denmark
	Ireland	Iceland	Switzerland	Vanuatu	Japan	Switzerland	Iceland	Finland
	Germany	Switzerland	Canada	Vietnam	Sweden	Denmark	Austria	Germany
	Iceland	Netherlands	Norway	Panama	Italy	Sweden	Dominica	Sweden
	Hong Kong	Canada	Mexico	Nicaragua	Finland	UK	Canada	Ireland
	Sweden	New Zealand	Finland	Bangladesh	Iceland	Canada	Switzerland	UK
	Singapore	Sweden	Sweden	Thailand	Belgium	Netherlands	Belize	Austria
	Netherlands	Australia	Australia	Ecuador	Norway	Ireland	Guyana	Norway
USA	13th	18th	24th	108th	39th	17th	27th	25th
Canada	12th	7th	5th	85th	25th	8th	7th	14th
Bottom Ten	Mozambique	Malawi	Congo	Burundi	Afghanistan	Burundi	Sudan	Eq Guinea
	Liberia	Haiti	Niger	Swaziland	Niger	Angola	India	Syria
	Mali	Liberia	Cameroon	Sierra Leone	Sudan	Mauritania	Un Arab Emir	Angola
	Burkino Faso	Syria	DR Congo	Turkmenistan	Uganda	Iraq	Mauritania	Mali
	Sierra Leone	Rwanda	Mozambique	Cote d'Ivoire	Nigeria	DR Congo	Tonga	Mauritania
	Burundi	Yemen	Benin	Mongolia	Somalia	Sudan	Saudi Arabia	Chad
	Chad	Tanzania	Sierra Leone	Benin	Yemen	Chad	Uganda	Yemen
	South Sudan	South Sudan	Burundi	Togo	Sierra Leone	Yemen	Afghanistan	Iraq

	Cent Af Rep	Cent Af Rep	Tanzania	Luxembourg	Chad	Cent Af Rep	Syria	Libya
	Niger	Burundi	Togo	Chad	Cent Af Rep	Afghanistan	Iraq	Afghanistan
Year	2018	2018	2014	2016	2018	2018	2001	2017

recall that the structure of the HPI disdains any measure of economic wealth and puts great emphasis on a country's ecological footprint, so it is perhaps not surprising that its rankings have their own flavor. More surprising, perhaps, is the fact that the other index that gives great weight to ecosystem wellbeing, Prescott-Allen's Wellbeing Index, does not differ nearly as much from the rest as does the HPI. All eight indexes are consistent at the bottom end, where countries from Africa and the Middle East dominate. They are also consistent in ranking Canada above the USA on the North American scorecard.

There are many other sources of country rankings of a more-detailed nature. Wikipedia's International Rankings [49] include over 200 such listings, providing data on such diverse topics as beer consumption per capita, number of Olympic medals, vehicles per capita, rates of incarceration, levels of wine production, literacy rates, suicide rates, and proven oil and gas reserves. The Economist offers a website called The World in Figures which provides hundreds of country rankings in 51 different categories [50]. In just one of those categories, for example, the one that covers inflation, country-ranked lists are provided for the annual change in commodity prices for 29 different commodities including wheat, corn, rice, sugar, tea, coffee, oil and gas, gold, lead, timber, beef, wool and hides. The world's largest free integrated global database is run by the Knoema Corporation. It contains 2.8 billion time series, from more than 1200 sources, on over 1000 topics [51].

The Questions of Normalization, Aggregation, and Weighting: Reprise

Some issues and questions about composite indexing that have already received some attention in this and earlier chapters are so significant that they deserve further mention. The remainder of this chapter addresses such questions. First up are the issues associated with normalization, aggregation, and weighting that were introduced in Chap. 7 in some detail. They are reprised here simply as a reminder of their importance in the application of composite indexes.

All of the multi-dimensional nationwide indexes involve a wide variety of indicators with very different units of measurement (think *dollars* for economic indicators, *years* for longevity, and perhaps *pollutant concentrations in streamwater* or *bird counts* in environmental modules). *Normalization* is the process by which these varied units are brought into dimensionless unity (usually onto a [0,10] scale or as [0,100] percentages). The process requires the setting of minimum and maximum values, which may be straightforward, or may involve decisions that invite bias or cloud the calculations. Care and transparency are needed.

Aggregation of normalized indicators across sub-dimensions and dimensions can be carried out in a variety of ways, the most common being *additive* (add the values together and take the arithmetic average) or *geometric* (multiply the n values together and take the nth root). The choice of aggregation method can lead to significant differences in results.

The primary question about aggregation is whether to do it at all. Back in Chap. 7, Table 7.5 outlined the advantages and disadvantages of trying to arrive at a single-valued overall measure for a composite index, as opposed to leaving the end-product in the form of a matrix of dimensional or sub-dimensional results. The decision rests on the perceptions of the index developers of the trade-off between the effectiveness of a single-valued result as a communication tool and the possible loss of transparency that is engendered. The main support for a single-valued index comes from those who see it as a necessary feature of any realistic competitor to the GDP as a measure of national wellbeing.

Weighting of one or more indicators relative to others is popular with index designers because of the perceived differences in the importance of specific indicators to the composite index as a whole. The problem is that different index designers may have different opinions on the impacts of, say, access to medical care, the dangers of climate change, freedom of the press, or the value of military preparedness. Given that most host organizations develop their indexes as part of an overall mission, it may be difficult for developers to avoid introducing bias into weighting schemes if the weights are set in-house on an *a priori* basis. To avoid such bias, many agencies use panels of external experts to help in the process. It is an important issue because many sensitivity studies have shown that large influences can be exerted on results by changes in weighting.

Index developers use a variety of methods to set weights, among them *equal weighting* (the so-called value-free choice), *normative weighting* (where weights are hardwired into the methodology), and more-advanced *multivariate statistical methods*. A review of the various national indexes described in this chapter indicates examples of all of these methods. The Canadian Index of Wellbeing uses equal weighting. The Bhutanese Index of Gross National Happiness and Prescott-Allen's Wellbeing Index use weights specified by the developers. The Legatum Prosperity Index uses expert advisors in part, but also admits to a weighting scheme that is "compatible with the Legatum Institute's view of prosperity." The Weighted Index of Social Progress and the US News and World Report Rankings use statistically-based weighting. The Better Life Index uses equal weighting as its default, but also allows users to set their own weights.

The Question of Information Content Relative to the Per-Capita GDP

There is no question that the results of multi-dimensional indexing on a country-by-country basis show a strong correlation with per-capita GDP. This should not be a huge surprise given that per-capita GDP is a major input into most of the calculations. It is also likely that many of the other indicators (like expenditures on education, housing status, food security, cultural participation, community vitality, and so on) are themselves positively correlated with GDP.

Having said this, it is apparent from most comparative studies that the annual increases in per-capita GDP that have been experienced by most first-world countries over the past several decades have not been matched by similar percentage increases in overall wellbeing. Wellbeing has increased, but not as much as per-capita GDP. This finding can be found anecdotally in the above discussions of the Human Development Index and the Canadian Index of Wellbeing, but it has also been put forward on the basis of a more encompassing analysis carried out by Ruut Veenhoven using the data for many countries from the World Database of Happiness [52].

The reasons for this lack of synchronicity are many and varied, but at the top of the list is the fact that the benefits of economic growth in the financial sector are often countered by serious social costs that must be borne by society as a whole, and which are not included in GDP calculations. It is also true that economic benefits often accrue primarily to a favored few, and in many countries rising per-capita GDP has been accompanied by a deteriorating Gini coefficient, indicating growing inequality in personal outcomes. Furthermore, those multi-dimensional indexes that emphasize an environmental component (like the Sustainable Human Development Index, the Happy Planet Index, and Prescott-Allen's Wellbeing Index) clarify the long-term environmental costs that are being engendered to maintain current levels of economic growth. The per-capita GDP metric simply does not capture these various externalities as well as a multi-dimensional wellbeing index.

Moreover, sole reliance on an economic measure does not allow the identification of the specific sectors of society that are performing well or badly, as can often be gleaned from the workings of a multi-dimensional index. In short, it seems clear that there is considerably more information content in the results of composite nation-wide indexing than can be found in the GDP alone.

The Question of Diversity

Population diversity is a commonly-used indicator in nation-wide composite indexes. In most cases it is treated as a boon to wellbeing, but the question arises as to whether increased diversity in a nation's social makeup actually leads to greater societal happiness, or could it in some cases be a drag on it? Is the social cohesion produced by a population that is relatively homogeneous in ethnicity, religion, and language, a positive influence on wellbeing or is it a stultifying negative? Are the people in a country with more open immigration policies and a more diverse citizenry really happier? Or if not necessarily happier, are they somehow the better for it in the context of national wellbeing?

For the developers of multi-dimensional indexes, the answers to these questions seem to lie in the timing of index development. The earliest indexes like Estes Weighted Index of Social Progress were developed in a period when many "homogeneous" nations like Australia, New Zealand, and Spain seemed to have the best of all worlds, and the indexes of the day reflected this apparent evidence by treating homogeneity as a plus and diversity as a minus. There then followed a period where indexes tended to be developed by more liberal think tanks where population diversity was valued positively, and the demands of political correctness came into greater play. Most of the indexes currently in use date from this latter period.

However, not all happiness researchers agree. Alberto Alesina, an Italian political economist based at Harvard University, has been the leader of those who question the positive influence of diversity on communal happiness [53]. He recognizes that many countries base their immigration policies on a belief that increased ethnic and cultural diversity are beneficial to national wellbeing. However, he argues that the evidence has not supported this view. He points to the negative public response to the massive migrations of refugees and asylum seekers in most first-world countries, the failure of migrants to adapt to their new homes, the development of ethnic enclaves, and the growth in racism, intolerance, exclusion, and conflict. He presents statistical evidence that such "fractionalization" weakens economic performance, and he points to the results of recent international polling of subjective wellbeing that show much greater levels of happiness and life satisfaction in more-homogeneous, less-fractionalized countries.

The host organizations of composite indexes feel caught in the middle of this controversy. The changing mores with respect to population diversity have brought stress to their indexing teams, most of whom want their calculations to be value-free and politically independent. Time will tell whether the structures that are currently in place in these long-established indexing procedures can withstand the winds of change.

The Question of Cultural Bias

Anyone who peruses the summary results of Table 9.7 cannot help but be struck by the similarity in the listing of countries at the top of the heap in the various indexes. The Scandinavian countries, the rest of Europe, and the British Commonwealth countries of Canada, Australia and New Zealand, always seem to lead the pack. The USA and the UK are usually not far behind. The question arises whether life is truly better in these Western democracies, or whether the rankings reflect the cultural biases of the index developers, most of whom reside in these same favored nations. Certainly the issue has been raised on many occasions over the years by representatives of lower-ranked countries who feel that the indexes give too much credit for material comforts and not enough for the wellbeing that is generated by a harmonious communal society [54]. They see a bias toward a Christian, individualist, capitalist ethic; an unfair disdain for Buddhist and Muslim beliefs; and a failure to recognize the positive features of more collectivistic or ecumenical societies. As an extreme example of a countervailing view, a 2011 magazine article reported that a Global Happiness Index developed in North Korea produced a ranking with China, North Korea, Cuba, Iran and Venezuela in the top five positions, and the USA last [55]. Clearly, bias is not a one-way street.

Shigehiro Oishi of the University of Virginia has been a leader in laying out the conceptual and methodological issues associated with culture and wellbeing [56]. It is his view that there are diverse concepts of wellbeing across cultures, and that national differences in the levels, correlates, and consequences of wellbeing should be interpreted with this diversity in mind. As evidence of this viewpoint he reports studies showing that self-esteem and personal freedom have much stronger impact on global life satisfaction in individualistic nations than they do in collectivist nations, and that relationship harmony plays a greater role than financial security in Asian nations whereas the reverse tends to be true in Western nations.

The keeper of the faith with respect to the applicability of national rankings is Ruut Veenhoven. In a classic paper, he puts out four strawmen and then knocks them down [57]. Among the "qualms" that he feels some observers might have about such ranking exercises are the following: (1) Are happiness and wellbeing "Western" concepts that are alien to non-Western nations? (2) Is there a language or translation issue? Do the terms "happiness" and "wellbeing" have a direct analogue in all languages? (3) Are there differences in social norms? In countries where happiness is "morally desirable" might respondents over-report their levels of life satisfaction? In societies that value modesty and humility might respondents under-report? (4) Might there be a difference between individualistic societies where respondents might over-report their happiness in an attempt to appear successful, and collectivistic societies where respondents might under-report in order to appear average?

Veenhoven used the extensive data of his World Database of Happiness to dismiss each of these hypotheses in turn. With respect to the first one, he posited that if true, there would be more "don't know" and "no answer" responses in non-Western nations than in Western nations, but he found that this was not the case. For the second question, he compared responses to questions on happiness and life satisfaction from the two linguistic groups in two bilingual countries, and found no evidence of linguistic bias. With respect to the third and fourth items, he carried out many tests on response statistics from countries with apparently-different social norms and different mixes of individualism and collectivism, and found that the data did not support any of the qualm-based hypotheses. He concluded that the impacts of cultural differences on national assessments of happiness and wellbeing are at worst very small and probably non-existent.

A similar conclusion was reached by the development team of the Good Country Index. They claim to have been initially surprised by the dominance of the Western European countries in their rankings of do-gooders. After carrying out a careful review of their methodology and results, they conclude that, based on the available data, the European Union member states "do appear to contribute more to the international community at this point in history;" that they have a "long habit of international collaboration;" and that on the whole they have "made the greatest effort to correct the risks and imbalances" of globalisation.

Comparative Analyses

Researchers in happiness modeling have shown far greater interest in developing and promoting their own indexes than in carrying out comparative studies of the growing number of indexes that already populate the happiness literature. However in recent years there have been a few such efforts.

Alex Michalos and Maurine Hatch compared five indexes over 105 countries at national scale. The indexes were the Human Development Index (HDI), the Weighted Index of Social Progress (WISP), the Social Progress Index (SPI), the Sustainable Society Index (SSI), and the World Happiness Report (WHR). The first four of these are objective indexes, the WHR is subjective. They found "good convergent validity" among the five, and strong correlations between the results [58].

A team of Australian researchers at Deakin University led by Rebecca Patrick compared 12 composite indexes from the specific point of view of whether they could effectively bond human wellbeing with the health of the environment. Among those that failed the test were the OECD Better Life Index (BLI), the Social Progress Index (SPI), and the Genuine Progress Indicator (GPI). They reserved their strongest recommendation for the Happy Planet Index (HPI) which they claim can be used to "mobilise conversations and drive actions towards achieving the UN Sustainable Development Goals (SDGs) where human wellbeing and health of the environment are conceptually linked." [59].

By far the most widely quoted comparative study of composite indexes was carried out in 2001 by a committee of experts from the social indicators movement led by Michael Hagerty of the University of California at Davis and including leading lights Robert Cummins, Kenneth Land, Alex Michalos and Joseph Sirgy. They identified 14 criteria for determining the validity and usefulness of such indexes, and assessed 22 national-scale quality-of-life indexes from around the world against these criteria. They concluded that "many of the indexes are potentially very useful," but that many "fall short" on a variety of criteria. None of the indexes in the suite that they examined had assessed convergent validity against any of the others. They were unable to choose any particular index or any particular group of indexes as the "best," probably in part because most of the participants had their own oar in the water [60].

A Summary of Critical Issues

It is probably clear to the reader by now that the design and application of a multidimensional index of happiness and wellbeing is a complex endeavor. Alex Michalos has recently published a list of the critical decisions that must be made by the designer of such an index [61]. He notes that "different individuals, institutions, or communities may prioritize different developmental aims depending on their particular mandates, purposes, circumstances, and resources ... so one cannot know a priori if one's own perspective is appropriate for everyone." Although his list was presented in the context of indexes for "sustainable development," it clearly has relevance to the broader suite of indexes that one finds in the happiness movement as a whole. Table 9.8 is adapted from Michalos' list, and while it has been massaged somewhat to meet our broader needs, it retains a very close resemblance to the original. It outlines 23 decision points that every modeller must

Table 9.8 Critical issues in the design and application of multidimensional indexes of happiness and well-being. (Adapted from the source material listed in [61])

	Critical issue	Example
1.	Individual or group basis	Per capita incomes apply to individuals, while unemployment rates apply to groups.
2.	Spatial coordinates	A representative area for understanding air pollution may be very different from that for understanding crime statistics.
3.	Temporal coordinates	The optimal timeframe for understanding the impact of resource depletion may be very different from that for understanding the impact of housing availability.
4.	Population composition	Emphasis on specific populations in order to uncover the impacts of language, sex, age, education, ethnicity, or income, might suggest different agendas for action
5.	Domains of life composition	Emphasis on different domains like health, family, or the environment, might suggest different agendas for action.
6.	Objective vs. subjective indicators	Subjective appraisals of community wellbeing based on responses by individuals who live in the community may be different than "expert" appraisals based on objective datasets of external influences.
7.	Positive vs. negative indicators	In the health domain, negative measures of morbidity and mortality may crowd out positive measures of wellbeing.
8.	Input vs. output indicators	Expenditures on teachers and school facilities may give a different view of the quality of an education system than that based on student performance on standardized tests, or on some more encompassing measure of whether the populace at large is becoming more literate, knowledgeable, educated and wise.
9.	Benefits and costs	Different measures of value or worth may yield different evaluations. Consider the market value of child care versus the social value of having children well cared for.
10.	Recipient populations	Who should be included as a recipient for particular benefits and costs?
11.	Measurement scales	Different measures of wellbeing may lead to different outcomes.
12.	Research personnel	Different stakeholders often have very different views about what is important to monitor and how to evaluate what is monitored.
13.	Target audiences	Different target audiences may need different reporting formats and media.
14.	Aggregation	Different methods of aggregating indicators in an index may lead to different results.
15.	Indicator distributions	Average values of indicator variables can conceal important information, so appropriate representations of their statistical distributions are needed. Different methods of representing these distributions can lead to different results.
16.	Distance impacts	Indicator data taken from an individual's home jurisdiction may underestimate their ability to take advantage of facilities in nearby jurisdictions at various distances from their place of residence.
17.	Causal relations	Correlations among variables need to be explored with a view to discovering possible evidence of dependence or independence, redundancy, or double-counting.

(continued)

Table 9.8 (continued)

	Critical issue	Example
18.	Rates of change	Design of indexes that track over time need to have some a priori idea of the potential rates of change of indicator variables.
19.	Discount rates	How much should one discount costs and benefits delivered to generations sometime in the future compared to those delivered to people today?
20.	Nesting levels	Indicator variables may be available at the level of families, cities, regions, states, countries, or the world at large. These different levels may have interactions with one another leading to different causal effects. What levels and interactions should be examined?
21.	Confidence levels	What level of confidence should be required to accept any particular claim or measure?
22.	Auditors	Who should decide if any assessments are adequate or appropriate?
23.	Auditing criteria	What criteria should be used to assess the adequacy of auditors' assessments, the adequacy of the procedures used for audits, and even the adequacy of answers to the questions raised in this list of critical issues?

address, and gives an example for each one. Almost all of these items have received some level of discussion in this or earlier chapters. The list is presented here, at the end of this rather overwhelming chapter, as a summary of the critical issues that must be faced by designers and users of multidimensional indexes of happiness and wellbeing.

References

1. Bauer, Raymond A., ed., *Social Indicators*, MIT Press, 1966; Andrews, Frank M. And Stephen B. Withey, *Social Indicators of Well-Being*, Plenum Press, 1976; *Social Indicators: Selected Data on Social Conditions and Trends in the United States*, U.S. Office of Management and Budget, 1973; U.S. Bureau of the Census, 1977,1980
2. Nordhaus, W. And J. Tobin, Is growth obsolete?, *Economic Growth*, National Bureau of Economic Research, 1972.
3. Morris, M.D., *Measuring the World's Poor: the Physical Quality of Life Index*, Pergamon Press, 1979.
4. Estes, R.J. and J.S. Morgan, World social welfare analysis: A theoretical model, *International Social Work*, 19(2), 29-41, 1976; Estes, R.J., *The Social Progress of Nations*, Preager, 1984.
5. Ul Haq, M., The Birth of the Human Development Index, Chapter 4, in *Reflections on Human Development*, p. 46-66, Oxford University Press, 1995.
6. Sen, A., *Commodities and Capabilities*, North-Holland/Elsevier, 1985.
7. [www.nobelprize.org/prizes/economics/1998/sen/auto-biography]
8. Ul Haq, op. cit.
9. [www.worldbank.org/en/programs/icp]

10. Klugman, J., F. Rodriguez, and H-J. Choi, The HDI 2010: *New Controversies and Old Critiques*, UN Development Program, Human Development Research Paper 2011/01, 2011.
11. [www.un.org/development/desa/en]; [https://data.worldbank.org]; [www.imf.org/en/Data]; [https://unstats.un.org]; [uis.unesco.org]; [mics.unicef.org]; [www.oecd.org/education/education-at-a-glance]; [www.icf.com/resources/projects/research-and-evaluation/demographic-and-health-surveys]; [www.barrolee.com]
12. Anand, S. and A. Sen, *Human Development Index: Methodology and Measurement*, UN Human Development Report Office, Occasional Paper 12, 1994; Klugman et al, 2011, op. cit.; [http://hdr.undp.org/site/default/files/hdr2018-technical-notes.pdf]
13. UN Development Programme, *Human Development Indices and Indicators, 2018 Statistical Update*, 111 pp., 2018; [hdr.undp.org/en/2018-update]
14. Kovacevic, M., *Review of HDI Critiques and Potential Improvements*, Human Development Research Paper 2010/33, 44 pp., 2011.
15. [https://ourworld.unu.edu/en/the-2010-human-sustainable-development-index]
16. Alkire, s. and M.E Santos, *Acute multidimensional poverty : A new index for developing countries*, Working Paper 38, Oxford Poverty and Human Development Initiative, 2010
17. Herrero, C., R. Martinez and A. Villar, Population structure and the Human Development Index, *Social Indicators Research*, 141, 731-763, 2019
18. Land, K.C., The human development index, Chapter 7 in *Global Handbook of Quality of Life: Exploration of Well-Being of Nations and Continents*, edited by W. Glatzer, Springer, 2015.
19. Michalos, A.C. and P.M. Hatch, Good societies, financial inequality and secrecy, and a good life: from Aristotle to Piketty, *Applied Research in Quality of Life,* 15(4), 1005-1054, 2020.
20. Helliwell, J.F., R. Layard and J. Sachs, *World Happiness Report*, Sustainable Development Solutions Network, 2018 ; [worldhappiness.report/ed/2018].
21. Anonymous, The Economist Intelligence Unit's Quality of Life Index, *The World in 2005*, The Economist, 2005.
22. Veenhoven, R., Happy life expectancy : A comprehensive measure of quality of life in nations, *Social Indicators Research*, 39, 1-58, 1996 ; Veenhoven, R., Happy life years : A measure of gross national happiness, *Proc. First Intern. Conf. On Operationalisation of GNH*, 2004.
23. Veenhoven. R., *Average happiness in 158 nations 2005-2014.* [worlddatabaseofhappiness.eur.nl]
24. Veenhoven, R. and W. Kalmijn, Inequality-adjusted happiness in nations: Egalitarianism and utilitarianism married in a new index of social performance, *Jour. Happiness Studies*, 6(4), 421-455, 2005.
25. Jeffrey, K., H. Wheatley and S. Abdallah, *The Happy Planet Index : A global index of sustainable well-being*, New Economics Foundation, 2016.
26. [happyplanetindex.org]
27. Daly, H., Beyond Growth : *The Economics of Sustainable Developmen*t, Beacon Press, 1989 ; Daly, H. and J. Cobb, *For the Common Good : Redirecting the Economy Toward Community, the Environment, and a Sustainable Future*, Beacon Press, 1994.
28. Redefining Progress, *Genuine Progress Indicator : Summary of Data and Methodology*, 1995.
29. Cobb, C., T. Halstead and J. Rowe, If the GDP is up, why is America down? *Atlantic Monthly*, 59-78, October 1995.
30. Talberth, J., C. Cobb and N. Slattery, *The Genuine Progress Indicator : A Tool for Sustainable Development*, Redefining Progress, 2006.
31. Lawn, Philip A., A theoretical foundation to support ISEW, GPI, and other related indexes, *Ecological Economics*, 44, 105-118, 2003.
32. Max-Neef, M., Economic growth and quality of life : A threshold hypothesis, *Ecological Economics*, 15, 115-118, 1995.
33. Talberth, J. and M. Weisdorf, Genuine Progress Indicator 2.0 : Pilot accounts for the US, Maryland, and the City of Baltimore, 2012-2014, *Ecological Economics*, 142, 1-11, 2017.
34. [https://uwaterloo.ca/canadian-index-wellbeing]

35. Michalos, A. et al, *The Canadian Index of Wellbeing: Technical Paper*, 73 pp., 2011.
36. Canadian Index of Wellbeing, *How are Canadians Really Doing?*, The 2016 CIW National Report, University of Waterloo, 2016.
37. Estes, R.J., The world social situation: Development challenges at the outset of a new century, *Social Indicators Research*, 98(3), 363-402, 2010; Estes, R.J., The social progress of nations revisited, *Social Indicators Research*, 144, 539-574, 2019.
38. Estes, R.J., 2010, op. cit.
39. [www.miqols.org/toolbox/isp.html]
40. [www.iim-edu.org/grossnationalhappiness/index.htm]
41. Munro, L.T., Where did Bhutan's Gross National Happiness come from? The origins of an invented tradition, *Asian Affairs*, 47(1), 71-92, 2016.
42. Ura, K., S. Alkine, T. Zangmo and K. Wangdi, *A Short Guide to the Gross National Happiness Index*, Centre for Bhutan Studies, 2012. [www.grossnationalhappiness.com]
43. Organization for Economic Cooperation and Development (OECD), *How's Life? Measuring Well-Being*, 4th edition, 2017; [www.oecdbetterlifeindex.org]
44. Legatum Institute, Prosperity Index, *Methodology Report*, 2018; [www.prosperity.com]
45. [www.usnews.com/news/best-countries]
46. Prescott-Allen, R., *The Wellbeing of Nations: A Country-by-Country Index of Quality-of-Life and the Environment*, Island Press, 2001; [www.iied.org]
47. [www.goodcountryindex.org/results]
48. Anholt, S., *Places: Identity, Image, and Reputation*, Palgrave Macmillan, 2010.
49. [https://en.wikipedia.org/wiki/List_of_international_rankings]
50. [https://worldinfigures.com/rankings]
51. [https://knoema.com/atlas/ranks]
52. Veenhoven, R., What we have learnt about happiness, Classic qualms in the light of recent research, in *A Life Dedicated to Quality of Life*, Social Indicators Research Book Series, vol. 60, 151-170, 2015.
53. Alesina, A., Fractionalization, *Journal of Economic Growth*, 8(2), 155-194, 2003.
54. Noorbakhsh, F., The human development index: Some technical issues and alternative indices, *Jour. International Development*, 10, 589-605, 1998.
55. *Business Insider*, May 3, 2011; [https://www.businessinsider.com]
56. Oishi, S., Culture and well-being: Conceptual and methodological issues, Chapter 3, in Diener, E., J. Helliwell and D. Kahneman, eds, *International Differences in Well-Being*, Oxford University Press, 2010.
57. Veenhoven, R., op. cit., 2015. See also: Veenhoven, R., Cross-national differences in happiness: Cultural measurement bias or effect of culture, *International Journal of Wellbeing*, 2(4), 333-353, 2012.
58. Michalos and Hatch, 2020, op. cit.
59. Patrick, R. et al, Human wellbeing and the health of the environment: Local indicators that balance the scales, *Social Indicators Research*, 146,651-667, 2019.
60. Hagerty, M.R., et. al., Quality-of-Life indexes for national policy: Review and agenda for research, *Social Indicators Research*, 55(1), 1-96, 2001.
61. Michalos, A.C., Corporate social responsibility in universities and sustainable development, in D.C. Poff, ed., *Corporate Social Responsibility and University Governance*, Springer Nature, 2022.

Chapter 10
The Livability of Cities

Livable Cities

In the year 2000, there were 3646 cities on the planet with a population greater than 100,000, and the world's total urban population was estimated to be just over 2 billion people. It is predicted that these numbers will double over the next 50 years. Today, roughly 50% of the world's population lives in cities. By 2050 it is expected to be 66% [1]. Over the past half century, interest in urban issues has intensified. Concern about the growth in the spatial footprint of urbanized areas, the increased population and density of cities, and the challenges faced by urban citizenry, has led to the development of a large and active urban studies community. This community involves a coming together of specialists in such diverse fields as land-use planning, landscape architecture, transportation studies, civic infrastructure, and the psychology and sociology of people living in close proximity to one another.

The American Planning Association (APA) is the premier urban planning group in the USA. It was formed in 1978, but dates its precursor organizations back to 1935. The Journal of the APA provides a primary outlet for academic research papers in urban studies. In addition to its academic wing, the APA is also home to planning practitioners through its affiliated organization, the American Institute of Certified Planners. One of the APA's most visible programs is one that identifies the Great Places, Great Neighborhoods, Great Public Spaces, and Great Streets of America. This program provides public recognition to the cityscapes "that make communities stronger and bring people together through good planning." [2]. In 2018, the APA highlighted the Canalway Cultural District in Lowell MA and the Aspa Pedestrian Mall in Stamford CT.

There are many other national and international planning organizations. The International Society of City and Regional Planners (ISOCARP) dates to 1965. It sponsors an annual World Planning Congress and publishes the *International Manual of Planning Practice* [3].The American Sociological Association includes

R. A. Freeze, *The Metrics of Happiness*, Social Indicators Research Series 86,
https://doi.org/10.1007/978-3-031-10913-3_10

a section on Urban Sociology. The Association of Metropolitan Planning Organizations, the Urban Affairs Association, and the National League of Cities each represent different sets of players in the urban planning community.

On the academic side, Wikipedia lists 52 professional journals under the rubric of urban studies. They include Urban Studies (launched in 1964), Urban Affairs Review (1965), Landscape and Urban Planning (1974), the International Journal of Urban and Regional Research (1977), the Journal of the American Planning Association (1978), the Journal of Urban Affairs (1979), Urban Geography (1980), Cities: The International Journal of Urban Policy and Planning (1983), City and Community (2002), and the International Journal of Community well-Being (2018).

An organization called Urban Insight based in Los Angeles publishes a *Guide to Graduate Urban Planning Programs*. In the most recent sixth edition, they identify 97 graduate programs in the USA. The five schools that rate most highly in their assessment are MIT, Berkeley, Rutgers, UCLA, and the University of North Carolina [4]. Most of these graduate programs are housed within separate research institutes associated with each university. The one at MIT is called the Centre for Urban Studies and Planning; at Berkeley, the Institute for Urban and Regional Studies; at Rutgers, the Center for Urban Research and Education. Other university-based institutes zero in on Urban Policy, Community Studies, Civic Engagement, and Urban Innovation. One of the most-widely recognized international efforts is the Global Cities Research Institute at the Royal Melbourne Institute of Technology in Australia.

There are also many non-university-based research centers that focus on the livability of cities. One of the most impactful has been the Washington-based Urban Institute which was founded over 50 years ago as part of the Johnson administration's war on poverty. It hosts a widely-referenced blog called the Urban Wire, a publishing outlet under the name of the Urban Institute Press, and 12 Policy Centers (dealing with such civic issues as Education, Labor, Health, Housing, Income, Justice, and Philanthropy). The Institute delivers "fact-based solutions to civic problems that are trusted by decision-makers across the ideological spectrum." It uses "the power of evidence to support the economic security of families, promote racial and economic justice, and revitalize communities." [5].

Another private institute of interest is the Ross Center for Sustainable Cities, which has provided an online resource since 2007, publishing reports on such issues as electric bus adoption, bike sharing, and urban water access. They claim that world-wide sustainable-cities initiatives in 2016–2017 alone reduced CO_2 emissions by 3.2 million tons, saved 665 million hours of commuter travel time, saved 1776 lives, and leveraged 9.1 billion dollars in civic investments [6]. The Philips Center for Health and Well-being based in San Diego CA produces a set of graphical presentations called the Insight Series on Livable Cities [7]. Among the topics that are highlighted are civic resilience, inclusiveness, and the development of a sense of pride in a community's history and heritage. They also give out an annual Livable Cities Award for simple solutions that improve the health and wellbeing of cities. The most recent winner was a rainwater aggregation scheme in Yemen. The

Washington-based Pew Research Center is a non-partisan think tank that carries out polls on where Americans most want to live [8]. The delightfully-named Future Cities Catapult is a non-profit organization based in London, England that acts as a collaborative hub for business, academics, and city leaders to develop and market products and services that help build healthy cities [9]. The Happy City is a small UK-based non-profit that provides training and consultant services to local civic governments [10]. The Center for the Living City has offices in both New York NY and Portland OR. It develops programs that emphasize "participatory planning, equitable engagement, community-generated solutions, and the integration of social, economic and environmental systems in addressing urban challenges." [11]. The Atlantic Media Group (publishers of *The Atlantic* magazine) host an online research center called CityLab, which funds and reports on issues of urban concern [12].

The United Nations has also been active in urban studies. Its Programme for Human Settlements, known as Habitat, was launched in 1978 "to advance sustainable urbanization as a driver of development and peace to improve living conditions for all." It produced one of the first lists of urban indicators, a set of 41 of them, based on the UN Millennium Development Goals [13]. Habitat sponsors a World Cities Day on October 31 each year, as well as being the lead agency for the annual World Urban Forum, the most recent of which was held in Abu Dhabi in 2020. It also publishes a bi-annual report on the State of the World's Cities (renamed the World Cities Report in 2016).

In due course, some of these organizations will be encountered again in their role as sponsors of city-scale livability indexes that are the focus of this chapter.

A Little History

Before presenting these indexes, it is perhaps appropriate to look at a little recent history. Prior to the 1960s, urban planning efforts tended to emphasize the more practical aspects of the urban environment, things like city layouts, transportation grids, urban architecture, and city infrastructure. That all changed in 1961 with the publication of two books that now hold an honored place in the history of urban design. The first was *The Death and Life of Great American Cities* by Jane Jacobs [14], and the second *The City in History: Its Origins, Its Transformations, and Its Prospects* by Lewis Mumford [15]. Neither Jacobs nor Mumford were trained urban planners: Jacobs was a journalist, author, and activist; Mumford was an historian. Both questioned the consensus among urban planners of the day toward what they saw as heartless technological solutions to urban problems. Both decried the trend toward sweeping high-rise urban-renewal programs that destroyed neighborhoods and gave no thought to people-based cultural vitality. They abhorred urban sprawl and argued for the value of a vibrant downtown core. They emphasized the deep-seated relationship that exists between people and their living spaces. Jacobs, especially, fought for the empowerment of citizens to become advocates for their own communities. From the perspective of this book, Jane Jacobs and Lewis

Mumford should be recognized as the founders of a new school of urban thought that recognizes the happiness and wellbeing of city dwellers as the ultimate goal of urban planning. Certainly, improved civic infrastructure can contribute to this happiness and wellbeing, but it must be coupled with recognition of the need for cultural vitality and livability.

The paradigm shift encouraged by Jacobs and Mumford is now pretty much fully endorsed by the modern-day planning community. Most of the academic research labs and private institutes that are mentioned above study and promote the livability of cities, and they do so with a clear recognition of the primary importance of strengthening the social, psychological, and environmental wellbeing of the people who call cities their home. These points were further driven home in the turn-of-the-millennium best-seller by Harvard political scientist Robert Putnam: *Bowling Alone: The Collapse and Revival of American Community* [16]. In his book, Putnam decried the decline in participation in political parties, public meetings, civic organizations, parent-teacher associations, service clubs, and fraternal groups, and highlighted the threat to democracy posed by growing distrust in science and government. The "revival" that he envisages in the book's title is based on strong support for the livability movement, and for people-based solutions to civic ills.

Dimensions and Indicator Variables for the Livability of Cities

Back in Chap. 7 an eight-dimensional structure was developed that has served us well in the discussions on the measurement of happiness and wellbeing at a country-wide scale. Table 7.2 outlined the types of issues that might be considered under each dimension. Chapters 8 and 9 presented detailed coverage of many of the most widely-used single-dimensional and multi-dimensional indexes, and included a full listing of the individual indicator variables for several of them.

The question now arises as to whether the same dimensional structure that was used at a national scale can also serve in the discussion of happiness and wellbeing at city and community scale. The short answer is that it probably could. However, an examination of a wide suite of studies of the livability of cities reveals that many of the contributors in this area tend to highlight more than eight dimensions. In effect, they have promoted some of the sub-dimensions listed in Table 7.2 to full dimensional status. For the purposes of discussion in this chapter, the following set of 12 dimensions are proposed to meet the needs of the civic-scale analyses: Economic Vitality; Education and Learning; Environmental Sustainability; Security and Safety; Mobility and Transportation; Governance and Public Infrastructure; Housing and Urban Planning; Health; Recreation, Arts, Culture, and Amenities; Technology, Industry, and Innovation; People and Community; and Place and Character [17].

Furthermore, and also unlike Chaps. 8 and 9, it is not the intention here to provide repetitive detailed lists of the indicators used in the various indexes and projects discussed in this chapter. Rather, Table 10.1 (on two pages), presents a relatively comprehensive list of the types of indicator variables that are often invoked in these studies. Some of these indicators will be familiar from the earlier nation-scale treatments (like life expectancy, GDP per capita, and violent crime rates); others really only apply at civic or community scale (like proximity of neighborhood schools, voter turnout rates in civic elections, and number of art galleries, museums, and libraries). This chapter will discuss both comparative studies that rank a large number of cities, and more-focused projects designed specifically for one individual city. In both cases, it can be assumed that the indicator variables that are used consist of some subset of those listed in Table 10.1, or at the very least, indicators that are very close in concept and definition to those listed there.

There is a problem that can arise in the application of city-based indexes in areas of urban sprawl. The indicator statistics that are available from geographically-defined civic jurisdictions may not reflect the full availability of cultural, social or economic support that is open to citizens in these types of urban areas. Significant cross-border usage of recreational facilities, regional shopping malls, educational institutes, medical centers, museums and art galleries provide many more options than might appear from counts of facilities in individual jurisdictions. Those assessing the livability of cities and regions must be aware of the complexities of interpreting urban statistics.

Where Do the Data Come From?

The incredible diversity of the indicators listed in Table 10.1 clarifies the need for an equally-diversified set of databases that can be mined to produce the necessary information to feed the calculation procedures of the various city-based indexes. If the developers of each index had to develop their own sources of data, progress on the indexing and ranking of the worlds' cities would probably have ground to a halt long ago. Luckily there are several organizations that have taken on the task of identifying, organizing, listing, and providing links to city-scale datasets. Ruut Veenhoven's World Database of Happiness, which has received much attention in earlier chapters for its country-by-country coverage also provides information on city-scale sources [18]. In the USA, there are at least three programs that provide lists and links for city-scale datasets. The first is the State of the Cities Data System (SOCDS) run by the federal Department of Housing and Urban Development [19]. The second is the Community Indicators Consortium [20]. And the third is the American Community Survey administered by the US Census Bureau, the data from which are published in the Community Facts section of the American Fact Finder website [21]. All three of these sources can be of direct use in locating datasets that are pertinent to the calculation of city-scale indexes.

These meta-data sites also played a role in the development of the more comprehensive listing of data sources in Table A.1 in Appendix to this book. This table, first introduced in earlier chapters with respect to countrywide indexes, will also prove

Table 10.1 Selection of sample city indicators

Economic vitality	**Education and learning**
Per capita GDP	Kindergarten readiness
Average annual wages	Proximity of neighborhood schools
Household income	High-school graduation rate
Household income on mortgage or rent	Per-pupil public school expenditures
Property tax rates	Standardized test scores in math, science, reading
Consumer price index, cost of living	Rates of student truancy/expulsion/dropout
Percent population home owners	Adults with bachelors degree or higher
Percent population living in poverty	Number of colleges and universities in city
Job availability	International students in colleges and universities
Percent population unwillingly unemployed	Number of vocational schools in city
Business-friendly tax and regulatory climate	Availability of workplace education and training
Availability of commercial space	Registered apprenticeships completed
Availability of banking services	Library card holders
Bankruptcy and foreclosure rates	
Health	**Environment and sustainability**
Life expectancy at birth	Air quality, particulate matter
Self-reported health status	Water quality public water supplies
Access to health care	Water quality recreational waters
Number of health professionals per capita	Per capita water consumption
Percent population with health insurance	Per capita energy consumption
Hospital wait times	Percent renewable energy use
Infant mortality rate	CO_2 emissions
Prevalence of illicit drugs	Climate-change readiness
Percent population smokers	Proper waste disposal facilities
Percent population obese	Proper care of brown-field sites
Teen pregnancy rate	Residential recycling programs
Mortality rate due to heart disease	Limitations on pesticide use
Percent adult population with diabetes	Disaster readiness
Percent population with mental health issues	Percent population exposed to noise pollution
Suicide rate	Number and volume of bird species
Number of fitness centers	Ecosystem protection programs
Percent population regular active exercise	
Work/leisure balance	
Security and safety	**Governance and public infrastructure**
Crime severity index, total crime rate	Stable democratic civic government
Violent crime rate	Representativeness and diversity of elected leaders
Property crime rate	Strong citizen input to city planning decisions
Perceptions of gang activity	Regular use of referendums
Annual number of 911 calls	Voter turnout rates in civic elections

(continued)

Table 10.1 (continued)

Prevalence of domestic abuse	Publically-available and transparent city records
Properly funded/staffed law enforcement	Number of civic/neighborhood associations
Percent population feel safe after dark	Participation rate in civic associations
Lighted streets program	Percent population feel can influence public policy
Free from foreign threats and terrorism	Well-managed public services and utilities
Percent population satisfied public safety	Percent population satisfied with public services
Percent population who trust neighbors	
Mobility and transportation	**Housing and urban planning**
Commuting times	Affordable housing
Quality of roads	Ratio of home price to income
Level of traffic congestion	Level of average mortgage debt
Per capita daily miles traveled by car	Percent population home ownership
Extent of public transit system	Rental vacancy rates
Percent workers commuting by public transit	Rate of homelessness
Ride sharing programs	Rate of population growth
Dedicated bus lanes	Vibrant downtown core
Bicycle-friendly city streets	Urban tree canopy
National and international air links	Number and/or area of parks, plazas, greenbelts
Percentage of hybrid vehicles	Walkability
Number of traffic accidents	Appealing streetscapes, flowers, sculptures
Deaths due to traffic accidents	Percent of city area permeable surfaces
	Walk-to-work neighborhoods
	Well-funded urban land-use planning
Recreation, arts, culture, and amenities	**People and community**
Playground accessibility	Positive relationships with friends and family
Sports and fitness facilities	Positive relationships with neighbors
Professional sports teams, stadiums	Sense of community spirit
Youth activity programs	Tolerance for diversity
Number of movie theaters and live music venues	Presence of racism, sexism, bullying
Number of live theaters, performances	Presence of ethnic or religious intolerance
Number of art galleries, museums, and libraries	Level of community volunteerism
Number of heritage sites	Number of linguistically isolated communities
Cultural participation rates	Participation rates in local clubs and societies
Number of non-fast-food restaurants	Participation in church or spiritual groups
Number of major shopping centers	Workplace satisfaction
Technology, industry, and innovation	**Place and character**
Percent population internet participation	Population
Students per computer in public schools	Population density
Enrollment in post-secondary tech programs	Percent population living downtown
International conferences held	Percent seniors, adults, youth, children

(continued)

Table 10.1 (continued)

Number of research labs	Percent single, married, separated
Number of patents granted	Annual days rain and snow
Civic spending on R&D	Annual days >90° and <20°
Tech employment as percent of total employment	Natural beauty of city setting
	Presence of oceans, mountains, lakes
	Distance to camping/hiking wilderness

useful at city scale. The reader is directed there as a reminder of the impressive diversity of organizations that house data that is useful in the calculation of levels of happiness and wellbeing, both subjective and objective, and on both the world stage and in the USA itself. Sources of city-scale data developed for cities in countries other than the USA are not listed in Table A.1, but the reader can rest assured that similar databases to those listed for the USA exist for most of the other developed countries of the world. For Canada, for example, data can be gleaned from Statistics Canada, the Canadian Census, the Canadian General Social Survey, the Canadian Centre for Health Information, Environment Canada, Elections Canada, Parks Canada, Childcare Canada, and specific government-generated surveys on the labor force, household spending, ethnic diversity, living costs, community health, giving patterns, and resident travel.

Some Single-Dimensional City-Scale Indexes

As with the national-scale indexes, it is likely that the reader's interest at city scale lies mainly with multi-dimensional indexes that produce an overall integrated score that takes into account all the various component dimensions of happiness and wellbeing in the urban environment. But, as at national scale, there are many indexes that are scored on the basis of a single urban issue. It is probably safe to say that there are single-dimensional indexes available for each and every one of the 12 civic dimensions that have been identified. Sometimes these indexes are promoted alone; in other cases they form the building blocks for more inclusive indexes. This section briefly reviews four areas where single-dimensional city-scale indexes are widely referenced: economic performance, housing affordability, sense of community, and safety and security.

There are many single-dimensional indexes that track the comparative economic performance of cities. As an example, consider the Milken Institute's annual listings of Best Performing Cities [22]. This Santa Monica-based think tank publishes research findings and hosts conferences that "apply market-based principles and financial innovations to social issues." They offer the Best Performing Cities Index as a way to measure which American metropolitan areas "offer the greatest opportunities for prosperity and innovation." They use statistics on job growth, wage growth, and high-tech GDP growth, to identify tech hubs with attractive business climates and solid economic development strategies. These same metro areas tend to have a highly-educated workforce, and are well-placed to reap the rewards of a modern knowledge-based economy. The most recent ranking of American cities was topped by Provo-Oren UT, followed by two California metro areas (San Jose-Sunnyvale-Santa Clara, and San Francisco-South San Francisco-Redwood City), and two from Texas (Austin-Round Rock, and Dallas-Plano-Irving).

Looking at housing affordability next, one can start by introducing Demographia, a public policy firm that specializes in urban issues. It is based in Belleville, IL, a suburb of the greater St. Louis metropolitan area. The sole owner of Demographia is Wendell Cox, an urban planner who is well-known for his somewhat contrary views on the value of massive investments in public transportation in American cities. He holds fellowships at several conservative think tanks in the USA and Canada, including the Heritage Foundation and the Heartland Institute. Demographia publishes two documents every year that are widely circulated and have proven valuable to urban planners as a source of useful information. The first is the *Demographia World Urban Areas* report, which provides up-to-date data on the urban land areas, population, and population densities of the major cities of the world. The second, and the one that interests us here, is the *Demographia International Housing Affordability Survey* [23].

The results of Demographia's housing affordability survey have been offered annually since 2004. The survey currently covers 406 metropolitan areas in 9 first-world countries: Australia, Canada, Hong Kong, Ireland, Japan, New Zealand, Singapore, the United Kingdom, and the United States. Emphasis is placed on middle-income home affordability, not on the luxury market, or on housing issues in underdeveloped or developing countries.

Results are presented in terms of the "Median Multiple Scale." The median multiple for a given city is defined as the *median house price* divided by the *median household income* for that city. Historically, the value of the multiple median for most cities has been in the range 2.0–3.0, but in recent years it has been rising in most of the cities covered in the survey. Demographia considers values below 3.0 as "affordable," those between 3.1 and 4.0 as "moderately unaffordable," those between 4.1 and 5.0 as "seriously unaffordable," and those above 5.0 as "severely unaffordable." In the 2016 survey, of the 262 US cities covered, 82 were in the affordable category, and 94, 50, and 36 cities, respectively, fell into the 3 unaffordable categories. The most affordable city in America is Racine, WI. The most affordable larger cities (population greater than a million) are Rochester and Buffalo, NY. The least affordable US cities are Santa Cruz and Santa Barbara, CA. On the international front, the three cities with the least affordable housing are Hong Kong, Sydney Australia, and Vancouver Canada.

The data for the study are all taken from easily-accessible public-domain databases. For median house prices, these include real estate data, national sales transaction registries, and other government sources. For median household incomes, the main sources are national census figures. The Demographia website lists 59 sources in all for the 2 types of data for the 9 countries. In Canada, for example, data sources include the Bank of Canada, the Canada Mortgage and Housing Corporation, the Canadian Home Builders Association, the Canadian Real Estate Association, the Conference Board of Canada, Statistics Canada, and the Real Estate Boards for several of the Canadian cities in the study.

The Demographia survey has been criticized by some urban experts because it zeroes in on price and income, and does not include consideration of the financing costs of home purchase. No one ever buys a house outright these days, they argue, so the real issues of housing affordability revolve around interest rates and the availability of mortgage money. Demographia has answered its critics by crediting the simplicity of their index, highlighting the relative difficulty of obtaining credible mortgage information, and pointing out that the multiple-median approach that they use is the one recommended by both the United Nations and the World Bank.

Turning now to the third of the single-dimensional examples, the Sense of Community Index (SCI), is put out by a social research organization based in Gaithersburg MD called Community Science (formerly the Association for the Study and Development of Community) [24]. The CEO of Community Science is a former psychology professor from Rutgers University named David Chavis who was a coauthor of the seminal paper on sense of community published in the Journal of Community Psychology in 1986 [25]. The SCI is now in its second incarnation (SCI-2) and is held to be applicable to communities of any type, whether they be cities, towns, neighborhoods, workplaces, schools, or organizations. The SCI-2 score for a community is based on answers provided by members of the community to a survey, in which the questions are designed to address in equal measure four aspects of a sense of community: (1) the degree of participation by the responder in community affairs, (2) the influence of the community on the responder's life, (3) the fulfillment of the responder's needs provided by the community, and (4) the level of shared emotional connection in the community. Respondents are asked to rate their level of agreement with each of 24 statements (e.g. Being a member of this community makes me feel good) on a 4-point Likert scale (not at all, somewhat, mostly, completely). The answers are awarded values of 0, 1, 2, and 3, so that the final SCI-2 score has a numerical value between [0, 72]. Community Science uses the SCI-2 scores in their work with local governments, NGOs, and foundations, in helping to solve urban social problems through planned community change.

Of all the city-scale dimensions listed in Table 10.1, the one that receives the greatest attention as a stand-alone issue is that of Safety and Security. There are a host of safety and security indexes on the web, each of them ranking the cities of the world from a variety of different perspectives. Three of them will be highlighted here.

The Economist Intelligence Unit's Safe Cities Index is probably the gold standard [26]. It ranks 60 international cities on 4 areas of security using 49 indicators. The four areas are: (1) personal security, (2) cyber security, (3) infrastructure security, and (4) health security. The safest cities in the world in the EIU ranking are almost all in Europe or the Asia-Pacific region (Tokyo, Singapore, Osaka, Toronto, Melbourne, Amsterdam, Sydney, Stockholm, Hong Kong, and Zurich). Toronto is the only North American city to crack the top ten. San Francisco is the highest US city at number 20. The most dangerous cities are Karachi, Jakarta, and Ho Chi Minh City. The EIU rankings are used primarily by business personnel in staffing foreign offices and deciding on appropriate remuneration for those on foreign assignment.

Numbeo is the largest crowd-sourced global database in the world [27]. It publishes statistics on crime, pollution, health care, traffic, and cost of living for 334 international cities. Numbeo publishes a Crime Index with values in the range [0, 100] based on answers to a survey completed by online visitors to the Numbeo website. The Numbeo Safety Index is the inverse of the Crime Index. If the Crime Index for a City is 25, then the Safety Index is 75. According to Numbeo, the five safest cities in the world are Abu Dhabi, Doha (Qatar), Quebec City, Taipei, and Munich. The five most dangerous are Caracas, Port Moresby (New Guinea), San Pedro Sulo (Honduras), and two cities in South Africa (Pretoria and Pietermaritzburg). The Numbeo results are used by the magazine CEOWorld in their World's Safest Cities Rankings [28]. CEOWorld is aimed at an upscale market of "high-level executive professionals, business leaders, and high net-worth individuals." Presumably their interest in safe cities is related to their concerns over far-flung subsidiary offices, global expansion, and international trade.

SafeAround is a website aimed at travelers in the tourism market [29]. The SafeAround team rank 148 cities in the world on their safety and security record, with emphasis on cities that are common tourist destinations. In developing their city scores they use an eclectic set of sources, including other established indexes like the EIU Safe Cities Index and OECD's Better Life Index, websites like Tripadvisor and travel books like the Lonely Planet Guides. Their top-ten safest cities are Andorra, Zurich, Niagara Falls, Vienna, Seoul, Munich, Rhodes, Oslo, Calgary, and Prague. Interestingly, their list of the bottom-ten, least-safe cities in the world includes four US cities (Philadelphia, Memphis, New Orleans and Dallas).

A Selection of Multi-dimensional Composite Indexes on the Livability of Cities

Table 10.2 provides a selection of composite indexes that measure and rank the livability of cities based on a full analysis of multi-dimensional scope. These are the indexes that use some subset of the civic indicators listed in Table 10.1. The actual number of indicators used in the various indexes ranges from 28 to 162. The top four indexes listed on the table cover a large suite of international cities. The next five are limited to cities in the USA. The final three cover cities in the UK and Canada. The number of cities that are covered by the various indexes ranges from 50 to 500. The remainder of this section provides brief comments on each of the indexes listed in Table 10.2. More details can be gleaned from the websites provided on the table for each index. At the end of the section, a summary is presented of the most-livable and least-livable cities as determined from the comparative rankings carried out with these indexes.

Table 10.2 A selection of multi-dimensional composite indexes of livability of cities

Name	No cities	Coverage	Dims	Inds	Website
Economist Intelligence Unit Global Livability Index	140	World	5	30	[www.eiu.com]
Mercer Quality of Living Index	231	World	10	39	[www.mercer.com/qualityofliving]
Innovation Cities Index	500	World	3/31[a]	162	[www.innovation-cities.com]
Numbeo Quality of Life Index	206	World	8	50	[www.numbeo.com/quality-of-life]
WalletHub Best Big Cities to Live In	62	USA	5	56	[www.wallethub.com/edu/best-worst-large-cities-to-live-in]
Resonance Consulting America's Best Cities	100	USA	6	28	[http://resonancecs.com/reports/2019-americas-best-cities]
Sperling's Best Places to Live	331	USA	[b]	[b]	[https://bestplaces.net]
Richard Florida's Place Finder	200+	USA	[b]	[b]	[www.creativeclass.com/_v3/whos_your_city/place_finder]
Sustainable Development Solutions Network	100	USA	16	44	[unsdsn.org]
Happy City Thriving Places Index	372	UK	Jul-27	62	[www.happycity.org.uk]
MoneySense Magazine Best Places to Live	415	Canada	10	39	[www.moneysense.ca]
Conference Board of Canada City Magnets	50	Canada	7	43	[www.conferenceboard.ca]

[a] x/y indicates dims/sub-dims
[b] Proprietary

We have encountered the Economist Intelligence Unit twice before, once in Chap. 9 as the developers of the one-off, country-by-country Quality of Life Index produced in 2005, and again earlier in this chapter as the architects of the Safe Cities Index. Now, at the top of Table 10.2, one finds their highly-regarded and widely-quoted Global Livability Index. It is a city-based index that is structured with 5 dimensions: Stability (with 5 indicators, and 25% weighting), Healthcare (6 indicators, 20%), Education (3 indicators, 10%), Infrastructure (7 indicators, 20%), and Culture and Environment (9 indicators, 25%). Each indicator is given a value between 0 and 100, where zero is "intolerable" and 100 is "ideal," as determined by a combination of qualitative judgments by in-house analysts (26 indicators) or quantitative calculations based on external data sources (4 indicators). The individual scores are then weighted, summed, and converted onto a [0,100] scale to produce a single composite score for each of the 140 cities in the study. In the 2018 analysis, Vienna, Austria, was the highest-ranked city, and Damascus, Syria, the lowest.

Table 10.3 Sectors used in Innovation Cities Index. (Adapted from source material on Innovation Cities website listed in [17])

Architecture, History and Planning	Information, Media and Publishing
Arts and Culture	Labor, Employment and Workforce
Basic Services	Law and Governance
Business	Logistics, Freight and Ports
Commerce and Finance	Military and Defense
Cultural Exchange, Travel and Tourism	Mobility, Autos, Cycling and Transport
Diplomacy and Trade	Music and Performance
Economics	People and Population
Education, Science and Universities	Public Safety
Environment and Nature	Resources, Mining, Oil and Gas
Fashion	Retail Shopping
Food and Hospitality	Spirituality, Religion and Charities
Geography	Sports and Fitness
Government and Politics	Start-Ups and Entrepreneurs
Health and Medicine	Technology and Communications
Industry and Manufacturing	

Continuing down Table 10.2, one encounters the Mercer Quality of Living Index. It is produced by Mercer Human Resources Consulting, a private New-York-based company with an international presence in over 40 countries. Mercer markets their index to governments and multinational corporations who use it to set compensation levels for their internationally-mobile employees. The 39 indicators used in calculating the index are weighted "to reflect their importance to expatriates." The city of New York is assigned a score of 100, and cities under analysis are scored relative to New York City. The 2019 ranking was the 21st annual inventory, and included 231 cities. The highest score (for Vienna, Austria, again) was 108; the lowest (for Baghdad, Iraq) was 14. There were 43 international cities with scores greater than 100, the great majority of them in Europe.

The Innovation Cities Index is produced by 2thinknow, a "city benchmarking agency" based in Melbourne Australia. It measures the "pre-conditions for an innovation economy" in 500 international cities. It classifies cities as *Upstart Cities* (cities moving toward being globally competitive), *Node Cities* (globally competitive cities), *Hub Cities* (challenger cities, innovating in key segments of the economy), and *Nexus Cities* (cities in the top few percent of global innovation). The index is calculated using 162 indicators in 31 sectors, grouped under 3 over-riding dimensions (Cultural Assets, Human Infrastructure, and Networked Markets). These 31 sectors provide such an all-encompassing portrayal of the character of a city that they bear detailed listing in Table 10.3. Sydney, Australia, leads the innovation parade. Kinshasa, in the Democratic Republic of the Congo ranks last.

The Numbeo crowd-sourcing website mentioned earlier as the home of the Numbeo Safety Index also features a more-encompassing livability index known as the Numbeo Quality of Life Index. It uses 50 indicators to rank 206 cities, based on data provided primarily by users of the Numbeo website. The Numbeo results are also cited by Deutsche Bank in their widely-circulated Livability Survey, although they are accompanied by the disclaimer that the Numbeo rankings are "not the definitive guide on the matter but a good starting point for debate." [30]. The highest-ranked city in the Numbeo index is Canberra, Australia, the lowest, Caracas, Venezuela.

Turning now to the five livability indexes in Table 10.2 that are limited to American cities, one notes that the first four of them are all produced by private companies with methodologies that are largely proprietary. WalletHub is a personal finance website owned by Evolution Finance Inc. It uses 56 indicators, all based on data taken from publically-available databases, to arrive at its ranking of the Best Big Cities to Live In. The analysis is structured under 5 dimensions: Affordability (5 indicators), Economy (12 indicators), Safety (4 indicators), Quality of Life (24 indicators), and Education and Health (11 indicators). The Quality of Life dimension includes consideration of such diverse issues as public transport, traffic congestion, walkability, shopping, playgrounds, restaurants, music venues, fitness centers, sports facilities, museums, beaches, weather, and air quality. The city of Virginia Beach VA tops the WalletHub list, Detroit MI is at the bottom.

Resonance Consulting uses "business strategy and marketing creativity" to advise city authorities on real estate, tourism, and economic development. Its ranking of America's Best Cities is carried out on the basis of 6 Key Categories (Place, Product, Programming, People, Prosperity, and Promotion), using 28 indicators that are determined largely from online ratings and reviews (such as Trip Advisor, Google searches, and Facebook check-ins). Two sets of rankings are provided, one for "large" cities (population greater than one million) and one for "small" cities (population less than one million). New York tops the list of large cities, Honolulu the small-cities.

Sperling's Best-Places-to-Live rankings are the brainchild of author and researcher Bert Sperling of Portland OR. They are designed to help those folks who are planning a move to find their perfect urban match [31]. His website is interactive, allowing prospective relocators to take a Best Places Quiz and to carry out comparative analyses of competing cities. The site also offers a Best Places App which allows users to build their own list of best cities to their own specifications. One can generate lists that identify cities that are energetic, romantic, or green, or on the flip side, those most prone to stress, respiratory infections, or cybercrime. There is even a Best Places Board Game. In addition to his Best Places to Live, Sperling also presents listings of the Best Cities to Retire, Best Cities for Singles, Best Places to Raise Your Family, Safest Places from Natural Disasters, Best Baseball Cities, and somewhat tongue-in-cheek, America's Manliest Cities. Also tongue-in-cheek is his "adult-themed" list of American cities with "quirky, weird, bizarre, or unusual" names, which includes Buttzville NJ, Intercourse PA, and Weed CA.

Richard Florida is an economic geographer now at the University of Toronto and the author of the best-selling book "Who's Your City: How the Creative Economy is Making Where You Live the Most Important Decision of Your Life." His book is designed to help young professionals pick the best locations to live and work "to match their personalities and aspirations." [32]. He provides lists of Best Cities that are categorized by lifestyle (Young Singles, Mid-Career Professionals, Gays and Lesbians, Empty Nesters, Retirees, and Families with Children). His indicators tend to be catchy and trendy. For his Best Cities for Families with Children, for example, one of his indicators is the Trick-or-Treat Index which is defined as how far from home parents are willing to allow their children to go door-to-door for Halloween treats. For his online presence, he provides a Place Finder which allows interactive comparisons of American cities on over 20 factors. For young singles he identifies San Francisco CA, Madison WI, and Boulder CO as the best American cities in each of three size ranges (large, medium, and small); for mid-career professionals, San Jose CA, Bridgeport CN, and Durham NC; and for retirees, San Francisco, Bridgeport, and Santa Barbara CA.

The Sustainable Development Solutions Network (SDSN) is a United-Nations-sponsored international agency based in New York and Paris. The *raison d'etre* of SDSN is to assess various jurisdictions around the world as to how well they are performing with respect to the United Nations' Sustainable Development Goals (SDGs). Hopefully the reader will recall earlier discussions of the 17 SDGs back in Chap. 4 and the listing of them in Table 4.3. (No Poverty. Zero Hunger. Good Health and Well-being. Quality Education. And so on.) The US branch of SDSN has taken on the task of ranking the 100 most-populous metropolitan areas in the country on their SDG performance. They do so using 44 indicators spread across 15 of the 17 SDG goals. (Data are insufficient to assess the other two.) Scores for each indicator are scaled from [0, 100] where zero implies no progress toward the goal in question, and 100 is defined as an "ambitious aspirational target." Data are obtained from a large suite of publically-available databases. Findings indicate that the best-performing cities have achieved over 65% compliance, while over two-thirds of large American cities still languish below 50%. The top metropolitan area in the SDSN analysis is San Jose-Sunnyvale-Santa Clara CA, the worst performance is that of New Orleans LA [33].

The Happy City Initiative is a British NGO based in Bristol, England, that develops wellbeing tools for use by municipal authorities. Their Happiness Pulse is based on input to a survey from individual responders. Their Thriving Places Index, which is listed in Table 10.2, analyses conditions for wellbeing at the community level. Their 2019 report provides results for 373 cities, towns, and "rural councils" in England and Wales [34]. The index is structured on a 4-level scheme (3 "headlines," 7 "domains," 27 sub-domains, and 62 indicators). Raw indicator data are gathered from national-agency datasets, standardized to mean zero and standard deviation one, capped on either end at +/− five standard deviations, and scaled onto a [0, 10] scoring range. Indicators are averaged over their sub-domains and domains, but left as a threefold score with respect to the three "headlines" (Local Conditions, Sustainability, and Equality). The highest ranking communities, taking all three elements into account (but not integrating them into a single score), are Devon, Kingston Upon Thames, and Bath.

The first of two Canadian rankings listed in Table 10.2 is published by MoneySense magazine based on an analysis carried out by Environics Analytics.

The ranking of 415 Canadian cities and towns is carried out with 10 dimensions using 39 indicators. Data are from publically-accessible sources like Statistics Canada, Environment Canada, and the Canada Revenue Agency. In keeping with the name of the magazine, the indicators are strongly weighted toward affordability, taxes, wealth, and economy. Results indicate that 25 of the top 50 cities are in Ontario, 11 in Alberta, 10 in Quebec, and only 4 in the remaining 7 provinces.

The Conference Board of Canada is "Canada's foremost evidence-based applied research organization." A 2014 report benchmarked the attractiveness of 50 Canadian cities to potential residents [35]. Their analysis used a seven-dimensional structure with a balanced suite of several indicators per dimension. The top five cities in the CBC ranking are Waterloo ON, Calgary AB, Ottawa ON, Richmond Hill ON, and Vancouver BC.

There are many other analyses and indexes of city livability that are not listed in Table 10.2. A recent paper critically evaluates a more encompassing suite of 26 such models [36].

Summary of City Rankings

Table 10.4 provides a summary of the top-ten and bottom-ten cities from seven of the multidimensional urban analyses discussed above. The first four columns present the results for indexes with international coverage; the final three columns for indexes limited to cities in the USA.

There are several cities that appear on more than one of the top-ten international lists in Table 10.4. They include Vienna Austria, Zurich Switzerland, Tokyo Japan, Copenhagen Denmark, Toronto and Vancouver Canada, and Sydney and Adelaide Australia, all of them large cosmopolitan cities in first-world countries in beautiful natural settings. There are no American cities on the EIU or Mercer top-ten listings, but several appear on the Innovation Cities Index, which places high value on technological capabilities, and on the Numbeo Index, which may reflect wider participation on crowd-sourcing websites by American respondents relative to those from Europe. The bottom-ten listings are populated with cities from the developing world that are rife with poverty, instability, and diminished choices. The countries that are represented (Senegal, Nigeria, Chad, South Sudan, Yemen, Syria, and Bangladesh, for example) mirror those that populated the bottom-ten lists in the country-wide analyses reported in Table 9.6 back in Chap. 9.

The listings for the 3 US-based indexes do not show much consistency, in large part due to the difference in coverage of the 3 listings (from 62 "big cities" in the WalletHub analysis, to over 300 cities of widely-divergent sizes in the Sperling analysis). Apart from Atlanta, most of the cities that are highlighted in Sperling's top-ten ranking are small-to-mid-sized cities that are not included in either the Wallethub or SDSN analyses. Despite these distinctions, three west-coast cities (Seattle, San Jose and San Francisco) make multiple appearances on the three

Table 10.4 Summary of city rankings from multi-dimensional composite indexes of urban wellbeing

Index	EIU Global Livability Index	Mercer Quality of Living Index	Innovation Cities Index	Numbeo Quality of Life Index	WalletHub Best Big Cities	Sperling's Best Places	Sustainable Development Solutions Network
Coverage	World	World	World	World	USA	USA	USA
Cities	140	231	500	206	62	331	100
Top Ten	Vienna	Vienna	Tokyo	Canberra	Virginia Beach	Charlottesville	San Jose
	Melbourne	Zurich	London	Raleigh	Austin	Santa Fe	Seattle
	Osaka	Vancouver	San Francisco	Adelaide	Seattle	San Luis Obispo	Boston
	Calgary	Munich	New York	Madison	San Diego	Santa Barbara	San Francisco
	Sydney	Auckland	Los Angeles	Wellington	Las Vegas	Honolulu	Madison
	Vancouver	Dusseldorf	Singapore	Zurich	San Francisco	Ann Arbor	Manchester
	Tokyo	Frankfurt	Berlin	Brisbane	New York	Atlanta	Albany
	Toronto	Copenhagen	Toronto	Eindhoven	San Jose	Asheville	Bridgeport
	Copenhagen	Geneva	Paris	Austin	Honolulu	Reno	Oxnard
	Adelaide	Basel	Sydney	Dallas	Portland	Corvallis	Provo
Bottom Ten	Dakar	Conakry	Simferopol	Rio de Janeiro	Albuquerque	Fort Smith	Tulsa
	Algiers	Kinshasa	Luanda	Jakarta	Fresno	Anniston	Lakeland
	Douala	Brazzaville	Dar es Salaam	Ho C M City	New Orleans	Gadsden	Memphis
	Tripoli	Damascus	Addis Ababa	Mumbai	Indianapolis	Pine Bluff	Houston
	Harare	N'Djamena	Dakar	Beijing	Milwaukee	Lawrence	Cleveland
	Port Moresby	Khartoum	Port Harcourt	Dhaka	St Louis	Kankakee	Jackson
	Karachi	Port au Prince	Duala	Tehran	Baltimore	Merced	Indianapolis
	Lagos	Sana'a	Dushanbe	Manila	Cleveland	Newburgh	Bakersfield
	Dhaka	Bangui	Khartoum	Lagos	Memphis	Stockton	Baton Rouge
	Damascus	Baghdad	Kinshasa	Caracas	Detroit	Laredo	New Orleans
Year	2018	2019	2018	2019	2019	2019	2018

top-ten lists. In the bottom-ten listings, several cities appear more than once (New Orleans, Indianapolis, Cleveland and Memphis).

City Ranking Skeptics

There is no question that there is a large subjective component in these city rankings. Results are impacted and skewed by the selection of dimensions and indicators, by the datasets that are mined, by the weightings that are used, by the purposes for which the rankings are carried out, and by the limitations introduced by the different levels of coverage. If direct evidence is needed of the somewhat intangible nature of the game, consider the case of Albuquerque NM, which has the peculiar distinction of making both a top-ten list (the Resonance Consulting Rankings) and a bottom-ten list (the WalletHub analysis).

It is also clear that the issues of cultural bias and changing mores that were discussed with respect to national rankings in Chap. 9 could also be important in the city rankings presented in this chapter.

Adam Okulicz-Kozaryn of Rutgers University has written two papers that raise the question of whether city rankings that are based on objective datasets match up well with data from life satisfaction surveys [37]. A comparison of the Mercer city rankings with subjective wellbeing scores for a suite of European cities showed only a weak correlation (correlation coefficient = 0.4). He identified many cities like Belfast Ireland that are "unlivable" but "happy" (which he dubbed "fool's paradise"), and others like Paris France that are "livable" but "unhappy" ("fool's hell").

Meg Holden of Simon Fraser University in Vancouver Canada and Andy Scerri of the Global Cities Research Institute in Melbourne Australia use the friendly rivalry of Vancouver and Melbourne (which at one point traded places as top dog in the EIU Global Livability Index) to question the relevance of these livable-city indexes [38]. While they acknowledge that such rankings may describe the urban conditions of life for the "luckily-satisfied few" (those who actually get to experience a city's vaunted livability), they question whether such indexes have much meaning to the disadvantaged members of a community who cannot even meet their daily needs let alone experience the livable city. They accuse such efforts of creating a self-fulfilling prophecy, "one that sets its own measures of success while casting failure simply as failing to live up to the measures set by the prophecy itself." They decry the absence in most civic indexes of a sufficient emphasis on social equity, which they see as the primary "big-picture" issue facing cities today and into the future.

The strongest attack on city rankings comes in a widely-quoted article in Forbes Magazine by Joel Kotkin, a professor of Urban Studies at Chapman University in Orange, California, entitled "Why the Livable Cities Rankings are Wrong." [39]. He argues that the choice of indicators in most index calculations favors "compact cities in prosperous regions; well-manicured older European cities with lovely facades and ample parks; and wealthy cities with a limited underclass." All this peace and quiet, he says, is very nice, but hardly the measure of true urban vitality. These "most-livable" cities generally have high taxes and are among the most-expensive places to live on the planet. The average person who is trying to make a little money and improve his or her status in life is unlikely to settle in one of them. Better for them is one of the new-world metropolises with all their cultural diversity, bustle and chaos, their "yeasty confrontations" and social dynamics. Think about the great cities in history, Kotkin argues, like ancient Rome, or Islamic Baghdad, or nineteenth-century London, or twentieth-century New York. These are the cities that drove global culture and commerce. The livable-city rankings may be useful for "corporate executives, academics, or urban researchers," he says, but they don't reflect the messy complexities of the truly livable city.

The Community Indicator Movement

Most cities now host a publically-accessible website that provides a data-rich portal into living conditions within their jurisdiction. Data are usually presented first on a city-wide basis, and are then broken down by districts or neighborhoods. Information is provided for a wide suite of indicator variables, generally grouped under a set of overarching dimensions, targets, or goals. Most of these sites are information rich, but also pleasing to the eye, making use of the latest tricks of graphic design, with colorful, often-interactive, graphs and maps. Most of them offer some analysis of the data, clarification of year-to-year trends, correlations with demographic factors, comparisons with other jurisdictions, and an assessment of the degree to which civic targets and goals have been met. They are a source of valuable insight for city planners, corporate decision makers, civic politicians, and the public at large.

There are at least three national organizations that help to develop these community indicator projects, and then provide a link to them from their own websites. The largest of these is the Community Indicators Consortium (CIC) based in Issaquah, WA, which has been in business since 2005 [40]. Its sponsoring partners include the Organization for Economic Cooperation and Development (OECD), the Rutgers University School of Public Affairs and Administration, and the federally-funded program on the State of the USA. The CIC produces a Community Indicators Development Guide, training webinars on the use of community indicators, and a registry of state and national sources of civic information. They also host an annual Community Indicators Impact Summit to bring together interested parties from across the country, at which they hand out one or more Impact Awards for "projects that demonstrate the power of community indicators to drive positive community change." Their website lists 298 "partners" and provides links to 31 foreign indicator projects and 162 such projects in the USA (20 at state level, 73 for counties or other regional jurisdictions, and 69 for cities).

The National Neighborhood Indicators Partnership (NNIP) is even older than the CIC having launched in 1996. It is hosted by the Urban Institute, a non-profit research organization based in Washington, DC, that describes its staff as "truth seekers, problem solvers, and strategic advisors." They hope to lead cities to make "decisions based on facts rather than ideology." The NNIP website provides links to 31 partner cities, a list that includes most of the major metropolitan areas in the US. They also provide a link to a guidebook for building and operating neighborhood indicator systems [41].

The third organization that provides a central clearinghouse for community indicator projects is the Institute for Innovation and Social Policy (IISP) at Vassar College in Poughkeepsie NY [42]. This is the same group, led by Marque-Luisa Miringoff, that produces the Index of Social Health which was highlighted back in Chap. 8. The IISP was established in 1985, well before either the CIC or the NNIP, but now appears to be less active than the other two. Most of the city indicator projects linked through the IISP can also be reached through the CIC or the NNIP websites.

A Roster of City-Based Community Indicator Projects

Table 10.5 provides a listing of 20 large-city community indicator projects from the USA, and 4 from Canada. All of them are website-based, publically-available, and user-friendly. Some have traditional names like the Boston Indicators site or the Albuquerque Progress Report. Others use catchier titles like Atlanta's Neighborhood Nexus, the Portland Pulse, New Haven's DataHaven, and Milwaukee's Data You Can Use. All of them provide multiple datasets for a variety of civic indicator variables, usually organized under an umbrella of dimensional headings, and usually specified on a neighborhood-by-neighborhood basis. Tables, graphs, and interactive maps abound. Some of the sites with large numbers of available datasets, like Boston's (with 285 indicators) and Atlanta's (with 400+) further organize their presentations by using sub-dimensional headings (as noted in Table 10.5: 75 in Boston's case, 64 in Atlanta's). Two of the sites listed in Table 10.5 (the New Orleans Prosperity Index, and the Santa Monica Wellbeing Index) perhaps imply the calculation of a single-valued overall measure of livability in their cities, but this is not the case. Like the other websites in Table 10.5, they produce great swaths of useful information, organized in the form of dashboards and scorecards, but not a single-valued overall index.

The granddaddy of civic indicator projects is the one listed in Table 10.5 for Jacksonville, Florida. It started in 1985 under the auspices of the Jacksonville Community Council Inc. (JCCI), a civic engagement group that was launched in 1974, but traces its history back to 1883 when the citizens of Jacksonville formed a committee to confront a smallpox epidemic. The JCCI has already been introduced back in Table 7.4 in Chap. 7 where their guidelines were presented for the selection of indicator variables. Using these guidelines, the JCCI set up a dashboard of 27 indicators grouped under 9 dimensions. The dimensions were cast as goals (Achieving Educational Excellence, Growing a Vibrant Economy, Moving Around Efficiently and Safely, Keeping the Community Safe, Promoting Social Well-Being,

Table 10.5 A selection of community indicator projects

City Indicator Project	Dims	Inds	Website
Albuquerque Progress Report	8	59	[http://abqprogressreport.sks.com]
Atlanta Neighborhood Nexus	5/64	400+	[www.neighborhoodnexus.org]
Baltimore Vital Signs	8	138	[www.bniajfi.org/vital_signs]
Boston Indicators	Oct-75	285	[www.bostonindicators.org]
Charlotte-Mecklinburg Quality of Life Explorer	9	80	[www.mcmap.org/qol]
Denver Community Facts	Not specified	92	[www.denvermetrodata.org]
Data Driven Detroit	10	210	[www.datadrivendetroit.org]
Houston Community Data Connections	8	57	[www.datahouston.org]
Indianapolis Social Assets and Vulnerabilities Indicators	9	52	[www.savi.org]
Jacksonville Community Council Quality of Life Progress Report	10	58	[www.jaxpact.org]
Kansas City Metro Dataline	7	24	[gis2.marc2.org/metrodataline]
Milwaukee Data You Can Use	4	19	[www.datayoucanuse.org]
New Haven DataHaven	10	50	[www.ctdatahaven.org]
New Orleans Prosperity Index	6	19	[s3.amazonaws.com/gnocdc/reports/ProsperityIndex.pdf]
New York City Social Indicators Report	9	51	[www1.nyc.gov/assets/operations/downloads/pdf/Social-Indicators-Report-April-2016.pdf]
Pittsburg Today	11	66	[www.pittsburgquarterly.com/pittsburgtoday]
Portland Pulse	12	45	[www.portlandpulse.org]
San Antonio SA2020	11	61	[www.sa2020.org]
San Francisco Bay Area Vital Signs	5	41	[www.vitalsigns.mtc.ca.gov]
Santa Monica Wellbeing Index	6	42	[www.wellbeing.smgov.net]
Calgary Vital Signs	5	17	[www.calgaryfoundation.org/initiatives/vitalsigns]
Edmonton Citizen Dashboard	6	66	[www.dashboard.edmonton.ca]
Montreal Vital Signs	4/13	73	[www.fgmtl.org/en/signesvitaux_arch.php]
Vancouver Vital Signs	12	44	[www.vancouverfoundation.bc.ca]

Preserving the Natural Environment, Sustaining a Healthy Community, Maintaining Responsive Government, and Enjoying Arts, Culture, and Recreation), and every year for over 30 years each indicator was judged in light of these goals and identified as Getting Better, Getting Worse, or Staying the Same. In 2016, the JCCI was disbanded and replaced by a multi-organization Citizen Engagement PACT. The PACT has updated the civic indicators project with a new website, a new set of

10 dimensions, and an expanded set of 58 indicators. In addition to the objective indicators based on hard data from the original formulation, the new dashboard includes the subjective results of several questions asked on civic surveys. (e.g. Do you feel safe in your neighborhood? Do you feel you can have influence on local government? Are you satisfied with the quality of your elected leaders? Do you volunteer? Are you satisfied with your health insurance? Do you engage in recreational activities on the river?) The identification of year-to-year trends as Better, Worse, or the Same, is continued. The Quality of Life reports which have had such significance in the history of the indicators movement continue to be produced by one of the lead sponsors of the new PACT, the United Way of Southeast Florida [43].

The San Antonio 2020 project listed in Table 10.5 also charts year-to-year progress for its 61 indicators. Targets for each indicator are identified as Met and Exceeded, On Track, Showing Progress, Flat, or Getting Worse. Graphic results are displayed using the website's "viz-a-lyzer."

The Albuquerque Progress Report differs from most other indicator projects in that it provides a comparison of Albuquerque's livability progress with that of five other comparable southwestern cities (Colorado Springs, El Paso, Oklahoma City, Tucson, and Salt Lake City).

Some of the indicator projects have more specific goals than just charting annual gains and losses. The New Orleans Prosperity Index is specifically targeted on the city's recovery from the ravages of Hurricane Katrina, and with the success or failure of this recovery experienced by the different racial groups and ethnicities in the Greater New Orleans region.

Regional and Statewide Indicator Projects

Many indicator projects are designed to cover areas that are much larger than neighborhoods, or individual towns and cities. They are often developed by metropolitan planning authorities that have multi-city or multiple-county jurisdiction with respect to regional growth and land-use planning. Three of the most-highly-regarded regional projects will serve as examples here: the Long Island Index, the Silicon Valley Index, and the Cascadia Scorecard. All three provide (or have provided in the past) a similar public service to the city indicator projects, but for a larger region of interest [44].

The Long Island Index (LII) functioned from 2004 to 2018. It included data for 2 cities, 13 towns, and 95 villages in Nassau and Suffolk Counties on Long Island, New York. These municipalities have a total population of almost three million people. The LII was organized under 5 dimensions (Economy, Communities, Health and Education, Environment, and Governance), which were further subdivided into 12 sub-dimensions expressed in the form of goals (Vibrant Communities, Affordable Homes, Natural Resource Conservation, and so on). It is now in the process of transitioning into a new and improved "digital toolbox" to be known as nextLI.

Table 10.6 Cascadia Scorecard, 2007. (Adapted from source material on Sightline website in [44])

Dimension	Indicator	Target	Source of target	Cascadia score	Years to reach target
Health	Life expectancy at birth (years)	81.3 years	Japan	79.5 years	11
Population	Total fertility rate (births per woman)	1.7 births	Netherlands, Sweden	1.8 births	12
Energy	Per capita use of fuel for highway driving (gal/week)	7.4 gal/week	Germany	14.5 gal/week	91
Wildlife	Population of 5 key indicator species as percent of historic abundance	43%	None specified	18%	69
Sprawl	Percent of metropolitan area residents in compact transit-friendly neighborhoods	62%	Vancouver	33%	57
Economy	Composite index of unemployment rate, median income, and poverty rate	108.6	Some US states	100.2	20
Pollution	Median concentrations of PBDEs and PCBs in breastmilk (ppb)	1.3 ppb PBDEs[a] 5.1 ppb PCBs[a]	None specified	50 ppb 134 ppb	Unknown

[a] *PBDEs* polybrominated diphenyl ethers, *PCBs* polychlorinated biphenyls

The Silicon Valley Index covers the technological heartland that runs from San Francisco down to San Jose, CA. The data on its website come from 39 separate municipal jurisdictions. It has been administered by the Silicon Valley Institute for Regional Studies since it was launched in 1995. It features 5 dimensions, 17 sub-dimensions, and 93 indicators.

One of the most original regional indicator projects is the Cascadia Scorecard, which apparently (and unfortunately) disappeared from the scene back in 2007. It was put out by the Sightline Institute, a non-profit, non-partisan research center in Seattle, WA. The Scorecard was based on data from a large swath of the Pacific Northwest that encompassed the Canadian province of British Columbia, the American states of Washington, Oregon, and Idaho, and parts of Alaska, California and Montana. As outlined in Table 10.6, the Scorecard was based on a 7-dimensional dashboard with just one representative indicator for each dimension. *Health* was represented by life expectancy at birth; *Population* by the fertility rate; *Energy* by the per-capita use of fuel; *Wildlife* by the populations of five key indicator species as a percent of historic abundance; and *Sprawl* by the percent of metropolitan-area residents in "compact transit-friendly neighborhoods." The final two dimensions were also defined by just one indicator, but that indicator was a compound calculation of sorts. *Economy* was represented by a composite index that included the unemployment rate, median income, and poverty rate. *Pollution* was based on the median concentration of two toxic chemical groups (PBDEs and PCBs) in breast milk.

The designers of the Cascadia Scorecard then took the highly original step of defining a target for each indicator, one that they held to be achievable, because it was based on values that had already been achieved in other worldwide jurisdictions. As indicated on the two right-hand columns of Table 10.6, the Cascadia score determined from an analysis of the available data was then compared with the target, and an estimate was made of the number of years it would take to reach the specified target, given current trends and assuming the feasibility of bringing online a viable suite of policy interventions that would lead in the right direction.

Most American states also maintain websites that allow public access to statewide datasets of interest to wellbeing researchers. As examples, and to give a flavor of the titles that are used to identify these sites, consider the Connecticut Data Collaborative, Delaware Focus, Georgia Community Indicators, Hawaii Quality of Life, Indicators Idaho, Stats Indiana, Maine Measures of Growth, Minnesota Compass, Ohio Social Indicators, Oregon Benchmarks, South Dakota Dashboard, Virginia Performs, and the Utah Community Data Program.

The Smart Cities Movement

The past few decades have seen an exponential growth in information and communication technology (ICT). The world has become "connected" to a degree that was unimaginable just a few years ago. This connectedness has been fueled by technical advances in digital technology, lower costs of computing, the increased availability of digital storage, advances in data analytics, and the growth of the so-called "knowledge economy." Accessibility to the ICT world takes place by means of an ever-increasing suite of electronic devices that are controlled through direct links to the Internet: computers, cell phones, GPS devices, fitness trackers, heart monitors, security cameras, thermostats, appliances, home security systems, drones, fiber-optic networks, and so on; the so-called Internet of Things (IoT) [45]. It is thought that connected devices now outnumber people worldwide. It has been estimated that their number will reach 40 billion by 2025, and the market for such devices and their support could reach $2.5 trillion [46].

Smart cities are so called because they tap into the ICT world using many different types of IoT sensors to collect and analyze a vast array of data that can be used to manage a city's assets, resources and services in an efficient manner [47]. Applications of digital technology abound in many areas of urban governance: transportation grids, water supply networks, waste management systems, energy utilities, healthcare delivery, policing and crime prevention, community services, information systems, citizen interaction, and numerous other aspects of city infrastructure. Specific apps have been designed to optimize such nitty-gritty urban tasks as scheduling bus routes, controlling garbage collection and recycling programs, siting electric-vehicle charging stations, optimizing traffic lights, providing "smart" street lighting, controlling irrigation systems in city parks, enhancing traffic ticket collection, automating heat and lighting systems in public buildings, and providing online parking information.

The smart cities movement has fostered its own subculture for the benefit of urban administrators. There are academic centers of excellence like the MIT Smart Cities Lab, the Boston University Center for Information and Systems Engineering, and the IGLUS program (Innovative Governance of Large Urban Systems) at the Ecole Polytechnique Federale in Lausanne Switzerland. There are specialty journals such as the *Journal of Urban Technology*, which actually began publication back in 1992 on a broader front, but now caters largely to the smart cities movement, and the online journal *Smart Cities* launched in 2018 by the Multidisciplinary Digital Publishing Institute in Basel Switzerland. The UK Institution of Engineering and Technology has recently opened a Smart Cities Digital Library [48]. The US National Science Foundation set aside $60 million for a Smart Cities Initiative. Another US federal agency, the Network and Information Technology Research and Development Program (NITRD), has published the *Federal Smart Cities and Communities Programs Resources Guide* [49]. In 2015 the US Department of Transportation issued its Smart Cities Challenge which eventually led to a $50 million grant to the winning entrant, Columbus Ohio [50]. A London-based blog entitled Smart Cities World "provides a centralized source of intelligence about the infrastructure required to create a smart city." It also provides smart city profiles for a large number of the world's major cities, and a webinair called "*Smart Cities: Beyond the Hype.*" [51]. The Smart Cities Council is a network of private consulting companies that provide "trusted, neutral advice" to city managers. They do so in part through their Smart Cities Activator, "an online collaborative platform for the discovery of a city's needs, assets, and stakeholders," and their Readiness Guides "to help make a city smart." [52]. One of Google's so-called Alphabet companies is Sidewalk Labs which "imagines, designs, tests, and builds urban innovations to help cities meet their biggest challenges." [53]. All of these various groups undoubtedly sent representatives to take part in the Smart City Expo World Congress held in Barcelona Spain in November 2019. The Congress was attended by 21,000 participants representing 844 global organizations and companies. The stated goals of the congress were to "empower cities and collective urban innovation across the globe … and create a better future for cities and their citizens worldwide." [54].

It will probably come as no surprise to readers that there are indexes available to rate municipal jurisdictions on their level of "smartness." A recent article reviews several of them [55]. One of the leading examples is the Smart City Index put out under joint sponsorship of the International Institute for Management Development in Lausanne Switzerland and the Singapore University of Technology and Design [56]. It emphasizes the "technological provisions and services available to inhabitants" in five key areas: Governance, Activities, Mobility, Opportunities at Work and School, and Health and Safety. Rankings of cities are based on citizen polls in which responders are asked to agree or disagree with 18 positive statements about their city and its use of smart technology. Under the Governance heading, for example, there are four such statements: (1) Online public access to city finances has reduced corruption; (2) Online voting has increased participation; (3) An online platform where residents can propose ideas has improved city life; and (4) Processing documents online has reduced waiting times. Similar statements appear for the other four key areas. Respondents are also asked to agree or disagree with three general statements that register their attitude toward civic technology: (1) You are willing to concede personal data in order to improve traffic congestion; (2) You are comfortable with face recognition technologies to lower crime; and (3) You feel the availability of online information has increased your trust in authorities. On these bases the Smart City Index has been used to rank 102 major cities of the world. Despite the difference in emphasis of this index relative to those reported in Table 10.4, the usual suspects appear at the top and bottom of the list: Singapore, Zurich, Oslo, Geneva and Copenhagen at the top; Bogota, Cairo, Nairobi, Rabat, and Lagos at the bottom. It appears that livable cities tend to be smart and vice-versa.

The question still arises as to whether smart cities really lead to increased happiness and wellbeing for the folks that live there. Are smart-city systems truly advantageous to citizens, or just to city administrators?

Not all urban experts are enamored of the smart city concept. One of them, writing in *The Guardian* in 2012, complained that smart cities are too-planned, and that they "deaden and stupefy the people who live in their all-efficient embrace." [57]. Another, in a contribution to the online journal *Places*, argued that "a city is not a computer," that it is much more than "an apparatus for record keeping and information management." Furthermore, a city has history, and memory, and "happenstance." One can feel it in the "sign of wear on a well-trodden staircase, or the creaks in a battered bridge." [58]. More specific objections have been raised by the Internet Society and the World Economic Forum (WEF), who zero in on security issues, the vulnerability to cyber attack, questions of citizen privacy under possible over-surveillance by municipal authorities, and the proper balance between law enforcement and civil rights [59]. At the Osaka Summit in 2019, the G20 countries established a Global Smart Cities Alliance to establish standards of use for the implementation of smart technology, with special focus on promoting transparency, privacy and security [60]. Others worry about a possible lack of inclusivity for citizens with disabilities. On this front, the UN launched a Global Initiative for Inclusive ICT (G3ICT) in 2006 with one of its goals being the elimination of the "digital divide for persons with disabilities and older persons in smart cities around the world." One of the lynchpins of the G3ICT program is a Smart-Cities-for-All-Toolkit designed to help cities focus on ICT accessibility [61].

Having noted all these caveats, the overwhelming conclusion of most urban experts is that smart cities are a boon to the man on the street. It is felt that issues of privacy, security and inclusivity are solvable. In addition, many cities now make available smart-cards that allow citizens to tap directly into municipal services, a feature that should reduce the bureaucratic snafus that so bedevil municipal administrations. It is an unquestioned tenet of the smart-cities movement that the "smart" approach to city management has the potential to reduce costs, reduce taxes, reduce energy consumption, enhance the quality of city services, and improve the life of a city's citizens. According to one blog: "Smart cities are more than a trend. They are the wave of the future. They improve and impact people's lives. Period. End of story." [62].

Happy Cities

The connection between "smart" cities and "happy" cities has been tackled directly by Charles Montgomery in his book *Happy City: Transforming Our Lives through Urban Design* [63]. His book is the first to explore the intersection between urban design and the new happiness studies. He and many others draw particular attention to the value of green spaces, pleasing streetscapes, and walkable downtowns. Adrienne Brown, a Vancouver landscape architect sings the praises of "civil spaces": the country lane, the front porch, grassy knolls, cloisters, central plazas, fountains, medians, parks with shade trees, sculpture parks, walking paths, cycling lanes, and pedestrian malls [64]. Eric Klinenberg, a professor at New York University points out that it is in shared spaces like libraries, child-care centers, churches, and parks where critical connections are made, and that such social infrastructure helps fight "inequality, polarization, and a decline in civic life." [65]. Another recent article defines these non-home, non-work environments as "third places" and touts their importance in enhancing "social sustainability." [66].

The reader may recall references to the World Happiness Reports in earlier chapters. The publisher of those reports, the Sustainable Development Solutions Network, also produces a series of companion pieces known as the Global Happiness and Well-Being Policy Reports [67]. The 2018 report includes a chapter on "Happy Cities in a Smart World," and the 2019 version a chapter titled "A Happy Cities Agenda." Both these chapters differentiate between the *design* of happy cities and the *enablers* of citizen happiness. Design involves tangible, action-oriented interventions in city governance. The enablers of happiness are the intangible policy outcomes that result from the interventions. Design interventions night include any of the practical steps suggested earlier in this section, things like bike lanes, citizen-services platforms, cultural hotspots, walkable downtowns, well-lit public spaces, green areas, and health and fitness programs. The enablers of happiness are the outcomes: the feelings of trust, meaning, and belonging that develop within citizen groups; the increase in perceptions of safety and security; the creation of an environment of sociability, tolerance and inclusivity; improved affordability; and the generation of better health habits and life balance.

In his *Happy City* book, Montgomery outlines his basic recipe for happiness in cities. He argues that a city must: (1) meet our basic needs of food, shelter, and security; (2) strive to maximize joy and minimize hardship; (3) lead us toward health rather than sickness; (4) offer us freedom to live, move, and build our lives as we wish; (5) build resilience against economic and environmental shocks; (6) be fair in the way it apportions space, services, mobility, joys, hardships, and costs; and (7) enable us to build and strengthen the bonds between friends, families, and strangers that give life meaning. Cities that follow this recipe, he argues, "that acknowledge and celebrate our common fate, that open doors to empathy and cooperation, will help us tackle the great challenges of this century."

Many of these challenges are outlined in Richard Florida's recent book on *The New Urban Crisis* [68]. Some are longstanding: our inability to wean ourselves from dependence on the automobile, the unaffordability of inner-city housing, the flight to ever-expanding suburbs with their long commute times and inefficient infrastructures, the growth of inequality and segregation, by race, by income, by class, by occupation, and by like-mindedness. The elephant in the room is the potential impact of climate change, and its possible implications for city infrastructure, availability of affordable insurance, and potentially deleterious effects on citizen health. Few cities (indeed few countries) have yet to wrestle realistically with this fast-tracking threat to happiness and wellbeing.

The Civil Society Movement

Smart cities provide the infrastructure; walkable cities provide the settings for human interaction; but it is the nature of these interactions that provides the final key to human happiness and wellbeing in the urban milieu. A civil society is one in which human discourse is friendly, cooperative, respectful, orderly, and compassionate. Those who help build a civil society are tolerant of racial and religious diversity, and inclusive of those who are often forgotten: immigrants, indigenous peoples, the disabled, the homeless, the poor. The Ford Foundation's Center for Social Justice states that a civil society is simultaneously a "goal to aim for, a means of achievement, and a framework for engaging with one another." [69]. One of the best definitions comes from Geoff Plant, Commissioner of Project Civil City in Vancouver Canada, who defines a civil society as "a vibrant and diverse community of individuals adhering to the basic standards necessary for life together in a crowded place: social order, mutual respect, and responsibility for one's fellow citizens." [70].

The Centre for a Civil Society at the London School of Economics (now disbanded, but which has morphed into the Conflict and Civil Society Research Unit) has noted that the institutional structures of a civil society are distinct from those of the state, the family, or the market [71]. They fall into that part of the social network that lies between family ties and top-down city-wide governance. A civil society thrives at the scale of churches, schools, service clubs, and sports organizations where friendships are made and ideas are debated in a constructive respectful fashion.

The civil society movement owes much to the concept of social capital, introduced back in Chap. 3, and made popular by Harvard political scientist Robert Putnam in his best-selling book *Bowling Alone: The Collapse and Revival of American Community* [72]. Putnam argues for cooperative social behavior, economic production that benefits the common good, and the value of social networks. With respect to the latter, he differentiates between networks that promote "bonding" social capital and those that promote "bridging" social capital. He is less enamored of bonding groups, wherein most members share similar beliefs, values and backgrounds, including shared prejudices that may lead to distrust of those who don't share the beliefs of the group. Better are bridging groups that foster mutual understanding, negotiation, tolerance, and inclusivity. Civil societies are those that are well-populated by the bridging social networks that may develop through registered charities, community groups, women's organizations, faith-based communities, professional associations, trade unions, self-help groups, social movements, business associations, advocacy groups, volunteer activities, and non-governmental organizations.

The Ends of the Earth

It is in the cities that populate the top-ten lists in Table 10.4, most of which are situated in the economically-strong Western democracies, that one might expect to find the growth of smart-city technology and the communal striving for a civil society. In the cities that appear on the worlds' bottom ten lists, and sadly, even many of the cities that avoid the bottom ten but just lie in the bottom half, civic concerns run more to survival than to the niceties of a vibrant urban milieu. Many of the city indicators that appear in Table 10.1, things like the number of library card holders, or the accessibility of fitness facilities, or the presence of an urban tree canopy, would gain little purchase in the concerns of citizens of Lagos or Sana'a or Kinshasa. The citizens of the least happy cities in the world would have little interest in our prissy, compulsive assessments and rankings.

In his book *The Ends of the Earth*, Robert Kaplan, a deft analyst of international realities, takes a "journey to the frontiers of anarchy," and reports on conditions in many of the worlds' most unfortunate cities [73]. Almost all of them are ravaged by poverty, homelessness and drug addiction; many of them are racked by civil war; and others suffer from failing infrastructure and rampant disease. Roughly one-third of the world's urban population lives in "mega-slums:" vast tracts of tumbledown subsistence dwellings with scant municipal servicing. Only 54% of city dwellers in all of Africa have access to the kind of functional sanitation that is taken for granted in the West. In sub-Saharan Africa, two-thirds of the population does not have electricity. In Conakry, Guinea, for example, which appears on one of the bottom-ten lists in Table 10.4, Kaplan describes a never-ending shantytown with "scabrous walls coated with black slime," streets that are "a long puddle of floating garbage," a "perspiration-soaked bedlam" overrun with armed teenage gangs, malaria, and destitute refugees from other nearby African disasters. In Karachi, which also appears on our bottom-ten listings, he bemoans the gulf between rich and poor, with the small minority of rich living in guarded luxury villas protected by barbwire-topped walls and iron-grille gates, while the teeming masses live in hopeless, dysfunctional misery in unstable neighborhoods of "cinder block, burlap and cardboard." Other cities on his tour are riven by a "bewildering complexity of ethnic and religious divisions." They are often disturbed by gunfire and nightly violence, and many have an economy that is based almost totally on drug smuggling and weapons sales.

When those of us who live in happier climes find ourselves obsessing over whether Melbourne or Vancouver provide the best quality of life, or when we succumb to road rage over some minor traffic congestion, it would behoove us all to take a deep breath and think about our fellow citizens in Damascus or Dhaka or Bangui, and their never-ending challenges to put clothes on their back and food on their table.

References

1. Angel, S., *Making Room for a Planet of Cities*, Policy Focus Report, Lincoln Institute of Land Policy, Cambridge, MA, 2011.
2. [www.planning.org]
3. [www.isocarp.org]
4. [www.planetizem.com]; *Guide to Graduate Urban Planning Programs*, 6th edition, Planetizem Press, 2019.
5. [www.urban.org]
6. [www.thecityfix.com]
7. [www.philips-thecenter.org]
8. [www.pewresearch.org]
9. [www.futurecities.catapult.org.uk]
10. [www.happycity.org.uk]
11. [http://centerforthelivingcity.org]
12. [www.citylab.com]
13. [undp.org.un.habitat]
14. Jacobs, Jane, *The Death and Life of Great American Cities*, Random House, 1961. (Reprinted by Vintage, 1992).
15. Mumford, Lewis, *The City in History: Its Origins, Its Transformations, and Its Prospects*, Harcourt, Brace and World, 1961. (Reprinted by Mariner Books, 1972).
16. Putnam, Robert, *Bowling Alone: The Collapse and Revival of American Community*, Simon and Schuster, 2000.
17. The proposed list of civic dimensions is a composite of those found in many sources including: Sirgy, M.J. et al, Developing a measure of community wellbeing based on perceptions of impact in various life domains, *Social Indicators Research,* 96(2), 295-311, 2010; Richard Florida's Place Finder [www.whosyourcity.com]; the 2019 Global Happiness and Well-Being Policy Report [www.happinesscouncil.org]; the Thriving Places Index [www.thrivingplaces.org]; the Mercer Quality of Living Index [www.mercer.com/qualityofliving]; the Innovation Cities Index [www.innovation-cities.com]; the United Nations Habitat urban indicators [undp.org/un/habitat]; and the indicator projects for the cities of Jacksonville, Pittsburg, Charlotte-Mecklinsburg, Boston, and Albuquerque. (See Tables 10-2 and 10-5 for the internet addresses for these projects).
18. [www.worlddatabaseofhappiness.eur.nl]
19. [www.huduser.gov/portal/datasets/socds]
20. [http://communityindicators.net]
21. [data.census.gov]
22. Jackson, J, J. Lee, M.C.Y. Lin, and M. Ratnatunga, *Best Performing Cities: Where America's Jobs Are Created and Sustained*, Milken Institute, 2018; [www.milkeninstitute.org/taxonomy/term/rankings]

23. [www.demographia.com/dhi.pdf]
24. [www.senseofcommunity.com]; [www.communityscience.com]
25. McMillan, D.W. and D.M. Chavis, Sense of community: a definition and theory, *Jour. Community Psychology*, 14(1), 6-23, 1986.
26. [www.safecities.economist.com/safe-cities-index-2019]
27. [www.numbeo.com]
28. [https://ceoworld.biz]
29. [https://safearound.com]
30. [dbresearch.com]
31. Sperling, B. and P. Sander, *Cities Ranked and Rated: More than 400 Metropolitan Areas Evaluated in the US and Canada*, Wiley and Sons, 2007.
32. Florida, R., *Who's Your City? How the Creative Economy Is Making Where You Live the Most Important Decision of Your Life*, Basic Books, 314 pp., 2008.
33. Espey, J., H. Dahmm and L. Mandarino, *Leaving No US City Behind: The US Cities Sustainable Development Goals Index*, Sustainable Development Solutions Network, 2018.
34. *Thriving Places Index: Full Report*, Happy City, 2019.
35. *City Magnets III: Benchmarking the Attractiveness of 50 Canadian Cities*, Conference Board of Canada, 153 pp., 2014.
36. Mittal, S., J. Chadchan and S.K. Mishra, Review of concepts, tools and indices for the assessment of urban quality of life, *Social Indicators Research*, 149, 187-214, 2020.
37. Okulicz-Kozaryn, A. City life: Rankings (Livability) vs Perceptions (Satisfaction), *Social Indicators Research*, 110(2), 433-451, 2013; Okulicz-Kozaryn, A. and R. Valente, Livability and subjective well-being across European cities, *Applied Research in Quality of Life*, 14(1), 197-220, 2019.
38. Holden, M. and A. Scerri, More than this: Livable Melbourne meets livable Vancouver, *Cities*, 31, 444-453, 2013.
39. Kotkin, J., Why the livable cities rankings are wrong, *Forbes Magazine*, Aug. 11, 2009.
40. [http://communityindicators.net]
41. [www.neighborhoodindicators.org]; Kingsley, T., ed., *Building and Operating Neighborhood Indicators Systems: A Guidebook*, Urban Institute, 1999; [http://www2.urban.org/nnip/pdf/guidebook.pdf]
42. [www.iisp.vassar.edu/socialindicator.html]
43. [www.jaxpact.org]
44. [www.longislandindex.org], [www.siliconvalleyindicators.org], [www.sightline.org/research_item/cs07]
45. [weforum.org/platforms/shaping-the-future-of-technology-governance-iot-robotics-and-smart-cities]; [internetsociety.org]
46. [ww2.frost.com]
47. Picon, A., *Smart Cities: A Spatialized Intelligence*, Wiley, 2015; Allwinkle, S. and P. Cruikshank, Creating smart-er cities: An overview, *Journal of Urban Technology*, 18(2), 1-16, 2011; Albino, V., U. Berardi and R.M. Dangelico, Smart cities: Definitions, dimensions, performance, and initiatives, *Journal of Urban Technology*, 22(1), 3-21, 2015.
48. [https://digitallibrary.theiet.org]
49. [nitrd.gov/apps/smartcity]
50. [transportation.gov/policy-initiatives/smartcity/smart-city-challenge-lessons-building-cities-future]
51. [smartcitiesworld.net]
52. [smartcitiescouncil.com]
53. [www.sidewalklabs.com]
54. [www.smartcityexpo.com]
55. Alderete, M.V., Exploring the smart cities indexes and the role of macro factors for measuring cities smartness, *Social Indicators Research*, 147, 567-589, 2020.
56. [smart_city_index_digital.pdf]

57. Sennett, R., *The Guardian*, Dec. 4, 2012.
58. Mattern, S., A city is not a computer, *Places*, Feb. 2017; [places.journal.org/article/a-city-is-not-a-computer]
59. [weforum.org] op.cit.; [internetsociety.org]
60. [https://globalsmartcitiesalliance.org]
61. [smartcities4all.org]
62. [techrepublic.com/article/smart-cities-the smart-persons-guide]
63. Montgomery, C., *Happy City: Transforming Our Lives Through Urban Design*, Anchor Canada, 2014; See also: Glaeser, E., *Triumph of the City: How Our Greatest Invention Makes Us Richer, Smarter, Greener, Healthier, and Happier*, Penguin, 2011.
64. Brown, A., Civil spaces, *Vancouver Sun*, April 5, 2008; See also: Speck, J., *Walkable City: How Downtown Can Save America, One Step at a Time*, North Point Press, 2013; Wey, W.M. and W.L. Wei, Urbanstreet environment design for quality of urban life, *Social Indicators Research*, 126(1), 161-186, 2016.
65. Klinenberg, E., *Palaces for the People: How Social Infrastructure Can Help Fight Inequality, Polarization, and the Decline of Civic Life*, Crown, 2018.
66. Goosen, Z. and E.J. Cilliers, Enhancing social sustainability through the planning of Third Places: A theory-based framework, *Social Indicators Research*, 150, 835-866, 2020.
67. [www.happinesscouncil.org/report/2018]; [www.happinesscouncil.org/report/2019]
68. Florida, Richard, *The New Urban Crisis*, Basic Books, 2017.
69. [fordfoundation.org]
70. [council.vancouver.ca/20080708/documents/a11.pdf]
71. [www.lse.ac.ik/ccs]
72. Putnam, Robert, *Bowling Alone: the Collapse and Revival of American Community*, Simon and Schuster, 2000.
73. Kaplan, Robert D., *The Ends of the Earth: A Journey to the Frontiers of Anarchy*, Vintage, 1996.

Chapter 11
Satisfaction in the Workplace

Work and Wellbeing

Most of us spend about half our waking hours of each working day on the job, so it should come as no surprise that the sum total of our personal wellbeing is strongly influenced by the satisfaction or dissatisfaction that we experience in the workplace. Neither should it surprise us that this facet of happiness and wellbeing has received a lot of attention from the academic world, the business world, and the popular media.

One can date the academic consideration of working conditions to at least 1935 with the publication of the book *Job Satisfaction* by vocational counsellor Robert Hoppock, based on his PhD dissertation at Columbia University. Actual measurement of job satisfaction is usually dated to 1951 when Arthur Brayfield, a counselling psychologist at the University of California (and later the chief executive officer of the American Psychological Association), and colleague Harold F. Rothe, published their Index of Job Satisfaction in the *Journal of Applied Psychology* [1]. Since that early date, there has been a huge and continuous outpouring of articles on workplace satisfaction, most of them from the perspective of employees, but many others from the perspective of their corporate employers. One review estimated that there had been 12,400 published articles in the field up to 1994 [2]. The numbers by now have probably multiplied tenfold.

The incredible breadth of workplace studies can be seen by a listing of journals in which widely-referenced articles have appeared. Our old standbys, *Social Indicators Research* and the *Journal of Happiness Studies* figure prominently, but so too do journals from specialized branches of psychology (*Journal of Occupational and Organizational Psychology, Journal of Applied Social Psychology, Journal of Occupational Behaviour, Journal of Managerial Psychology*), economics (*Journal of Economic Behavior and Organization, Journal of Labor Economics*), management (*Journal of Management, Management Science, Groups and Organization Management, Academy of Management Journal*), industrial relations (*Industrial Relations, Industrial and Labor Relations Review*), human resources (*Human*

R. A. Freeze, *The Metrics of Happiness*, Social Indicators Research Series 86,
https://doi.org/10.1007/978-3-031-10913-3_11

Resources Management, Journal of Career Assessment, Journal of Vocational Behavior), and occupational medicine (*American Journal of Public Health, Journal of Health Economics, Work and Stress*).

Many of the happiness and wellbeing compendiums referenced in earlier chapters of this book have chapters or sections dedicated to the workplace. See for example Chap. 6 of the 2017 *World Happiness Report*, and Chap. 5 in each of the 2018 and 2019 editions of the *Global Happiness and Well-Being Policy Reports* all of which are authored or co-authored by Jan-Emmanuel de Neve of Oxford University [3]. Oxford figures prominently in other ways. The *Oxford Handbook of Happiness* has nine papers on happiness in the workplace, and a more specialized treatment from the same source can be found in the *Oxford Handbook of Positive Psychology and Work* [4]. There are chapters on job satisfaction in the multi-authored treatises: *Well-Being: The Foundations of Hedonic Psychology* edited by Daniel Kahneman, Ed Diener and Norbert Schwartz, and *The Science of Subjective Well-Being* (the Diener Volume) edited by Michael Eid and Randy Larson [5]. The six-volume reference work *Wellbeing: A Complete Reference Guide* has one volume (Volume III) dedicated to *Work and Wellbeing*. Alex Michalos' 12-volume *Encyclopedia of Quality of Life and Well-Being Research* has many entries on the workplace and job satisfaction [6].

Three researchers that deserve special mention in this field are Peter Warr of the Institute of Work Psychology at the University of Sheffield, Joseph Sirgy of the College of Business at Virginia Tech, and Cary Cooper of the University of Manchester Business School. Warr summarized his lifetime of contributions in his 2007 book, *Work: Happiness and Unhappiness*. Sirgy did so as editor and contributor to a 25-chapter treatise on *Work and Quality of Life* published in 2012. Cooper has authored or coauthored several books on work-based wellbeing including *Well-being, Productivity and Happiness at Work* which came out in 2018 [7].

If you peruse the business aisle at your local bookstore, you will find that there is no shortage of authors who promise to interpret all these academic findings into digestible sound-bites for the entrepreneur-on-the-street. Their books are aimed at the owners and CEOs of small to mid-sized businesses who want to jump on the happiness bandwagon and ride it to higher profits and a healthier bottom line. Some are written by escapees from academia like Sean Achor, a former guru in Harvard's positive psychology program, who has promoted the findings of his book, *The Happiness Advantage: The Seven Principles of Positive Psychology that Fuel Success and Performance at Work,* in TED talks and on Oprah. Others are published by successful businessmen like Tony Hsieh, the CEO of the online retailer ZAPPO, who provides workplace advice in his book, *Delivering Happiness: A Path to Profits, Passion and Purpose*. Jennifer Moss, cofounder of the human-relations firm, Plasticity Labs, makes her case in *Unlocking Happiness at Work: How a Data-Driven Happiness Strategy Fuels Purpose, Passion and Performance*. Other titles include *The Progress Principle: Using Small Wins to Ignite Joy, Engagement and Creativity at Work* by T.M. Anabile and S. Kramer; *Happy @ Work* by Tim Donovan; *How to be Happy at Work* by Annie McKee; and *What Happy*

Companies Know: How the New Science of Happiness Can Change Your Company for the Better by Dan Baker [8].

And if all else fails, there is always Dilbert, who keeps us smiling in *The Joy of Work: Dilbert's Guide to Finding Happiness at the Expense of Your Coworkers* [9].

Workplace Satisfaction from the Employee Perspective

The movement to apply the tenets of positive psychology in the workplace is a relatively recent development. Old-school management practices, which are still prevalent in some companies and some industries, look only to production efficiencies to enhance the bottom line, and have historically given little attention to human values. The image of Charlie Chaplin strapped to a giant gearwheel in *Modern Times* captures the tenor of its time. The union movement, which reached its zenith in the USA in the 1950s and 1960s was a response by workers to the lack of concern by employers for the welfare of their workforce, and in some cases the outright exploitation of the workforce by management.

Even before the new science of happiness burst on the scene with the new millennium, far-sighted business leaders had begun to realize that a happier and more satisfied worker was likely to be a more productive worker, and that more-forward-looking human-resources policies could improve the bottom line. The happiness revolution that had its start in the world of psychology quickly spread to the hallways of commerce. Hopefully this move toward a more-humane workplace was not based solely on the bottom line. Surely we must give some credit to the business community for recognizing the intrinsic value of providing their workers with greater opportunities for personal fulfillment, a greater sense of purpose in their jobs, higher levels of trust and respect, and more recognition of their achievements.

The explosion in academic research studies, anthologies, textbooks, and self-help business manuals has led to a widely-accepted menu of workplace attributes that lead to greater employee satisfaction with their jobs, and a comparable menu of workplace no-nos that create employee dissatisfaction. Table 11.1 (in two pages) outlines a relatively-thorough suite of these positive and negative indicators of job satisfaction. The table is organized under nine dimensions of working life: (1) the job definition and its assigned tasks, (2) the physical working environment, (3) the status of occupational health and safety, (4) the social environment at the workplace and the nature of collegial interactions, (5) the characteristics of the organization including the leadership style and the nature of the supervisory climate, (6) the balance afforded between work and the private lives of employees, (7) job and career prospects, (8) the personal meaningfulness that is engendered by the job, and (9) the financial rewards. This framework was informed by the *Guidelines on Measuring the Quality of the Working Environment* put out by the Organization of Economic Cooperation and Development (OECD) but it is quite different in detail [10].

Table 11.1 Dimensions and indicators for assessment of job satisfaction and engagement from the employee perspective

Dimensions	Positive indicators	Negative indicators
Job Definition and Tasks	Interesting job.	Boring job.
	Clear definition of tasks, goals, deliverables, and deadlines.	Tasks too difficult for skill set.
	Reasonable goals and deadlines.	Unreasonable goals.
	Good match between job tasks and skill set of worker.	Tight deadlines.
	Good fit between job and worker personality, strengths, and interests.	
	Job offers some level of independence, responsibility, control, and influence.	
	Sufficient resources available to meet job demands.	
	Job offers a variety of tasks.	
Physical Working Environment	Ergonomic work stations.	Noisy. Dusty. Draughty.
	Glare-free lighting.	Too hot. Too cold.
	Temperature and humidity control.	Smoke, gases, fumes.
	Noise control.	Poor lighting.
	Attractive office design.	Tiring or painful working positions.
		Poor office design.
		Unreasonable physical demands. Heavy lifting.
Occupational Health and Safety	Strong management emphasis on health and safety.	Dangerous working conditions.
	On-site exercise facilities.	Unsafe tools or machinery.
	Healthy foods at workplace dining outlets.	Accidents and injuries common.
	Available therapy for alcohol or drug abuse, stress, smoking.	Improper protection against chemical hazards.
		Outbreaks of infectious diseases common.
		Stress over job conditions.
		Alcohol and drug abuse.
		Cardiovascular issues.
		Work Exhaustion. Burnout.
		Depression. Other negative impacts on mental health.
Social Environment and Collegial Interaction	Friendly, collaborative working environment.	Incivility, bullying, and harassment in the workplace.
	Good interpersonal relationships with colleagues.	Evidence of intolerance, prejudice, or discrimination on the basis of race, ethnicity, religion, gender, sexual orientation or age in the workplace.

(continued)

Table 11.1 (continued)

Dimensions	Positive indicators	Negative indicators
	Open, trusting interactions with supervisory personnel.	
	Sense of belonging.	
Organizational Characteristics, Leadership and Supervision	Clear communication pathways.	Old-school management practices that give inadequate attention to human values.
	Strong, fair, supportive leadership by supervisory personnel. Recognition of achievements by management.	Manipulative supervisory behavior.
	Respectful supervisory feedback.	Lack of useful feedback.
	Sense of value and attainment of status within organization.	Management policies that lead to conflict with personal values.
	Perceived fairness in pay, security, recognition, status.	Ability to do job well limited by oppressive rules and regulations.
	Ethical business environment.	Managerial use of intimidation, coercion, overt public criticism, blame, threats, humiliation, sarcasm, or contempt of worker.
	Fair and equitable process for handling grievances, disputes, and personality conflicts.	
Work-Life Balance	Structured working hours.	Long hours. Take-home work.
	Flexibility in working hours, vacation time, and family leave policies.	Unwanted overtime.
	Job-sharing programs.	Unwanted shift work.
	Work-from-home programs.	Need for more flexible hours and working arrangements.
	Day-care facilities available.	Difficulty in taking time off at short notice.
		Long commute.
Job and Career Prospects	Job security.	Fear of downsizing, reorganization, job loss, and unemployment.
	Potential for personal and professional growth and development on the job.	Fear of advanced technologies, computerization, robotics and artificial intelligence.
	Opportunities for advancement.	Underemployment. Undesired part-time or temporary work.
	Availability of mentoring, job training, financial support.	Dead-end job.
	Regular and fair performance.	
	Evaluations.	
Meaningfulness	Sense of purpose.	Lack of engagement.
	Opportunities for personal fulfillment and self-realization.	

(continued)

Table 11.1 (continued)

Dimensions	Positive indicators	Negative indicators
	Feeling of usefulness to society.	
	Ability to help others in job.	
	Overall happiness and wellbeing.	
Financial Rewards	Salary, wages, pay.	Gig economy.
	Fringe benefits.	
	Bonuses.	
	Availability of stock options.	

A perusal of the positive indicators in Table 11.1 reveals a suite of adjectives that ought not to come as any great surprise. Employees are happier when their work environment is fair, supportive, respectful, ethical, structured, flexible, secure, friendly, collaborative, trusting, and healthy; where their job tasks are clear, reasonable, and varied; and where their achievements are recognized and rewarded. While these positive job attributes may seem fairly self-evident to the modern observer, the reader can rest assured that each and every one of them has been the subject of academic analysis, and that their positive correlation with employee job satisfaction, and with overall levels of societal happiness and wellbeing, is well-established.

So, too, with the negative indicators in Table 11.1 that point to job dissatisfaction. They are riddled with adverse descriptors like boring, unreasonable, exhausting, demanding, dangerous, improper, stressful, depressing, unfair, intolerant, prejudiced, manipulative, oppressive, intimidating, unwanted and fearful. These, too, have all received independent attention from researchers on worker quality of life.

Table 11.1 clarifies the connection that exists between the working environment and management style created by the employer, and its impact on the physical and mental health of employees. Poor employee health leads to increased direct healthcare costs, lower productivity, increased absenteeism, and higher turnover rates.

Satisfaction and Engagement

The discerning reader may have noticed that the title of Table 11.1 refers not only to job satisfaction *per se* but also to "engagement." The first use of this term is usually credited to William Kahn of the Boston University School of Business who introduced it in a 1990 paper in the *Academy of Management Journal* [11]. Since then, the distinction between satisfaction and engagement has been highlighted in many articles on employee management, including a comprehensive review paper [12] and a multi-authored anthology [13]. It is now widely recognized that *satisfaction* reflects happiness and contentment in one's job, which is nice, but that it may not represent a high enough bar for employee (or employer) aspirations. A satisfied worker is likely to fulfill assigned tasks, meet specified deadlines, and comply with the organization's rules and regulations. Certainly, a satisfied employee is better than a dissatisfied one, but an employee who is merely satisfied rather than engaged is unlikely to go the extra mile for the company.

Engagement implies a more serious commitment. Engaged employees are enthusiastic, collaborative, and attuned to opportunity. They are much more likely to help others, provide mentoring services, and share innovative ideas. Engaged employees feel an emotional connection with their organization and its goals.

Almost all engaged employees are happy, but not all happy employees are engaged. Furthermore, the concept works both ways. It is up to management to design jobs that provide workers with opportunities for engagement, and it is up to the workers to accept the challenge when it is presented. Many research studies have found that engaged workers are both happier and more productive than those who settle for the lesser standard of satisfaction and contentment.

The Measurement of Employee Job Satisfaction and Engagement

The measurement of employee job satisfaction and engagement is carried out in the same manner as was presented for the assessment of overall personal happiness and life satisfaction in Chap. 6. Here too, results are brought to light by means of surveys based on carefully-developed questionnaires. Having recognized the job attributes that lead to a happy, satisfied, and engaged workforce, as outlined in Table 11.1, the designers of job satisfaction questionnaires zero in on these features of the workplace, asking individual responders to agree or disagree with questions or statements that highlight the various positive and negative attributes.

Many of the international happiness surveys that were referenced back in Chap. 6 include consideration of job satisfaction and engagement as part of their overall evaluations. The Gallup World Poll (GWP), for example, includes a 17-question work module. The International Social Survey Programme (ISSP) has a 25-item module. The European Social Survey (ESS) features a 28-item module. In addition, Round 5 of the ESS carried out in 2010 featured an expanded 93-question treatment of Family, Work, and Wellbeing. Other European surveys such as the Eurobarometer, the European Quality-of-Life Survey, the EU Labour Force Survey, and the European Working Conditions Survey all include questions on job satisfaction. So too do most national wellbeing surveys such as the US and Canadian General Social Surveys, and specialized national surveys like the British Skills and Employment Survey.

There have been a very large number of questionnaires developed for the measurement of employee satisfaction and engagement, some by academics, some by business gurus, and some by human-resources consulting companies. Table 11.2 provides a listing of a representative suite of some of the most widely-used, well-

Table 11.2 A representative suite of questionnaires used in the measurement of employee satisfaction and engagement

Questionnaire	Date	Developer	Number of dimensions or aspects	Number of questions or statements	Number of scale divisions
Index of Job Satisfaction	1951	A.G. Brayfield and H.F. Rothe, University of California, Berkeley		19 statements	5
Minnesota Satisfaction Questionnaire	1967	D.J. Weiss, et al., University of Minnesota	20	100 statements	5
Job Descriptive Index	1969	P.C. Smith et al., Bowling Green State University	5	72 statements	3
Job Diagnostic Survey	1975	J.R. Hackman and G.R. Oldham, Yale University	7	83 statements	5–7
Gallup Q^{12} Index	1996	Gallup Organization		12 questions	5
Job Satisfaction Survey	1997	P.E. Spector, University of South Florida	9	36 statements	6
Quality of Worklife Questionnaire	2002	National Institute for Occupational Safety and Health	9	76 questions and statements	3–5 (some yes/no)
Copenhagen Burnout Inventory	2005	National Institute of Occupational Health, Denmark	3	19 questions	5
Work-Related Quality of Life Scale	2007	S. Easton and D. Van Laar, University of Portsmouth, UK	6	24 statements	5
Work and Well-Being Survey	2011	American Psychological Association	15	138 statements	5
Brief Index of Affective Job Satisfaction	2012	E.R. Thompson, University of Bath, and F.T.T. Phua, University of Reading, UK		4 statements	5
Job Satisfaction Index	2015	KRIFA Job Satisfaction Knowledge Center; Happiness Research Organization, and Kantar/Gallup; Copenhagen, Denmark	9	47 questions	Percentiles 0–100
Workplace Wellbeing Questionnaire	2018	UK Department of Work and Pensions	4	45 questions	5

documented, and publically-available ones. They are listed in order of the date of their first appearance. Most of them are organized under a set of dimensions similar in number and topic to those suggested in Table 11.1. Some use questions, some use statements, and at least one uses both. Most responses are requested on a Likert scale with between 3 and 7 scale divisions. Some of the listed indexes have both a long and a short version. If so, only the long-version statistics are listed in Table 11.2.

The number of questions or statements used in the indexes listed in Table 11.2 varies widely, from a minimum of 4 to a maximum of 138. Obviously, the greater the number of questions or statements, the more detailed is the analysis with respect to the many workplace issues identified in Table 11.1. However, there is no consensus that those indexes using a greater number of questions or statements provide a better or more defensible analysis of job satisfaction and engagement in a specific workplace. In fact, the developers of each index tend to claim that they have utilized the optimal number, recognizing the tradeoffs that occur between more detail and the difficulties in administering a longer, more time-consuming questionnaire. There is much discussion in the literature about the likely correlations between many of the individual issues identified in Table 11.1 and the desirability of discarding redundant issues to reach the optimal mix.

We will now look briefly at each of the indexes in Table 11.2 in turn.

The original Index of Job Satisfaction developed in 1952 by Arthur Brayfield and Harold Rothe set the tone for later work [14]. The 19 statements in their questionnaire include 10 that are worded positively ("I find real enjoyment in my work."), and 9 that are worded negatively ("I am disappointed that I ever took this job."). Responders are asked to choose one of five responses to the statements, from "strongly agree" to "strongly disagree". Like many who came after them, Brayfield and Rothe remind responders that "there are no right or wrong answers." They implore responders to give their "honest opinion on each of the statements." The emphases in the questionnaire are on whether responders like or dislike their work, and whether they find it interesting or boring.

The Minnesota Satisfaction Questionnaire [15], the Job Descriptive index [16], and the Job Diagnostic Survey [17] were all developed in the late-1960s to mid-1970s by university researchers, and all include a large suite of statements for responders to address. The Job Diagnostic Survey (JDS) developed by psychologists J.R. Hackman and G.R. Oldham of Yale University is interesting on several counts. It is based on a Jobs Characteristics Model (JCM) put forward by the authors, which in itself had a large impact on the field (over 200 follow-up articles during the 10-year period 1975–1985). The JCM postulates relationships between the characteristics of a job (its variety, identity, significance, autonomy, and feedback) and the work-related outcomes they produce, both positive and negative (motivation, satisfaction, performance, absenteeism, and turnover). The 83 statements in the Job Diagnostic Survey are divided into 7 sections, 4 of which are quite traditional (job characteristics, job description, personal feelings about the job, and job satisfaction). The fifth section deals with the responders perceptions of the personal feelings of others in the organization with similar jobs, a consideration that is apparently unique to the JDS. The sixth section asks responders to judge the degree to which they desire specific job attributes, such as job security, high salary, friendly co-workers, opportunities for personal growth, and so on (on a 7-point scale from "moderately" to "extremely"). The seventh section is highly original. It asks responders to determine their level of preference between two jobs (on a five-point scale from "strongly prefer Job A" to "strongly prefer Job B"). Twelve pairs of jobs are differentiated on a variety of bases. For example, would you prefer Job A ("a job in which there is a real chance for you to develop new skills and advance in the organization"), or Job B ("a job which provides lots of vacation time and an excellent fringe benefit package")? Another example: Would you prefer Job A ("a job where you are required to make important decisions"), or Job B ("a job with many pleasant people to work with")?

One of the most popular workplace questionnaires is the Gallup Q^{12} Index [18]. It is usually administered by a team from the Gallup organization as part of a contracted assessment of a client company's work environment. Its popularity probably rests at least in part on its compactness and ease of administration. It consists of 12 questions "with proven links to vital performance outcomes." The first two questions cover "basic needs" to do the job. The next four ask what the responder "gives and gets" from the job. The next four examine issues of relationships and "teamwork," and the last two address "growth." Responders answer on a 5-point agree/disagree scale. The Q^{12} Index has been in use for over 25 years and has been administered to over 17 million employees.

The Job Satisfaction Survey [19] developed by Paul Spector of the University of South Florida is a straightforward, easy-to-administer 36-statement questionnaire in which positive and negative statements alternate. (No. 7: "I like the people I work with;" No. 8: "I sometimes feel my job is meaningless.") The 6-point scale goes from "agree very much" to "disagree very much." The statements cover such issues as pay, benefits, promotion, recognition, communication, supervisory style, work assignments, organizational goals, co-worker competence, and workplace environment.

The Quality of Worklife Questionnaire [20] developed by the National Institute for Occupational Health and Safety (NIOSH) differs from all the others in Table 11.2 in that it was not designed as a stand-alone tool to be used by companies to assess job satisfaction levels in their workforce, but rather as a module to be used in the U.S. General Social Survey (GSS) to assess employee job satisfaction on a national scale. It has appeared in the GSS at 4-year intervals starting in 2002. It features a mix of 79 questions and statements grouped under 9 dimensions (half of which were taken from an earlier Quality of Employment Survey carried out in 1977). Responders provide yes/no answers to many of the questions, while on others they are asked to use a Likert scale that varies from 3 to 5 scale divisions. The 9 dimensions are Job Level (41 questions, which include many that provide demographic data on the responder), Culture and Climate of Workplace (11 questions), Health Outcomes (9), Other Outcomes (7), Hours of Work (2), Work-Family Balance (4), Supervisor (3), Benefits (1), and Unionization (1).

The Copenhagen Burnout Inventory [21] by its very name identifies itself as something other than a straightforward job satisfaction tool. It is designed to identify those workers who are so physically and emotionally exhausted that they may actually be prone to some type of physical or mental illness. Its 19 questions are grouped under 3 headings: Personal Burnout (which is defined as "a state of prolonged physical and psychological exhaustion"), Work-Related Burnout (defined as "a state of prolonged physical and psychological exhaustion, which is perceived as related to the person's work"), and Client Burnout (defined as "a state of prolonged physical and psychological exhaustion, which is perceived as related to the person's work with clients"). A representative question under the first heading: "How often do you think that you just can't take it anymore?" Under the second heading: "Are you exhausted in the morning at the thought of another day at work?" Under the third: "Does it drain your energy to work with clients?" Responders are asked to reply on a 5-point Likert scale.

The Work-Related Quality of Life Scale (WRQoL) [22] is another widely-used tool with 24 statements grouped under 6 dimensions, with responders using a 5-point agree-disagree response scale. The six dimensions are General Well Being, Home-Work Interface, Job Career Satisfaction, Working Conditions, Stress at Work, and Overall Quality of Working Life.

The Work and Well-Being Survey [23] designed and circulated by the American Psychological Association (APA) is the most detailed of all the indexes in Table 11.2 with 138 statements grouped under 15 dimensions.

The Brief Index of Affective Job Satisfaction (BIAJS) [24] developed by two British management researchers represents the polar opposite of the 138-statement APA index. It uses only four statements. ("I find real engagement in my job." "I like my job better than the average person." "Most days, I am enthusiastic about my job." "I feel fairly well-satisfied with my job.") In an interesting twist on common practice, the BIAJS questionnaire actually features seven statements for the responder to consider, but three of them are "distracters" that are not taken into account in the calculation of the index score, and are only included to "distract" the responder into considering the four meaningful statements carefully and independently from one another. Perhaps surprisingly, the authors of the BIAJS claim that the results of their short, simple, highly-subjective questionnaire are highly correlated with the results of much more-detailed job satisfaction questionnaires, thus calling into question the need for a large and detailed suite of questions to uncover the state of satisfaction of a company's workforce.

The Denmark-based Job Satisfaction Index (JSI) [25] was developed cooperatively by three Danish organizations: The Job Satisfaction Knowledge Center, which is run by the trade union group KRIFA; the Happiness Research Institute, which is an independent think tank; and Kantar/Gallup, which is the Danish subsidiary of the Gallup polling organization. The JSI uses 9 general questions with respect to Overall Happiness and Overall Job Satisfaction, and 38 detailed questions grouped under 7 dimensions. The seven dimensions are *Influence* (the ability to participate in the design of work tasks and the making of key decisions affecting one's work), *Meaning* (the development of work tasks that are satisfying and fulfilling), *Mastering* (the opportunities for professional development), *Achievements* (work tasks that lead to a sense of accomplishment), *Leadership* (a workplace climate that allows for the development of positive relationships between workers and line managers), *Colleagues* (a workplace environment that breeds confidence in co-workers and presents opportunities for teamwork), and *Balance* (between work and personal life). All of the 47 questions are worded positively, and almost all of them begin with the words: "To what extent ..." (e.g. To what extent do you feel happy in your job?) The JSI does not use Likert scales, but rather asks respondents to signal their level of satisfaction as a percentile on a [0,100] scale. Furthermore, each dimension is weighted according to a set of values that have been determined by a quantitative analysis carried out by Kantar/Gallup. The score for each question is determined as its percentile value multiplied by its dimensional weighting. The final job satisfaction score is the sum of all the individual scores.

The final listing in Table 11.2 is the Workplace Wellbeing Questionnaire originally developed many years ago by the UK Department of Work and Pensions and recently updated in 2018. The 45 questions are presented to the responder in linear order without identifying which of the 4 dimensions are being addressed by each question, but the scoring is done with this knowledge in hand. The four dimensions are: Work Satisfaction (the degree to which you find your work fulfilling, and whether it provides your life with purpose and meaning), Organizational Respect (whether you see your senior management team as trustworthy and ethical), Employee Care (how well your boss treats you), and Intrusion of Work into Private Life (whether you feel pressured and stressed at work, and whether such pressures impact your private life) [26].

Consultant Services in Job Satisfaction

Most of the indexes and questionnaires listed in Table 11.2 are in the public domain. This is true for all those developed in the university milieu using federal grant monies, or by government agencies, or by not-for-profit institutes. However, these public domain systems are just the tip of a very large iceberg. There are thousands of private human-resources consulting firms around the world who offer job satisfaction services to their clients using their own proprietary job-satisfaction surveys and interpretive packages. All the major human resources giants, like Mercer LLC, Deloitte Consulting, Aon-Hewitt, Korn Ferry, and Willis Towers Watson provide full-service support to help client companies run their employee engagement programs. As an example from Table 11.2, consider the Gallup Q^{12} Index. The consulting wing of the Gallup organization provides the Q^{12} questionnaire to their clients as part of a package that includes not only the questionnaire itself, but also a numerical interpretation of the results that can be used by the client company to compare employee job satisfaction against past surveys or against industry standards.

There are also many consulting companies that specialize solely in employee engagement services. One of these is the Great Places to Work Institute (which is not an institute in the academic sense, but rather a fee-for-service provider). Job satisfaction levels at a client company are assessed with a proprietary 60-question questionnaire. These results are submitted to the Institute in the hopes of receiving certification as a "great place to work." If the results do not meet Institute benchmarks, the Institute provides the necessary guidance for the company to upgrade its program. Once a company meets specs, the Institute provides them with a media package that allows the company to announce its certification to maximum impact. The Great Places to Work questionnaire has been given to over 4.1 million employees in 50 countries [27].

In another twist, the whimsically-named firm, SurveyMonkey, offers to help a company's human resources team manage its employee engagement program, with the added perk that they will sweeten the pot by donating 50 cents per completed survey to a non-profit charity of their client's choice. In this way they hope to "use technology to champion human rights, empower the voiceless, and create a more inclusive, just, and sustainable world." [28].

Intriguing company names seem to be the norm in this corner of the human resources world. Plasticity Labs is a "people and culture consulting company on a mission to improve well-being, happiness, and performance." It uses a 20-question employee feedback questionnaire based on four HERO traits (hope/efficiency/resilience/optimism). The company co-founder is Jennifer Moss, a former colleague and co-author with Shawn Achor of Harvard positive psychology fame. In this sense, Plasticity Labs offers one of the most direct connections between the job satisfaction world and the positive psychology movement [29].

There are also many websites that offer software platforms that can spit out off-the-shelf or customized job satisfaction surveys on request, most of them also sporting new-age names like Bamboo Human Resources, Glint, TINYpulse, CustomInsight, and Amplitude Research [30].

Best and Worst Places to Work

Many of those who have tried to date the beginning of the turnaround in corporate policies from their paternal and patronizing past to the modern world of employee job satisfaction, have zeroed in on 1976, the year that a California business writer named Milton Moskowitz first published his list of "Best Places to Work" in Money magazine. His lists were based not on company bottom lines, but on employee feedback about the level of satisfaction with their working conditions. In 1984, in association with fellow business journalist Robert Levering, he published the first edition of his analysis in book form. That book, *The One Hundred Best Companies to Work for in America*, received wide circulation, and went through many updated versions in succeeding years [31]. In 1998, he and Levering provided the data that informed the first appearance in Fortune magazine of their 100 Best Companies to Work For, a collaboration that continued on an annual basis from 1998 to 2015. Milton Moskowitz died in 2019 at the age of 91. The University of California at Berkeley has established a Moskowitz Research Prize in his name.

Table 11.3 Industries with highest levels of workplace happiness (Kununu website, [33])

Tax consulting/auditing
Human resources
Consulting
Information technology (IT)
Research and development science
Arts and entertainment
Internet/media
Purchasing
Market research
Education

Table 11.4 Ten Best and Worst Jobs, 2019 (CareerCast website, [33])

Ten best jobs	Ten worst jobs
Data scientist	Taxi driver
Statistician	Logging worker
University professor	Newspaper reporter
Occupational therapist	Retail salesperson
Genetic counselor	Enlisted military personnel
Medical services manager	Correctional officer
Information secrecy analyst	Disc jockey
Mathematician	Nuclear decontamination technician
Operations research analyst	Advertising salesperson
Actuary	Broadcaster

Since 2015, the annual Fortune 100 Best Companies List has been prepared with the support of the Great Places to Work Institute. In the 2020 listing, the top-rated employer was Hilton Hotels. Among the names of companies that have appeared on the Fortune top-100 list on a regular basis are three grocery chains (Wegman's Food Markets, Whole Foods, and Publix), W.L. Gore (the makers of Goretex), Goldman-Sachs, the Mariott and Four Seasons hotel chains, the IT firm Cisco, and retail giant Nordstroms [32].

Rather than looking at lists of individual companies, it is perhaps more useful to identify the industries that are most often represented on these lists. One such industry list is presented in Table 11.3, based on the findings of the Kununu Workplace Happiness Index which is reported on Kununu's widely-used job placement website. Table 11.4 lists the ten best and worst jobs as determined by the career-guidance website CareerCast. Both best-ten lists are dominated by white-collar, number-crunching jobs in science, information technology, financial services, education, and human resources. For an alternative viewpoint see the results of the Career Happiness Index administered by the City and Guilds Group, a vocational education organization based in the UK. The best jobs on their list tend to be grey-collar positions like those held by florists, gardeners, hairdressers, plumbers and marketers [33].

Some Statistics on Workplace Satisfaction and Engagement

There have been many meta-studies of the results of widely-applied measurement tools such as Gallups' Q^{12} Index, the KRIFA Job Satisfaction Index, the Great Places to Work questionnaire, and the workplace components of various national General Social Surveys like the NIOSH Quality of Worklife Questionnaire. Some of these studies have appeared in academic research journals; some in review studies carried out by interested agencies like the Conference Board [34], the National Business Research Institute [35], and the Global Happiness Council [36]; some in reports prepared by job-satisfaction consulting firms like the Gallup Organization [37], and others on info-saturated blog sites like AccessPerks [38]. All of them include statistical information, much of which will be utilized in the next few sections without further attribution. The Access Perks site deserves particular mention; it comprises 15 pages of densely-packed statistical job-satisfaction stats gleaned from over 50 independent sources. Most of these statistics come from American studies of American workers. The numbers are probably representative for other Western countries like Canada, the UK, and Australia, but may not be appropriate for Asian economies, and certainly not for poverty-stricken or war-ravaged third-world countries.

So, to start with the primary question: How many first-world workers are satisfied in their jobs? The numbers from the various sources vary from a low just above 50% of the workforce to a high of almost 90%, with a median value that runs in the mid-to-high 70s. In short then, many more workers are satisfied in their jobs than are dissatisfied. The very large differences that are reported probably arise from the nature of the survey questions asked, the number and wording of the scale divisions offered to the responder, and the population of workers included in the survey. There are significant differences between different cohorts of responders: managers and workers, male and female workers, older and younger workers, self-employed and salaried employees, those in the public and private sectors, and full-time and part-time staff. More on this below but suffice it to say here that job satisfaction is highly correlated with job status, gender, generational attitudes, and employment situation.

At the upper end of the satisfaction scale, there are some surveys that give responders an opportunity to express great satisfaction rather than just ho-hum satisfaction. When given this opportunity on 4 independent polls, 7% said they had "a great job," 10% rated their work experience as "ten out of ten," 17% were "elated" on the job, and 25% were in "their dream job."

Unfortunately there is much evidence that those who are dissatisfied in their job are very dissatisfied. Only 12% of responders to the job-satisfaction module of the Gallup World Poll feel they have substantially higher overall wellbeing because of their jobs. In another study, 64% of workers claimed that their workplace had a negative effect on their lives. In another, only 42% of all workers rated their employee experience as positive, while 43% found it to be negative (presumably the remaining 15% were non-committal). In one study, less than 30% report having "a lot of fun" at work, and in another, 25% "dread going to work." The primary reasons given by those who hate their jobs are that it is boring (73%), that they are working under bad bosses (67%), that their coworkers are annoying (33%), and that their schedules are inflexible and unpredictable (30%). Among workers who had recently changed jobs, most did so to improve their pay grade (30%) or to escape a bad boss (29%), but others cited workplace harassment, inadequate opportunities for advancement, unfair performance reviews, a lack of respect and recognition, and dissatisfaction with their work-life balance.

With respect to employee engagement, the numbers show clearly that not all "satisfied" employees are actually "engaged" in their work. A meta-analysis of the 2018 Gallup Q^{12} results indicated that only 34% of American workers are truly engaged, 53% are not engaged, and 13% are "actively disengaged." A study by the National Business Research Institute found that only 11% of disengaged workers are "happy" in their job, compared to 86% of engaged workers. Engaged workers tend to be more innovative than there unengaged colleagues (59% to 3%), and more willing to advocate for the company (67% to 3%). Another study found that when supervisors empower workers to "take ownership, make decisions, lead, and innovate", there is a 78% increase in engagement.

Managers and professionals consistently show higher percentiles of job satisfaction (generally greater than 80%) than do salaried workers (generally less than 70%). This is perhaps unsurprising given that managerial and professional positions usually offer higher pay, better career prospects, stronger job security, more interesting assignments, a better physical workspace, greater scope for initiative and autonomy, and greater power to change things that are not working.

One disconcerting finding from the various meta-analyses is the considerable mismatch that is exposed in how managers see things relative to their workers. Consider the percentages of each group who agree with the following statements. "The organization has a sincere interest in the wellbeing of its employees:" (management—86%, workers—50%). "Employees are treated with dignity and respect:" (management—80%, workers—60%). "Workers are fairly paid:" (management—67%, workers—21%). "Management is transparent:" (management—39%, workers—22%). "Saying thank-you more would influence staff retention:" (management—22%, workers—70%).

There is no question that men and women experience the workplace very differently, and that women feel severely disadvantaged. Consider the following findings. On the question of whether they are paid less than a comparable colleague of the opposite sex, 19% of men workers feel that this is so, 54% of women. On whether everyone has a fair chance to advance, 59% of men agree, 43% of women. On whether their employer treats people fairly, 47% of men agree, 39% of women. On feeling unsupported by one's boss, 30% of men feel so, 45% of women. On whether their performance is properly rewarded, 51% of men feel it is, only 41% of women. Approximately one-quarter of the American workforce feels discriminated against on the basis of gender; of these, 25% are men, 75% women. A recent special issue of *Social Indicators Research* addresses the gender equity question [39].

There are less data on the respective levels of job satisfaction in older workers relative to younger ones. Presumably, the U-shaped curve described in Table 6.7, whereby life satisfaction levels are highest in youth and old age, and lowest in mid-life, also hold on the job. Certainly the concerns of the two groups probably differ, with younger workers perhaps more alert to nuts-and-bolts issues like salary, career opportunities, job safety, job security, and a work-life balance that allows them quality time with young families. Most older workers are probably less needy and more satisfied with their lot. Statistics show that recently-retired men in financially-stable situations are among the happiest of all people.

The job preference lists already presented in Tables 11.3 and 11.4 emphasize private-sector opportunities. However, there is much evidence in the literature that government employees working in the public sector have higher levels of life satisfaction than those in the private sector. This may be a reflection of the relative degrees of unionization in the two sectors, as there is also strong evidence that unionized employees are happier than their non-unionized colleagues, especially at lower income levels [40]. In both cases, the sources of satisfaction presumably lie in the higher levels of job security and the more generous nature of negotiated benefit packages in government service and in unionized shops.

Assessments of the relative levels of job satisfaction between salaried and self-employed workers, between permanent and temporary staff, and between full-time and part-time workers, have much in common with one another. The consensus viewpoint has always been that self-employed workers are happier than salaried wage earners, and that permanent, full-time staff are happier than temporary part-timers. A more nuanced reading of the data in recent years [41] has identified this conclusion as somewhat naive. Job satisfaction is not due to self-employment per se, or permanent or full-time employment, but rather being in the type of employment of first preference. Self-employed workers are more satisfied in their jobs only if they have a preference for self-employment. Many workers forced into self-employment are not happy about it. Many workers in third-world countries who are struggling to make a living on their own would far prefer to be salaried and secure. Conversely, there are many underemployed workers who have chosen this route, perhaps in order to spend more time with family, or to take on caregiver duties, or to upgrade their credentials through education and training. Such part-timers may have quite high levels of job satisfaction. There is a big difference in life satisfaction between those who *want* to work and those who *have* to work.

Stress in the Workplace

Four of the most prevalent drags on job satisfaction are stress in the workplace, employee harassment, failure to achieve a suitable work-life balance, and the insecurities of the gig economy. Let us look at each in turn.

Stress is definitely item one. Over 50% of all workers describe their work as somewhat stressful, 35% as moderately stressful, and 9% as highly stressful. Over 85% claim that they have been overwhelmed by their job at one time or another. A majority of stressed workers have experienced some level of burnout at some point in their careers. The most commonly reported causes of stress and burnout are unmanageable workloads, unreasonable demands from one's supervisor, looming organizational change, a toxic workplace culture, and long working hours that cut into family time. The most susceptible workers are hard-driving workaholics who place too much emphasis on reputation, status, and advancement. Stressed workers have difficulty concentrating on their work, have poor coping skills when problems arise, tend to be irritable and insecure, and suffer from lower productivity.

If not addressed, stress can decline into mental illness. According to one study, over 50% of all salaried workers in America have experienced a struggle with some form of mental illness in the workplace at some point in time, and over 20% have received dedicated mental health support from their employer. Of the latter group, 56% were diagnosed with stress disorders, 36% with disabling anxiety, and 25% with full-fledged depression. The average American worker claims 8.4 sick days per year for mental health issues. It has been estimated that depression costs the American economy over $200 billion per year.

Employee Harassment

Harassment in the workplace can take many forms: intimidation, coercion, humiliation, accusations, threats, innuendo, sarcasm, exclusion, dirty looks, or intemperate emails. It can come from supervisors or from co-workers. It often involves the misuse of an imbalance in power. It can be sexual in nature, or based on some other perception of weakness or vulnerability. If harassment and bullying are allowed to thrive, the result is a toxic workplace culture, with its open personality conflicts, productivity-sapping gossip, and added legal and mental-health costs. Some 20% of those who quit their jobs cite a toxic workplace as a contributing factor. Over 30% of American workers have observed at least one act of misconduct in their workplace, and 16% report "a severe disruption in their lives" from such misconduct.

Sexual harassment is the most common type of harassment for women. Over 40% of the female workforce has experienced some form of sexual harassment in the workplace. Over 30% of female employees who changed jobs report that they did so after "inappropriate behavior" in their former workplace. Roughly two-thirds of the unwanted attention came from co-workers, one-third from supervisory staff. Most women who experience sexual harassment don't feel comfortable reporting it (67% in one survey), largely because many of them have observed managerial retaliation for doing so (41% in the same survey). The only good news on this front is that 32% of American workers say that their employer has taken new steps to address and prevent sexual harassment since the start of the Me Too movement.

Work-Life Balance

Almost one-quarter of all workers express dissatisfaction with their work-life balance, and more than 12% of employees who quit their jobs do so out of frustration with the perceived imbalance. What these workers are searching for is a reduction in conflict between the requirements of their work and the demands of their family life. They want to establish a state of equilibrium between their professional life and their personal life, and a clear boundary between the two.

It is not purely a question of hours. John Robinson of the Department of Sociology at the University of Maryland has spent his life examining and interpreting the national time-use accounts collected by the US Census Bureau in their America Time Use Survey (ATUS) [42]. At first glance, the numbers do not look too bad. Americans between the ages of 18 and 64 spend an average of 34 h per week in paid work. Of course this number includes part-timers and the unemployed. For full-time paid workers, the number is 42.5 h per week. If one looks at data from 1965 to the present, these numbers show a steady decline of more than 6 h per week, with an equal and concomitant increase in leisure time. Despite these improvements, a 2014 study still found that respondents to a Cantril ladder-of-life questionnaire experienced much greater happiness on weekends than weekdays, with much lower levels of anxiety, sadness and anger [43]. The same study confirmed the reality of the "Thank God It's Friday" syndrome, and to a lesser degree the dread of "Blue Monday."

Work-life balance is not a new issue. In the United States the first reference to it can be dated to the 1977 book by the sociologist Rosabeth Moss Kanter on *Work and Family in the United States: A Critical Review and Agenda for Research* [44]. Her call to arms led to the formation of many dedicated academic research centers, among them the Wharton Work/Life Integration Center at the University of Pennsylvania, the Harvard Project on Global Working Families, and the Sloan Work and Family Research Network at Boston College. The Organization for Economic Cooperation and Development (OECD) produced a handbook on *Work-Life Balance* in 2014 as part of efforts associated with the Better Life Index [45]. The Harvard Business Review published its *HBR Guide to Work-Life Balance* in 2019 [46]. World at Work, an Arizona-based national organization for human-resources professionals, hands out an annual Work-Life Seal of Distinction to worthy companies [47]. The UK-based Working Families organization sponsors a National Work-Life Week in October each year [48]. There are lots of user-friendly self-help books on bookstore shelves, even including a *Work/Life Balance for Dummies* [49].

All of these studies have led to many hypotheses to explain the growth in dissatisfaction with work-life balance. The three most widely held ones place the blame on changes in workplace demography, the impacts of rapid technological change, and the vagaries of a long commute. The most obvious change in workplace demography over the past few decades has been the increasing role of women in the workplace and the resulting increase in dual-worker families. There is no question that the loudest voices against work-life imbalance come from working parents.

With both spouses suffering, there is less room for the kind of spousal support that is needed by both parties. The primary development on the technological front has been the now-almost-universal ownership of smart-phones and their aura of constant and immediate availability. Many employees feel tethered to their jobs, even in their leisure hours, by this unremitting connectivity. Lastly, there is the issue of increasing commute times, driven in part by unattainable house prices in city centers. A long commute is given as the main reason by 14% of those who hate their jobs. (Although there is one contrary study from Sweden [50] that claims that many commuters enjoy their commute as a time to prepare for their working day on the way in and unwind on their way home.)

It is now recognized that the "spillover" from one domain to the other can go in either direction, from work to family, or from family to work. Problems brought home from work might include work overload, collegial conflict, or a frenzied travel schedule. Problems brought to work from home might include marital conflict, parenting issues, or the strain of eldercare. The spillover may be time-based, due to competing time requirements, or it may be stress-based, due to the pressures in one role affecting performance in the other. Of course, spillover need not always be negative; positive spillover in either direction is also possible. Recognition at work might carry over to home life. The pleasures of a good marriage at home generally lead to greater happiness and satisfaction at work.

There have been several attempts to develop an index of work-life balance, some of them designed to measure balance or imbalance at an individual level and others at a national level. The earliest attempt at the individual level was the Work-Spillover Scale [51] developed in 1990 by the Child and Family Studies group at the University of Wisconsin. It included only negative spillover from work to family, using 20 indicators to identify impacts on 4 areas of family life: the marital role, the parental role, the leisure role, and the home management role. A later effort provided a 16-item scale that included consideration of both positive and negative impacts in both directions [52]. At the national scale, the OECD Work-Life Balance Index uses only two objective proxy variables: the percentage of workers in a country working long hours, and the average percentage time devoted by individuals to leisure and off-work personal endeavors. By far the most detailed index at national scale, the National Work-Life Balance Index, was developed in 2016 by a group of Spanish researchers [53]. It uses 23 indicators in 5 dimensions to assess 26 European countries, using objective data from European Union databases, the Eurobarometer, and the OECD. Among the primary indicators are country-wide estimates of average hours worked, average commuting times, employment rates (employed, unemployed, self-employed, and part-time), family earnings, child education levels, availability of paid maternity leave, and percentage GDP spent by government on family-friendly policies. The highest-ranked countries were Denmark, the Netherlands, Finland and Sweden; the lowest, Spain, Greece, Portugal and Bulgaria.

The Gig Economy

The gig economy is the natural extension of a long continuous trend in the nature of the U.S. workplace. The jobs that our grandparents held tended to be lifetime associations with a single employer, and that employer generally provided a fairly-inclusive benefits package and a generous retirement pension. In 1954, 35% of American workers belonged to a union that negotiated these issues on their behalf. Nowadays, union membership barely clears 10% of the workforce. In the dog-eat-dog world of today's business climate, the bottom line rules, and employment practices that feed the bottom line are still the norm in many industries.

A primary aspect of the current workplace is the increased use of gig workers who are paid on contract by the task or project rather than as salaried employees. The result is a growing freelance workforce of self-employed independent contractors. The numbers that are reported for the USA vary from source to source, but a 20% increase in the number of self-employed workers between 2005 and 2015 has been widely reported. A 2016 report from the National Bureau of Economic Research (NBER) estimated 15.8% of the workforce was involved in the gig economy, but this only included full-time workers, not the many who use self-employment as a supplementary source of family income [54]. The Gig Economy Data Hub, a joint effort between the Cornell University School of Industrial and Labor Relations and the Aspen Institute's Future-of-Work Initiative, reported a 25% participation rate in non-traditional work [55]. A 2018 Pew Research survey found 30% of the workforce to be self-employed in some sense (a total of 44 million workers) [56]. Of these, 29% counted on self-employment for "essential" income, 27% for "important" income, and 42% for supplementary income. A 2018 article in Forbes magazine quoted the Bureau of Labor Statistics as pegging self-employment at 35% of the workforce (55 million workers), with a projection of 43% by 2020 [57]. The Freelancer's Union, an advocacy group for the self-employed, claims that there are 56.7 million freelancers in the US [58].

In the early years, these gig workers tended to be concentrated in low-income jobs like delivery drivers, ride-hailing providers, handyman jobbers, home care workers, and residential cleaning services, but in recent years the gig world has become more ecumenical with many higher-income professionals joining the gig ranks in such fields as computer programming, web design, engineering, and management consulting.

There is a huge difference in attitude toward the gig economy between those who join it willingly and those who are forced into it. Those who choose self-employment willingly are often in the high-income end of the spectrum. They do so for the flexibility, the freedom, and the personal fulfillment. They are willing to trade the stability and security of salaried employment for the potential improvement in their finances, their mental health, and their work-life balance. There are now several self-help books on the market that are full of advice on how to parlay the gig life into greater financial return, more interesting work, more vacation time, and a happier family life [59].

However, this rosy picture does not apply to most gig workers. For those who are forced into it unwillingly, the gig economy has many negative aspects that can affect worker happiness and wellbeing [60]. There are no health benefits, no company pensions, no workplace protections, and no minimum-wage provisions or anti-discrimination laws. There may be uncertainty about financial security. There will almost certainly be added stress associated with the never-ending search for suitable gigs. Many newly-self-employed are very good at the work they do, but not necessarily good at generating the demand they need for their services. Despite the hopes and promises, the hours are often longer and the family time more precarious in self-employment, than in a salaried corporate setting.

Willingly or unwillingly the numbers climb, and there is no shortage of contract-job platforms like Freshbooks, UpWork, TaskRabbit and Gigworx.

The Employer Perspective: Job Satisfaction and the Bottom Line

From the employer's perspective, the issue is not so much whether employees are happy and satisfied (or at least not solely so), but whether all this effort to develop and maintain a happy job environment is actually reflected in improved productivity, profitability, and market success. It is the employers who fork out the money for job satisfaction surveys, and who bear the costs of making the changes recommended by their human resources team to improve employee wellbeing. They need confirmation that this modern-day, people-first paradigm actually improves the bottom line.

Researchers in the earlier years of the job-satisfaction paradigm shift were equivocal [61]. They recognized that the "happiness-productivity thesis," as it was then called, had "intuitive appeal" but they worried that a positive relationship had not really been confirmed in controlled studies.

They need not have fretted. Thousands of studies carried out since the turn of the new millennium by economists, workplace psychologists, and researchers of many stripes in business schools around the world have confirmed a strong correlation between the happiness, satisfaction, and engagement of employees, and the bottom-line performance of companies. Among the productivity-enhancing effects of a happy workplace are increased punctuality, reduced absenteeism, less shirking, greater cooperation among colleagues, lower turnover rates, fewer workplace accidents, fewer stress-related mental health issues, fewer health insurance claims, and less employee theft. A happier work environment also leads to higher-quality products and services, with fewer product defects or clerical errors. Enhanced performance in turn creates a stronger corporate reputation, greater customer satisfaction and loyalty, and better stock market performance [62].

The correlations and causal arrows are not in doubt. The only remaining questions relate to the degree of improvement that a company can expect to see when a people-first paradigm is introduced; or, recognizing the competitive nature of most business, how the bottom line of a people-first company compares with that of a company that has stayed with more traditional employer-employee relationships. To address these questions one can turn to the results of several meta-analyses that have appeared in review articles or books on job satisfaction.

The general approach has been to try to correlate job satisfaction scores from employee surveys with measures of a company's bottom-line success. A meta-study carried out by the Gallup organization on 339 independent proprietary studies involving almost 2 million employees in 49 industries in 73 countries is reported in the 2019 edition of the Global Happiness and Well-Being Policy Report [63]. It uses four bottom-line performance measures: (1) Employee Productivity (calculated as company revenue per employee), (2) Profitability (taken as the profit margin of company revenues), (3) Customer Loyalty (based on the percentage of repeat clients, the number of client referrals, and the results of customer satisfaction surveys), and (4) Staff Turnover Rates. The study found clear positive correlations between job satisfaction and productivity, profitability, and customer loyalty; and a clear negative correlation with staff turnover. The findings held for all industries including those from finance, retail, manufacturing and service.

The same report also references several studies that offer comparisons between companies. One such study found that a positive difference of one standard deviation in mean job satisfaction scores led to an average increase in productivity of 6.6%; another that a positive difference of one scale division (from 4 to 5, out of 6) in mean job satisfaction led to an average increase in productivity of 20%. Yet another study found that average stock market returns for companies listed on the "Fortune 100 Best Companies to Work For" were 2.1% greater than their industry averages.

A meta-analysis reported by Cary Cooper and coworkers in their 2018 textbook found that companies that placed in the top quartile of employee engagement scores were demonstrably more successful than those who fell in the bottom quartile: 16% higher profitability, 37% less absenteeism, 60% less product defects, 12% better customer ratings, 25% less turnover, and 27% less "shrinkage." [64].

A team of researchers from the University of Warwick in the UK have reported the results of a very interesting controlled trial. They report a 10–12% increase in productivity from a group of workers at a company who were given perks to make them happier, relative to a control group at the same company who did not receive the perks [65].

As a bottom line on the bottom line one can quote De Neve and coworkers from the Global Happiness and Well-Being Policy Report that "a meaningful increase in employee wellbeing yields, on average, an increase in productivity of about 10%" [66].

Workplace Wellbeing Programs

Given the apparently clear benefits of maintaining a happy, satisfied, and engaged workforce, most organizations now offer a variety of workplace interventions designed to enhance employee wellbeing. They tend to fall into four groups:

(1) those that are directly related to work tasks and work schedules; (2) those that address issues of physical and mental health; (3) those that involve training and education; and (4) those that emphasize the tenets of the positive psychology movement.

The first group includes programs that allow such worker-friendly policies as flexible scheduling, compressed work weeks, opportunities to work from home, and liberal leave policies for maternity, eldercare, or other personal matters. It also includes the opportunity for employees to exert greater autonomy over their work tasks and schedules through "job crafting." This latter concept has gained traction under the leadership of Amy Wrzesniewski of the Yale University School of Management [67]. As the title of one of her papers puts it, job crafting is the process of "turning the job you have into the job you want." According to its proponents, it is a "powerful tool for reenergizing and reimagining your work life." It is employee-driven in the sense that the ideas for change must come from the employee (although clearly, there has to be employer buy-in). There seem to be three strands to the concept: *task crafting* (adding or dropping responsibilities, and/or reframing one's role in the organization), *relationship crafting* (reshaping interactions with colleagues and supervisors), and *perception crafting* (changing one's mindset about the job). The goal is to enjoy and excel at the job, while simultaneously making the job more aligned to one's strengths, motives and passions.

Turning to the second group of interventions, those that address issues of physical and mental health, many companies now offer considerable support over and above their traditional medical insurance plans (assuming that such companies have not succumbed to the gig culture). On the physical health side, such support may include dental plans, eye-care plans, massage services, sleep clinics, injury-prevention programs, access to occupational therapy, on-site exercise programs or gym memberships, and healthy-living courses on nutrition, weight control, and stopping smoking. On the mental health side, many companies provide on-site or contract counseling services for anxiety, stress, depression, anger management, conflict resolution, alcohol abuse, drug abuse, gambling addiction, and other work-sapping personal crises and traumas.

In the third group, educational programs are no longer limited to traditional skills training and back-to-school opportunities, but now may include programs to help with personal financial difficulties, tax advice, and legal help.

And lastly there are the positive psychology programs, which usually involve seminars or courses based on one of the commercially-available strategies designed to fuel positivity and optimism in the workplace, enhance purpose and meaning in one's job, and foster employee engagement. The Emotional Intelligence (EI) movement has been particularly active in this sphere through the Consortium for Research on Emotional Intelligence in Organizations [68]. Yale University even offers a certificate for those trained to provide EI counselling.

All of these different types of programs have become immensely popular. In 2018, one US survey found that 82% of large firms and 53% of smaller employers offer some type of wellness program. Over 50 million American workers have access. In the USA, the Affordable Care Act allocates public funding to such programs. All of this activity is usually viewed as part of a society-wide move toward preventive rather than reactive health care.

Some companies run these support programs in-house but many others turn to the burgeoning industry that provides Employee Assistance Programs on a contract basis (known as EAPs in the trade). Among some of the better-known EAP firms are Lifeworks (out of Atlanta GA), Workwell (out of Duluth MN), and Mindwell U (which uses a mindfulness approach). Among those that emphasize a positive psychology spin are two that have been set up by Harvard Psychology alumni: Potentialife (by Tal Ben-Shahar) and Goodthink Inc. (by Shawn Achor). All these organizations provide self-standing courses, manuals, exercises, speakers, coaches, seminars, consulting services, an online presence, and support for the in-house human resources teams that act as facilitators. The courses are for employees, but the raison d'etre for employers is the bottom line. As Lifeworks promises on their website: "By improving lives, we improve business."

There have been many studies designed to assess whether these myriad types of workplace interventions actually do improve employee happiness and engagement, and whether they actually do improve a company's bottom line. The results over the years have been mixed, but it is possible to draw some conclusions from four meta-studies carried out in the past decade: the 2010 Harvard Study of Workplace Wellness Programs, the 2013 Rand Corporation Workplace Wellness Programs Study, the 2018 Illinois Workplace Wellness Study, and the 2019 update by the Harvard Workplace Wellness team [69]. The 2019 Harvard study is the biggest and most carefully-documented study to date. It involved 33,000 employees at 160 worksites, some with wellness programs and some without, 27 self-reported measures of health and behavior, 10 clinical measures of health, 38 measures of company spending on interventions, and 3 measures of employee performance.

One immediate finding is that employee participation in company-sponsored wellness programs is limited, ranging from 46% to 56% in the four studies, and that those who participate tend to be employees who are already healthier and happier than those who don't. Another finding common to all the studies is that employees who participate in interventions designed to improve lifestyle habits like fitness/exercise, smoking cessation, weight control, and nutritious food choices, do indeed show improvements in these areas. The question of whether these improvements lead to lower medical health costs for employers is more controversial. The earlier studies in 2010 and 2013 indicated a good return on investment ($3.27 saving per $1.00 invested in the 2010 study), but the later studies in 2018 and 2019 do not indicate any significant differences in health care spending rates between worksites with wellness programs and those without. Interestingly, none of the four studies was able to find a positive correlation between intervention spending and measurable improvements in job satisfaction or job performance. However most agreed that an active workplace wellness program acted as a strong incentive in hiring, and in that sense was more likely to lead to an engaged workforce.

The recent studies that seem to question the concept and value of workplace wellness are not going to go unanswered. Given the huge company investments, the entrenchment of the EAP industry, and the long-held views of the positive psychology movement, we can expect more studies and a strong counterattack. Stay tuned.

Values-Driven Business

Values-driven businesses are those that espouse a compassionate form of capitalism that is more humane, just, fair, and inclusive than the traditional business model. They are still about profits, but they like to see their profits distributed more equitably, and shared more fully for the common good. They believe in a market framework that will support a sustainable future. They favor the so-called triple-bottom line: people, planet, and profit, in that order. They are more likely to offer strong employee wellness programs, be involved in volunteerism and charitable giving, include ecological considerations in their product design and plant operation, and hold both employees and management to a high standard of ethical performance. They try to develop an organizational consciousness that features high performance, financial stability, a vibrant internal community, and a spirit of service to humanity and the planet [70].

Those companies that want to really walk the walk by publicly identifying themselves as values-driven businesses can do so by becoming corporate members of one of several organizations formed to promote corporate social responsibility. The Social Ventures Network (which has now morphed into the Social Ventures Circle) was launched in 1987 by "a raucous group of misfits" who were "impatient with an economic model that valued growth above all else." The Social Enterprise Alliance is "focussed on advancing the field of social enterprise and social entrepreneurship." The American Sustainable Business Council is a national coalition of mission-driven businesses, social enterprises, and sustainable business networks that "recognize the need to move to a new economy grounded in the principles of sustainability and equity." The Business for Social Responsibility is a global business network that "works with business to create a just and sustainable world." All of these organizations host conferences and workshops, distribute newsletters, and have a strong online presence through blogs and webinairs. All of them are regularly quoted on the Corporate Social Responsibility Newswire distributed by 3BL Media. Most of them also play a political role in lobbying for socially-conscious government policy, facilitating collaboration between member corporations, and raising consumer and investor awareness in issues of corporate social responsibility [71].

The academic world hosts many graduate programs that emphasize values-driven business principles, among them the Fowler Center for Business as an Agent of World Benefit at Case Western Reserve University, and the Wharton Social Impact Initiative at the University of Pennsylvania. The centerpiece of the Fowler Center program is an initiative on Business Innovations for Global Good which steers future business leaders toward meeting the United Nations Sustainable Development Goals. Research teams from these types of institutions have many possible publication outlets for their work. Corporate responsibility is closely aligned with the concept of business ethics, and there are at least six journals that highlight business ethics in their title (*Journal of Business Ethics, Journal of Academic and Business Ethics, Journal of Business Ethics and Organizational Studies, Business Ethics Quarterly, Business and Professional Ethics Journal, and the International Journal of Business Governance and Ethics*).

There are many private consulting firms that advise companies on how to become more socially responsible. The UK-based Barrett Values Centre, founded by British author and workplace visionary Richard Barrett, offers help to corporations in setting up a "thriving corporate culture with we're-all-in-this-together energy." The Spirit-at-Work counselling service out of Austin TX promises to "enhance workplace spirituality," not in a religious sense, but as an "alignment of personal and corporate values." The B Corporation hosts the B-Corp movement which provides certification of companies through an in-house impact assessment procedure. Companies must meet verified standards of social and environmental performance, legal accountability, and public transparency. They must prove that their business provides jobs with dignity and purpose, that it is a force for good, and that it creates benefits for all stakeholders through reduced inequality, lower levels of poverty, a healthier environment, and stronger communities [72].

The Educational Milieu

The educational workplace is the classroom, and in the classroom one can conceive of two types of workplace satisfaction, that felt by the teacher, and that felt by the students. Student satisfaction is a bit outside the focus of this chapter, but it is certainly worth noting that it has drawn much attention in educational circles. The Canadian social scientist Alex Michalos, whose name has figured prominently in earlier chapters, has written a four-volume *Global Report on Student Well Being*, the first volume of which centers on student happiness and life satisfaction [73]. The Oxford Handbook of Happiness includes a ten-article section on happiness in education [74]. The Global Happiness and Wellbeing Policy Reports which have been often quoted in these pages contain a chapter on Positive Education in each of their annual reviews [75]. There are several measuring tools, including the Students Life Satisfaction Scale (SLSS), the Personal Wellbeing Index – School Children (PWI-SC), and the EPOCH measure of adolescent wellbeing [76].

More apropos to current considerations is the question of teacher job satisfaction. A 1993 publication entitled *Instrumentation in Education: An Anthology* provides an exhaustive listing of measurement scales and indexes of job satisfaction to that date for many specific subfields of education and for a variety of educational positions (teachers, principals, counsellors, college faculty, etc.) [77]. Many of the same issues that control job satisfaction in other walks of life also apply to teachers, but these basic factors are then overlaid by the influences of education-specific input from state-level policy-makers, elected municipal school boards, individual school administrations, and parental interest groups. Whatever positive or negative impacts are impressed on a teacher's life by these groups, they are probably less important than the bittersweet day-to-day interactions that a teacher experiences with young people at various stages in their maturation process from children to adults.

There are several quantitative educational indexes that are quite widely quoted, all with very similar names: the Teacher Job Satisfaction Questionnaire (TJSQ) from 1987, the Teaching Satisfaction Scale (TSS) from 2002, and the Teacher Job Satisfaction Scale (TJSS) from 2011. Both the TJSQ and the TSS are based on relatively traditional questionnaires that do not differ much from job satisfaction surveys given to workers in other professions. The more recent TJSS is the most job-centric, consisting of nine questions under three headings that are directly related to teaching: (1) satisfaction with the support of principals and fellow teachers, (2) satisfaction with the interest and support of parents, and (3) satisfaction with the response and behavior of students [78]. Results from these studies and from statistics provided by the U.S. Department of Education National Teacher and Principal Surveys [79] show that roughly 40% of teachers are "very satisfied" with their jobs, and 70–90% "somewhat satisfied." On the flip side, there are as many as 25% who are looking to get out of the profession, or would do so if they could.

There are at least four international surveys that attempt to determine country-by-country trends in student performance. The first two, the TIMSS program (Trends in International Mathematics and Science Study), and the PIRLS program (Progress in International Reading Literacy Study), are run out of the Lynch School of Education at Boston College on behalf of the International Association for the Evaluation of Educational Achievement. The PISA program (Programme for International Student Assessment) and the TALIS program (Teaching and Learning International Survey) are administered by OECD. All of these programs include job satisfaction data for teachers along with their statistics on student performance. Surprisingly, attempts to correlate satisfied teachers with high student performance have not tended to uncover any clear relationships.

The Military

Another special case when it comes to job satisfaction relates to those who serve in the armed forces. The military lifestyle places demands on active service members, their spouses and families, and veterans of active service, that are not felt in a more traditional lines of work. These include frequent redeployments, assignments in faraway lands, family separations, long and unpredictable duty hours, and the ever-present risk of injury or death. Service personnel have to chart a route to personal happiness that can prevail in a structured and authoritarian work environment. Women in the military face the challenges of coping with a long-entrenched culture of masculinity. Military families often feel pressured to conform to a traditional model of military behavior.

Of course military service is not without its own special perks. The job offers camaraderie in a close-knit community with a common purpose. It offers built-in job security. Military bases usually abound with resort-style amenities in the form of gyms, pools, and theaters. Some have golf courses. Opportunities are generally provided to develop skills, get training, and attain credentials for post-service careers. Perhaps most important is the self-satisfaction of doing a job that has a meaningful impact in society, the feeling that one's job is making a difference.

Like more traditional workplaces, the military is not short on tools to assess job satisfaction and help recruits and re-trainees find an enlisted career path that matches their preferences and aspirations. There is the Air Force Work Interest Navigator (AF-WIN), the Armed Services Vocational Aptitude Battery (ASVAB), the Tailored Adaptive Personality Assessment System (TAPAS), and the Army Family Global Assessment Tool (AFGAT). The Walter Reed Army Institute of Research has carried out periodic Army Career Satisfaction Surveys (ACSS), and at a broader level the Pentagon has performed Surveys of Active Duty Personnel (SADP), both of which try to gauge satisfaction with military life. Results often appear in military newsmagazines like the *Military Times*, and they inform academic studies that appear in specialized journals like *Military Psychology*, and *Military Behavioral Health*.

One of the few indexes of job satisfaction designed particularly for military personnel was put forward in 2008 by Jennifer Lundquist, a sociologist at the University of Massachusetts. She used 5 "scales" with 19 individual variables. The scales were (1) Overall Quality of Life, (2) Employment Opportunities, (3) Career Commitment, (4) Family Benefits, and (5) Housing and Neighborhood. Data was taken from the most-recent SADP questionnaire. Many of the variables were based on answers to questions that asked responders whether such issues as pay, medical care, schools, or family support were better or worse than imagined at enlistment [80].

As for results, it depends on who you trust and when the purported data was collected. The 1999 SADP survey found 80% of all responders satisfied with military life to some degree. A 2014 article in *Military Times* entitled "A Force Adrift" reported a decline in those who claim their quality of life to be good or excellent from 91% in 2009 to 56% in 2014. An article in *USA Today* in 2015 based on the results of mandatory online "resiliency assessments" by the US Army found that only 28% of responders "felt good about their job." On the other hand, a 2010 survey by CareerBliss, an online resource "helping people find joy and success in their careers," listed the US Air Force, the Army National Guard, the US Marines, the US Navy, and the US Army all in the top 12 "Blissful Places to Work" alongside such multinationals as Google and 3M [81]. If there has been a decline in U.-S. military job satisfaction in recent years as some claim, the most common explanation apparently lies in the absence of a clear-cut global enemy, the unlikelihood of actual combat, and the questions that then arise in the ranks as to the societal value of their work.

References

1. Brayfield, A.H. and H.F. Rothe, An index of job satisfaction, *Jour. Applied Psychology*, 35(5), 307-311, 1951.
2. Brief, A.P., *Attitudes in and around Organizations*, Russell Sage, 1998.
3. de Neve, J-E and G. Ward, Happiness at work, Chapter 6, *World Happiness Report*, 2017; De Neve, J-E, Work and well-being: A global perspective, Chapter 5, *Global Happiness and Well-Being Policy Report*, 2018; Krekel, C., G. Ward, and J-E de Neve, Employee well-being, productivity, and firm performance: Evidence and case histories, Chapter 5, *Global Happiness and Well-Being Policy Report,* 2019.
4. David, S., I. Boniwell, and D. Ayers, *The Oxford Handbook of Happiness*, Oxford University Press, 2013; Linley. P.A., S. Harrington and N. Garcea, *Oxford Handbook of Positive Psychology and Work*, Oxford University Press, 2010.
5. Warr, P. Well-being and the workplace, in Kahneman, D., E. Diener, and N. Schwarz, eds., *Well-Being: The Foundations of Hedonic Psychology*, Russell Sage, 1999; Judge, T.A. and R. Klinger, Job Satisfaction: Subjective well-being at wotk, in Eid M. and R.J. Larson, eds, *The Science of Subjective Well-Being*, Guildford Press, 2008.
6. Chen, P.L. and C.L. Cooper, eds., *Wellbeing: A Complete Reference Guide*, vol. III, Work and Well-Being, 2014; Michalos, A.C., *Encyclopedia of Quality of Life and Well-Being Research*, in 12 volumes, Springer, 2014.
7. Warr, P., *Work: Happiness and Unhappiness*, Psychology Press, 2007; Reilly, N.P., J.M. Sirgy, and C.A. Gorman, eds., *Work and Quality of Life*, Springer, 2012; S. Johnson, I. Robertson, and C.L. Cooper, *Well-being, Productivity, and Happiness at Work*, Palgrave Macmillan, 2018.
8. Achor, S., *The Happiness Advantage: The Seven Principles of Positive Psychology that Fuel Success and Performance at Work*, Crown Business, 2010; Hsieh, T., *Delivering Happiness: A Path to Profits, Passion and Purpose*, Grand Central, 2010; Moss, J., *Unlocking Happiness at Work: How a Data-Driven Happiness Strategy Fuels Purpose, Passion and Performance*, Kogan Page, 2016; Anabile, T.M. and S. Kramer, *The Progress Principle: Using Small Wins to Ignite Joy, Engagement and Creativity at Work*, Harvard University Press, 2011; Donovan, T., *Happy @ Work: 60 Simple Ways to Stay Engaged and Be Successful*, New World Library, 2014; McKee, A., *How to be Happy at Work,* Harvard Business Review Press, 2018; and Baker, D. et al, *What Happy Companies Know: How the New Science of Happiness Can Change Your Company for the Better*, Prentice Hall, 2006.
9. Adams, S., *The Joy of Work: Dilbert's Guide to Finding Happiness at the Expense of Your Coworker*, Harper, 1999.
10. OECD, *Guidelines on Measuring the Quality of the Working Environment*, OECD Publishing, 2017.
11. Kahn, W., Psychological conditions of personel engagement and disengagement at work, *Academy of Management Journal*, 33(4), 692-724, 1990.
12. Shuck, B. and K.K. Woolard, Antecedents to employee engagement: A structured review of the literature, *Advances in Developing Human Resources*, 13(4), 429-446, 2011.
13. Truss, C. et. al., *Employee Engagement in Theory and Practice*, Routledge, 2013.
14. Brayfield and Rothe, 1951, op. cit.
15. Weiss, D.J. et al, *Manual for Minnesota Satisfaction Questionnaire*, University of Minnesota, 125 pp, 1967.
16. [bgsu.edu/arts-and-sciences/psychology/services/job-descriptive-index.html]
17. Hackman, J.R. and G.R. Oldham, Development of the Job Diagnostic Survey, *Journal Applied Psychology*, 60(2), 159-170, 1975.
18. Gallup Organization, Q^{12} *Implementation Guide*, 38 pp, 2018. [q12.gallup.com]
19. Spector, P., *Job Satisfaction: Application, Assessment, Causes and Consequences*, Sage, 1997.
20. [cdc.gov/niosh/topics/stress/qwlquest.html]
21. Kristensen, T.S. et al, The Copenhagen Burnout Inventory: A new tool for the assessment of burnout, *Work and Stress*, 19(3), 192-207, 2005. [nfa.dk/da]

22. Easton, S. and D. Van Laar, *User Manual of the Work-Related Quality of Life Scale*, University of Portsmouth, 2012. [www.qowl.co.uk]
23. [apaexcellence.org/assets/general/2017-work-and-wellbeing-survey-results.pdf]
24. Thompson, E.R. and F.T.T. Phua, A brief index of affective job satisfaction, *Group and Organization Management*, 37(3), 275-307, 2012.
25. [www.happinessresearchinstitute.com]
26. [whatworkswellbeing.org/product/workplace-wellbeing-questionnaire-methodology]
27. [greatplacestowork.com]
28. [surveymonkey.com]
29. [plasticitylabs.com]
30. [bamboohr.com], [glintinc.com], [tinypulse.com], [custominsight.com], [amplituderesearch.com]
31. A representative example of this series: Levering, R. and M, Moskowitz, *The 100 Best Companies to Work For in America*, Doubleday Business, 1993.
32. [fortune.com/best-companies]
33. [transparency.kununu.com]; [careercast.com/jobsrated]; [cityandguilds.com]
34. [www.conference-board.org]
35. [nbrii.com/infographics]
36. De Neve, J-E, 2018, op.cit.; Krekel, C., G. Ward, and J-E de Neve, 2019, op.cit.
37. Rath, T. and J. Harter, *The Economics of Well-Being*, Gallup Press, 2010.
38. [blog.accessperks.com/employee-engagement-loyalty-statistics]
39. Special issue on flexible working outcomes for gender equality and worker well-being, *Social Indicators Research*, 151(2), 2020
40. Flavin, P., A.C. Pacek and B. Radcliff, Labor unions and life satisfaction: Evidence from new data, *Social Indicators Research*, 98(3), 435-449, 2010; Pacek, A.C., B. Radcliff and M. Brockway, Well-being and the democratic state: How the public sector promotes human happiness, *Social Indicators Research*, 143, 1147-1159, 2019.
41. Kanhanan, M. and J. Natti, Involuntary temporary and part-time work, job quality and well-being at work, *Social Indicators Research*, 120(3), 783-799, 2015; Cueto, B. and G. Pruneda, Job satisfaction of wage and self-employed workers: Do job preferences make a difference?, *Applied Research in Quality of Life*, 12(1), 103-123, 2017; Bujacz,A., C. Eib and S. Toivanen, Not all are equal: A latent profile analysis of well-being among the self-employed, *Journal Happiness Studies*, 21, 1661-1680, 2020.
42. Robinson, J.P., ed., Special issue on time use and qualities of life, *Social Indicators Research*, 93(1), 2009; Fisher, K. and J.P. Robinson, Daily life in 23 countries, *Social Indicators Research*, 101(2), 295-304, 2011.
43. Helliwell, J.F. and S. Wang, Weekends and subjective well-being, *Social Indicators Research*, 116(2), 389-407, 2014.
44. Kanter, R.M., *Work and Family in the United States: A Critical Review and Agenda for Research and Policy*, Russel Sage Foundation, 1977.
45. [http://www.oecdbetterlifeindex.org/topics/work-lifebalance]
46. Harvard Business Review, *Guide to Work-Life Balance*, HBR Press, 2019; See also: Boushey, H., Finding Time: The Economics of Work-Life Conflict, Harvard U Press, 2016.
47. [www.worldatwork.org]
48. [workingfamilies.org.uk]
49. Lockett, K. and J. Mumford, *Work/Life Balance for Dummies*, 2012; Ring, J., *The Balance Point: Master the Work-Life Balance, Love What You Do, and Become an Unstoppable Entrepreneur*, Archangel, 2019; Bird, J., *Redefining Work Life Balance, Lifestyle Entrepreneurs Press*, 2019.
50. Olsson, L.E. et al, Happiness and satisfaction with work commute, *Social Indicators Research*, 111(1), 255-263, 2013.
51. Small, S.A. and D. Riley, Toward a multidimensional assessment of work spillover into family life, *Journal of Marriage and Family*, 52(1), 51-61, 1990.

52. Grzywacz, J.G. and N.F. Marks, Reconceptualizing the work-family interface, *Journal of Occupational Health Psychology*, 5, 111-126, 2000.
53. Fernandez-Crehuet, J.M. et al, The National Work-LifeBalance Index: The European Case, *Social Indicators Research*, 128(1), 341-359, 2016. See also: Noda, H., Work-life balance and life satisfaction in OECD countries: A cross-sectional analysis, *Journal Happiness Studies*, 21, 1325-1348, 2020.
54. Katz, L.F. and A.B. Kreuger, The rise and nature of alternative work arrangements in the United States, 1995-2015, *National Bureau of Economic Research*, Working Paper 22667, 2016.
55. [gigeconomydata.org]
56. [pewresearch.org]
57. Forbes Magazine, January 8, 2018.
58. Freelancers Union, *Freelancing in America*, 5th Annual Report, 2018; [upwork.com/i/freelamcing-in-america/2018]
59. Mulcahy, Diane, The Gig Economy: *The Complete Guide to Getting Better Work, Taking More Time Off, and Financing the Life You Want*, Amazon Books, 2016; Horowitz, Sara, *The Freelancers Bible*, Workman Publ., 2012.
60. Pfeffer, Jeffrey, *Dying for a Paycheck: How Modern Management Harms Employee Health and Company Performance – and What We Can Do About It*, Harper Business, 2018; Kalleberg, A., *Good Jobs, Bad Jobs: the Rise of Polarized and Precarious Employment Systems in the United States*, 1970s – 2000s, Russell Sage Foundation, 2011.
61. Iaffaldano, M.T. and P.M. Muchinsky, Job satisfaction and job performance: A meta-analysis, *Psychological Bulletin*, 97, 251-273, 1985; Ledford, G.E. Jr., Happiness and productivity revisited, *Journal of Organizational Behavior*, 20, 25-30, 1999.
62. Judge, T.A. et al, The job satisfaction – job performance relationship: A qualitative and quantitative relationship, *Psychological Bulletin*, 127, 376-407, 2001; Diener, E. and M.E.P Seligman, Beyond money: Toward an economy of well-being, *Psychological Science in the Public Interest*, 5(1), 3-31, 2004; Zalenski, J.M., S.A. Murphy and D.A. Jenkins, The happy-productive worker thesis revisited, *Journal Happiness Studies*, 9(4), 521-537, 2008; Weisbrod, M.R., Productive Workplaces, 3rd ed., Wiley, 2011; Oswald, A., E. Proto and D. Sgroi, Happiness and productivity, *Jour. of Labor Economics*, 33(4), 789-822, 2015.
63. Krekel, Ward and de Neve, 2019, op.cit.
64. Johnson, Robertson and Cooper, 2018, op. cit.
65. Oswald, A., E. Proto and D. Sgroi, 2015, op. cit.
66. Krekel, Ward and de Neve, 2019, op. cit.
67. Wrzesniewski, A., J.M. Berg and J.E. Dutton, Managing yourself: Turn the job you have into the job you want, *Harvard Business Review*, 88(6), 114-117, 2010.
68. [eiconsortium.org]
69. Baicker, K., D.M. Culter and Z. Song, Workplace wellness programs can generate savings, *Health Affairs*, 29(2), 304-311, 2010; Mattke, S. et al, *Workplace Wellness Programs Study: Final Report*, Rand Corporation, 2013; Jones, D., D. Molitor and J. Reif, What do workplace wellness programs do? Evidence from the Illinois Workplace Wellness Study, *National Bureau of Economic Research*, Working Paper 24229, 2018; Song, Z. and K. Baicker, Effect of workplace wellness program on employee health and economic outcomes, *Jour. Am. Med. Assn.*, 321(15), 1491-1501, 2019.
70. De Vos, R., *Compassionate Capitalism: Helping People Help Themselves*, Plume, 1994; Barrett, R., *Liberating the Corporate Soul: Building a Visionary Organization*, Butterworth-Heinemann, 1998; Sison, A.J.G., *Happiness and Virtue Ethics in Business*, Cambridge University Press, 2014; Bartlett, B. and D. Meltzer, *Compassionate Capitalism: Journey to the Soul of Business*, Tisn Media, 2016.
71. [svcimpact.org], [socialenterprise.us], [asbcouncil.org], [bsr.org]
72. [valuescentre.com], [spiritatworkatx.com], [bcorporation.net]
73. Michalos, A.C., *Global Report on Student Well Being, vol. 1, Life Satisfaction and Happiness*, Springer, 1991.

74. Boniwell and Ayers, 2013, op.cit
75. *Global Happiness and Well-Being Policy Reports*, op.cit.
76. Huebner, S., *Manual for Multidimensional Students Life Satisfaction Scale*, 2001; Cummins, R.A. and A.D.L. Lau, *Manual for Personal Wellbeing Index – School Children*, Deakin University, 2005; Kern, M.L. et.al., The EPOCH measure of adolescent well-being, *Psychological Assessment*, 28(5), 586-597, 2016.
77. Bishop, L. and P.E. Lester, *Instrumentation in Education: An Anthology*, Garland Publ., 1993.
78. Pepe, A., Measuring teacher job satisfaction, *Europe's Journal of Psychology*, 13(3), 396-416, 2017.
79. [nces.ed.gov/surveys/ntps]
80. Lundquist, J., Ethnic and gender satisfaction in the military: The effect of a meritocratic institution, *American Sociological Review*, 73(3), 477-496, 2008.
81. *Military Times*, Dec. 7, 2014; *USA Today*, Apr. 16, 2015; [www.careerbliss.com]

Part III
Nexus

Chapter 12
Policy, Politics and Happiness

The Social Indicators Creed

The political mantra of the social indicators movement can perhaps be traced back to Thomas Jefferson who said that "the only legitimate objective of good government is the care of human life and happiness." [1]. If people with higher levels of wellbeing function more effectively in life, are more likely to have meaningful relationships with others, are more engaged and productive in their work, are more likely to develop successful careers with higher incomes, and suffer less from the vicissitudes of poor physical and mental health, then surely it is a duty of government to develop policies that support and encourage greater happiness and wellbeing. Under this philosophy, the primary role of governance is to serve "the common good," and the good society is one that provides maximum satisfaction to its citizens.

This viewpoint is almost universally held by the leaders of the social indicators movement. Ed Diener and Martin Seligman state clearly in their influential article *Beyond Money* that "well-being should be the primary focus of policy-makers." In a paper written 12 years later with a different coauthor, Seligman declares that "well-being science is currently ripe and right to inform public policy." [2]. Richard Layard in his book *Happiness: Lessons from a New Science* says that "subjective well-being should be the main yardstick for public policy." [3]. Nic Marks in his TED talk on *The Happiness Manifesto* asserts that "the desired outcome of governance is the quality of people's experience of life." [4].

The point of departure for this philosophy of government is widespread dissatisfaction with economic constructs like the GDP as the measure of societal progress. As noted in another article coauthored by Seligman, "for almost a century, institutional architecture and public policy around the world have primarily revolved around maximizing GDP." [5]. The new happiness movement sees a need to challenge policy makers as to what "progress" really is, and how to better measure it. They argue that money and wealth are inadequate indicators of progress, and that those interested in maximizing society's welfare should shift their emphasis from

R. A. Freeze, *The Metrics of Happiness*, Social Indicators Research Series 86,
https://doi.org/10.1007/978-3-031-10913-3_12

increasing consumption to increasing social capital in the populace [6]. The populace seems to agree; in a BBC poll in the UK on what they see as the main objective of government, respondents came down at 19% for greater wealth, 81% for greater happiness [7].

The arguments for and against the use of GDP as the primary measure of national wellbeing were fully discussed back in Chap. 3. To briefly summarize, there are some advantages, but these tend to be more practical than philosophical. Supporters of the GDP point out that it is easy to measure, and that it can be viewed as a relatively objective indicator. On the flip side, the objections to its primacy are substantive. First and foremost, it must be recognized that the GDP is a measure of the economic production of goods in a country; nothing more, nothing less. The anti-GDP movement finds fault on two fronts: with those aspects of economic production that are included in the GDP but shouldn't be, and with those aspects that are not included but should be. In the first category are the increases in economic activity that arise out of events that are otherwise negative in their impacts on society, like wars and natural disasters. In the second category are non-market activities that nevertheless have great value to society like household work, volunteerism, and recycling. Furthermore, the GDP fails to properly account for the negative social impacts of environmental externalities like water pollution, climate change, and resource depletion. It is also felt that current methods of GDP calculation grossly underestimate the contributions to society of the arts, cultural activities, sports, and recreation; and the positive pleasures of leisure time. The GDP contains no feedback information to government policy-makers on many things that really matter, like a clean environment, crime-free neighborhoods, or minimizing the psychological distress engendered by unemployment, poverty, and mental illness. Lastly, the GDP gives no indication of the distribution of income and wealth. Gains at the top incorrectly imply bounty for all.

While dissatisfaction with the GDP is probably the primary pillar of the social indicators creed, an important secondary pillar is the need for measurement. If life satisfaction is to be an important driver of policy, then rigorous measurement of social indicators, both subjective and objective, should be a primary policy imperative. As one SI guru puts it: "If you treasure it, measure it." [8]. Chapters 6–11 of this book have attempted to summarize the current state of the art with respect to the measurement of social indicators and the use of such data in indexes that could inform policy decisions.

Of course, it is fully recognized that measures of life satisfaction are themselves far from perfect. As discussed in Chap. 6, subjective measures that are determined from polls and questionnaires are open to questions about the representativeness of the sampled cohort, the possible biases introduced by the wording and order of questions, the possible effects of cultural differences, the possibility of responder gamesmanship, and the overall validity, reliability, and internal consistency of the results. Nevertheless, as summarized there, it is widely held within the social indicators movement that such issues do not negate the evidential value of such data for use in the calculation of indexes, and by implication, with the use of such indexes in policy decisions.

Reservations

At a more fundamental level, the very idea that government policy should actively promote happiness is not held by all. There are many skeptics and dissenters. In addition to the practical issues of measurement noted above, they raise many deeper philosophical objections. Several such issues are introduced here, and then discussed more fully in the sections that follow [9].

First, and perhaps the most basic reservation of all, is the feeling by many that happiness and wellbeing are personal goals, and that their maximization is something for individuals to strive for on their own. In this life-view, such issues are private, and ought not to be the concern of government policy.

Second, even if raising the levels of happiness and wellbeing in the populace are thought to be suitable goals for government policy, there is the question of whether government legislation can actually be expected to succeed in such endeavors. Questions revolve around whether governments can define realistic societal goals and targets with respect to happiness and wellbeing, and whether they will be able to meaningfully measure the effectiveness of their policies.

Third, there is the question of political motivation. In a worldview dominated by us-and-them competition, policy is not designed to necessarily raise the happiness and wellbeing of the entire electorate, but rather to favor the supporters of the political party that brings it forward. It will follow the philosophical mantra of that party, and at least in that party's eyes, will offer the best chance for the party's re-election. From this viewpoint, which seems particularly relevant to the polarized political climate that currently exists in the USA and in many other countries, the fight for alternatives to the GDP becomes just one more issue on the polarized political battleground. Those of a liberal bent may have very different reactions to the social indicator movement than those of a conservative bent.

Fourth, even if social indexes are thought to be relevant as possible alternatives to the GDP, some supporters worry that there is still a lack of solid evidence as to whether they are of real value in the design and assessment of policy. They feel that serious consideration of practical policy options has lagged behind esoteric academic analysis. They see too many different indicators and indexes, and lots of conflicting results and interpretations. They wonder if these indexes are appropriate as a measure of policy-directed progress.

And lastly, at the farthest extreme of dissent, are the views of Helen Johns and Paul Ormerod of the UK-based Institute of Economic Affairs who have taken on the self-appointed role of lead skeptics of the happiness movement. They argue that most happiness research is just common sense. They believe that "we already know that stable family life and access to green spaces are good for us," and that current policy-makers already take this kind of thing into account. In fact, they say it is hard to imagine a government being elected if they did not offer some prospect of improved wellbeing. They agree that happiness and wellbeing are valid goals of government policy, but that such goals are already embedded in current economically-based approaches to policy analysis [10].

Some support for Johns and Ormerod come from a recent analysis carried out by researchers at the Gallup organization [11]. In a study based on 3 years of data from the Gallup World Poll for 153 countries in 10 geopolitical regions, they found that household income had far greater impact on the subjective wellbeing of responders than did non-economic factors like community functioning, governance, and altruistic behavior. They conclude, at least when looking at the full suite of the world's socioeconomic circumstances, that the policy agenda should remain on the economic front.

Let us now examine some of these reservations in more detail.

Can Government Policy Increase Happiness?

First off, let it be said that the foundational question as to whether the fostering of happiness and wellbeing in the populace is an appropriate role of government will not be debated here. It is unlikely that any readers of this book will have gotten this far without acceptance of such a credo. A more pertinent question is whether government policy can actually be expected to succeed in this role.

The populace is unsure. In polls, people often state that government contributes less to their happiness than any other potential source. Supporters of the social indicators movement usually ascribe this finding to the fact that most responders in western democracies take much for granted. Most such responders are probably thinking only of their own countries, where they accept many of the foundational roles of government as given. They may not be familiar with international statistics showing that happiness and wellbeing vary widely across countries and that they are highly correlated with issues of governance like accountability, transparency, stability, control of corruption, rule of law, and regulatory climate [12]. Around the world, good technical governance is almost always accompanied by higher levels of average subjective wellbeing. The implication of these data is that good governance *can* increase happiness and wellbeing (and that the findings of the Gallup study quoted above reflect the fact that those in economic hardship do not always recognize the importance that bad government plays in leading them to their lot in life).

Many observers dance around the question of the role of government in maintaining happiness and wellbeing by admitting that legislation probably cannot be credited with producing happiness directly, but that it does shape the economy, culture and society in which we live, and that these features feed our happiness and wellbeing [13]. By making decisions on how to spend finite resources, and by regulating the types of behavior that are and are not allowed, governments exert considerable influence over the milieu in which we live. Government legislation defines the fine line between freedom and control that allows happiness to thrive. In this sense then, government policy can be seen as a driver of citizen wellbeing.

Two other issues have received a full hearing in earlier chapters. First, some observers feel that policy prescriptions designed to increase communal happiness are unlikely to succeed because of the gene-related happiness set points of the individuals who make up the community. If such set points are common in the populace, happiness-driven policy would not be expected to have much permanent impact. As has been documented earlier, psychologists vehemently deny this theory, and the ongoing friction over this issue between psychologists and geneticists shows no sign of abating anytime soon.

Second, and also fully covered in earlier chapters, is the contention that the communal happiness of society cannot be significantly increased by top-down policy because personal individual happiness is relative. In this view, happiness does not depend on absolute wealth or social situation but on one's situation relative to others. It is argued that any government policy that claims to raise the boat for all of us will have little impact on overall happiness because it will produce little change in the relative situation of each of us.

Ruut Veenhoven, the founder of the World Database of Happiness, has taken it upon himself to be the official responder on behalf of the social indicators movement to the various "qualms" expressed by skeptics about the ability of policy to impact happiness. In a steady stream of papers over the years, he has addressed many of these doubts under the broad rubric of whether happiness is too "elusive and idiosyncratic" to be furthered by social policy. He argues that it is not, that it can be defined and measured, and that each and every one of the skeptics' qualms can be laid to rest [14]. It can certainly be argued that Veenhoven is far from a disinterested voice, but his papers are models of lawyerly logic.

Is Happiness Policy Ideologically Neutral?

There is little question that throughout its history the social indicators movement has tried to appear ideologically neutral, apolitical, and above the fray. However, many observers have argued that this has been a mistake, both because it is not really true, and because such a bland approach has been much less effective than if proponents had admitted that they are political activists fighting for an important goal.

The fiction of neutrality was recognized very early by Clifford Cobb, one of the developers of the Genuine Progress Indicator. "As soon as one wants to use the 'facts' to achieve a political purpose," he writes, "those facts become implicitly ideological. The evasion of ideology is simply not possible. In order to be taken seriously in public life, one must take sides." He argues that the ideological character of social indicators is "buried under a mountain of denial." In fact, social indicators are widely used by political parties, interest groups, and citizen activists to try to convince uncommitted citizens to join them in pushing for the "good" society. "Their use by partisans of particular policies is proof of their lack of neutrality." [15].

It should not be surprising that using indexes of wellbeing rather than the GDP to determine the value of government policies is much more likely to meet with the approval of liberals than conservatives. To some degree, the use of social indicators in policy-making is an attempt to redistribute the inequalities that exist in society. It is liberals who are generally more upset about inequality; conservatives are more likely to accept it as a natural outcome of a free, democratic meritocracy. Liberals are more likely to favor government actions that eliminate wealth as a control on outcomes in health care, legal disputes, and educational opportunities. These are also issues that tend to resonate with supporters of the social indicators movement. Conversely, conservative aversion to big government, the welfare state, and social engineering, and their tendency to favor market solutions over government action, makes them unlikely converts to the tenets of the social indicators movement. So not only is the social indicators movement not neutral, it is an active arena of liberal thought, and leads to policy that would generally be recognized as part and parcel of the canon of the left [16].

There are several other issues that identify the social indicators movement as an issue of conflict on the liberal/conservative battleground. For one thing, the development and interpretation of indexes of wellbeing are seen by many as requiring a significant reliance on experts. Liberals are more likely to accept a role for technical expertise. Conservatives often evince a fear of policy elites who claim to know what is best for people. These anti-elitist feelings that have been on the upswing in many Western nations in recent years find full voice when raised against the social indicators movement. As stated most pithily by Johns and Ormerod: "The logical conclusion of much happiness research—that an individual's own judgements about what is good for them can be overridden by experts wielding clipboards and regression models—is illiberal, undemocratic, and unattractively paternalistic." [17].

There is also the privacy issue. Liberals tend to be less threatened by the government bureaucracy that is required to run happiness-promoting programs. They are generally willing to suffer what they see as a minor invasion of their privacy for government agencies to collect the necessary data to fuel the calculation of wellbeing indexes. Conservatives are more wary of government intrusion into their lives.

A larger question concerns the long-contested trade-off between the welfare state and the putative undermining of responsibility and initiative. If reliance on social indicators to set and judge policy is seen as support for an enhanced welfare program, it may lead to fears on the right of a paternalistic "nanny state." [18]. These tradeoffs between freedom, privacy, opportunity, efficiency and equality lie at the very heart of liberal/conservative dialogue.

In Diener and Seligmans' classic treatise *Beyond Money* they recognize that many of the policy prescriptions that are based on maximizing happiness (or minimizing unhappiness) can be seen as associated with a liberal political agenda (the redistribution of wealth, a greater role for government, welfare for the poor, and so on), but they also note that many others might suit conservatives (support for strong families, the role of religious faith, support of marriage as an institution) [19]. Maybe so, but it seems that this muted argument of political neutrality has been overtaken by the times, and the consensus viewpoint now is that the social indicators movement is a value-laden enterprise. Its fundamental aims are to encourage morally-praiseworthy public policy that reduces inequalities and raises the levels of overall human happiness and wellbeing.

What Are the Appropriate Goals of Government Policy with Respect to Happiness and Wellbeing?

"The greatest good for the greatest number" has a nice ring to it as a policy goal, but what exactly does it mean? The simplest interpretation would lead governments to bring forth legislation that attempts to raise the average level of wellbeing in the entire populace. However such a hope flies in the face of one of the most influential books ever published on economic thought. The main point of *The Zero-Sum Society* by the MIT political economist Lester Thurow is that, despite the promises of elected parties, government legislation cannot create wealth. It can only redistribute it. Every piece of legislation helps some segments of society and hurts others. There is no raising the boat for everyone. There are always winners and losers [20].

The question arises whether happiness and wellbeing, like wealth, are also zero-sum, or can they be raised across the board? Certainly it has been shown in earlier chapters that there is a strong relationship between money and happiness, but it is also clear that there is considerable disconnection. Wellbeing rests not only on income and wealth, but also on many non-economic dimensions such as community vitality, safety and security, availability of health services, gender equality, educational opportunities, social capital, environmental preservation, freedom from persecution, a fair legal justice system, and a governance structure that is just and transparent. It is widely held in the social indicators movement that these aspects of wellbeing are not zero-sum, and that government action can increase wellbeing on these fronts, without causing a concomitant decline on other fronts elsewhere in the social fabric. They do so by enacting legislation that raises human capital, which is simply wealth by another name.

Of course, it must be recognized that there are distributional issues with respect to happiness and wellbeing just as there are with respect to income and wealth. Any attempt to increase happiness and wellbeing across the board does nothing to address these distributional effects. An alternative approach might be to try to raise the level of wellbeing of the least well-off? Either approach involves tradeoffs. In the first one, policy is designed in a *utilitarian* way, prioritizing an overall increase in the level of happiness in society, and accepting the continuing inequalities. In the second one, policy is designed in an *egalitarian* way, prioritizing the lessening of inequality, and accepting that many citizens may not benefit [21].

It appears that many policy makers are more comfortable with minimizing misery rather than maximizing happiness. They see happiness as a rather nebulous concept that is difficult to quantify. It is much easier for them to see the impact of legislation that improves the lot of those in trouble, than to chart any small marginal increase that may occur in the wellbeing of the general populace. To use the terms introduced by two social researchers from the Netherlands, governments generally prefer the role of "misfortune mitigator" to that of "happiness machine." [22]. From this perspective, the goals of public policy tend to focus on the minimization of unhappiness rather than the maximization of happiness.

There is a huge literature on the pernicious influence of societal inequalities in income and opportunity on happiness and wellbeing [23]. The poor suffer from increased mental health problems due to despair, lack of hope, self-doubt and shame. They experience job insecurity, lack of mobility, a lack of childcare options, and unsafe neighborhoods. The meagreness of their opportunities leads to more failed marriages, increased drug and alcohol addiction, more problem gambling, and higher rates of incarceration than in the population at large. The social indicators movement offers strong support for government policies that are designed to lessen these inequalities. On the taxation front, they favor progressive tax policies like the graduated income tax, which leads to some degree of income redistribution, rather than regressive tax policies like user-pay schemes or value-added taxes, which do not. On the social front, they favor policies that lead to the improvement of childhood education and care, the strengthening of communities, getting people into the workforce, and improving access to health care. Furthermore, they promote the use of indexes of happiness and wellbeing to identify and assess such policies [24].

Derek Bok, a former president of Harvard University, makes a strong case for income redistribution in his book *The Politics of Happiness* [25]. He argues that the poorest are the least happy and that even a small increase in their income is likely to bring added happiness, while a modest decrease in the income of the rich is unlikely to have much negative impact on this already-happy cohort. Viewed in this light, redistribution should have the net effect of increasing overall societal happiness.

Cost-Benefit Analysis

It is common for governments to invoke some form of cost-benefit analysis in assessing the worth of a set of alternative policies designed to reach some particular goal. This appears to be a reasonable approach, but as has been noted in earlier chapters, it requires placing a dollar value on many components of wellbeing that resist such monetization. Policy-makers who want to rely on cost-benefit analysis in its purest sense need to find some way to include the externalities, both positive and negative.

In this regard, there are often tradeoffs between short-term negative effects of a policy and long-term positive effects. Consideration of such issues in the design of legislation takes courage on the part of elected democratic governments because voters do not always respond well to upfront costs with delayed benefits, nor do they always see the benefits of protecting future generations from the negative impacts of current decisions. In a way, legislation of this type is asking the electorate to accept a discount rate for subjective wellbeing, and this is not something voters are necessarily prepared to do.

Layard and O'Donnell in their chapter in the 2015 edition of the *World Happiness Report* note that there are three types of governmental policy decisions: those that deal with *public expenditures*, those that set *taxation policy*, and those that create *regulations* against unacceptable behaviors. The first two are grist for cost-benefit analysis, in that it is the public expenditures that create the societal benefits, and it is the taxation policy that controls the money available for public expenditures. However, Layard and O'Donnell suggest an interesting twist on the cost-benefit concept [26]. They propose that costs be measured in monetary terms, benefits in units of happiness. Policy-makers would rank policy alternatives by weighing the increase in happiness that would be generated per dollar of expenditure against the decrease in happiness that would be caused by the increase in taxes needed to fund the policy. The predictions of increased happiness would be based on "social welfare functions," where the welfare gain per dollar of public expenditure must exceed some critical value, and the welfare loss per dollar of taxation must be below some critical value. The critical values would be set politically, and are in some sense a statement of the philosophy of the governing party. Distributional issues and zero-sum issues do not disappear; but they are perhaps taken into account in a fairer manner.

The third type of policy decision outlined by Layard and O'Donnell involves regulatory policy. Regulations set the constraints that must be imposed on the populace in order to have an orderly and just society. Clearly, every regulation should lead to a positive increase in overall societal happiness. Once again, however, there are distributional issues as to which segments of the population are made happier, and which less happy. Many regulations deal with contentious issues like abortion, drugs, or capital punishment, for which there is no consensus, and likely never will be. Others deal with externalities like environmental protection or climate change, for which consensus is growing but is still not universal.

The Role of Social Indicators in the Policy Cycle

The development of government policy takes place in a cycle with many steps. Martine Durand, the Chief Statistician with the Organization for Economic Co-operation and Development, has identified five steps: (1) agenda setting, (2) strategic planning, (3) policy formulation, (4) implementation, and (5) evaluation [27]. Data on communal happiness and wellbeing in the form of social indicator dashboards or multi-dimensional composite indexes have a role to play in each of these steps.

The first two steps involve identifying areas that require government intervention, setting the policy goals, and creating the necessary institutional structures. If one zeros in on municipal governance for example, it should be clear that the data collected in Community Indicator programs as described in Chap. 10 have much to offer municipal policy-makers. Indicator data are based largely on citizen feedback; they are usually set apart by district or neighborhood; and they usually provide comparative assessments of those aspects of city life most in need of municipal attention. The same reasoning applies at regional, state, or national levels.

The policy formulation and implementation steps are at the heart of the matter. Social indicator data can help policy-makers with the initial listing of available policy options, the assessment and prioritization of such options, feasibility studies, cost-benefit analyses, selection of a given policy instrument, identification of the appropriate public institutions to carry out the selected policy, allocation of the necessary resources to those institutions, and optimization of the methods of delivery of the benefits to the citizenry. At the budgetary level, for example, competing budget proposals can be assessed for their potential impact on communal wellbeing as part of the decision analysis. In the eyes of the social indicators movement, the concept of wellbeing must be hard-wired into the very machinery of government.

The final step involves selecting a performance framework, monitoring the impacts of policy interventions, and evaluating a given policy through to termination or continuation. If there is any skepticism over the value of social indicator data in the first four steps of the policy cycle, there is none at this final step. Measurement programs of the types that have been highlighted throughout this book are the meat of the policy appraisal step.

There are many mechanisms available for integrating happiness and wellbeing into government policy. At the highest level is actual constitutional change such as occurred in Bhutan with the enshrinement of gross national happiness into the country's very being. A more common approach is through legislation. In France, for example, there is a requirement by law that the ten leading indicators of wellbeing must be reported regularly to the National Assembly. Regulations that are embedded in legislation are often informed by social indicator data. Many countries have established government-supported happiness research centers to coordinate efforts at developing fair and effective regulations. Such centers are also usually an integral part of the policy appraisal process as well. There are also many steps short of legislation that governments can take to promote wellbeing, including media-based information campaigns directed at the citizenry, and the development of guidance documents for the civil service.

Many supporters of the social indicators movement feel that one of the most important roles played by happiness data is in the promotion of public debate. They see such debate as a valuable step in drawing attention to issues that affect the quality of people's lives, especially those issues that might otherwise fly under the radar. George Ward of MIT's Sloan School of Management notes that it is well-known that governments are much more likely to be re-elected if the economy is doing well, and this fact drives governments to focus on economic measures. If chances of re-election were tied to a broader set of outcomes, governments would focus more effort on these broader outcomes. To get government attention, supporters of the social indicators movement need to better popularize measures of these other outcomes so as to attract stronger media and political attention [28].

Sometimes parties in power seem to be trying to satisfy activists with symbolic gestures that let them avoid actions that would be politically untenable to vested interests or to their own party supporters (in labor-management issues, for example, or support of the petroleum industry). Where it is felt that government actions have been spurred by special interests rather than the public good, wellbeing data can prove useful in holding politicians to account.

The Political Power of Happiness

Political scientists have written tens of thousands of articles attempting to explain the mysterious ways of the electorate when it comes to election results. In recent years, while still recognizing the importance of economic factors like growth, unemployment, and inflation, more and more of these articles have begun to zero in on happiness and life satisfaction as a prime political motivator. It is now widely recognized that the outlook of the electorate in this regard is an important two-way street; not only can the state of individual and societal happiness affect political processes and outcomes, but political institutions and processes have the potential to impact happiness and life satisfaction.

Supporters of the social indicators movement have tried to take advantage of this situation by increasing their level of advocacy for policies and programs that fit their life-view. Such advocacy has been sporadically successful in getting governments to take a greater interest in monitoring the life satisfaction of the electorate, but it has not always been successful in achieving specific policy goals. Political strategists emphasize the need to get support on both ends of the game, from the voters, and from the legislators. Clifford Cobb argues that advocacy of a specific policy requires a "story" that appeals to the electorate. Proponents must be very clear on how the proposed policy will work, and how its adoption will positively impact individual citizens. "The absence of a story is a recipe for political failure," he says [29]. Other observers zero in on getting the politicians onboard. Advocates must realize that politicians need to get credit, and they are more likely to support policies where public credit will accrue. It must also be recognized that politicians will follow the course of action that is most likely to get them re-elected. Advocacy of unpopular positions is almost sure to fail. Policy advocates must win over the public first, then the legislators.

Looking at things from the perspective of a political party, it is clear that they need to carefully consider the impact of their policies on the life satisfaction of their party members and of the electorate as a whole. Studies have shown that party members with higher levels of subjective wellbeing are much more likely to take part in all aspects of supportive political action, including campaigning, contributing, and voting. A European study also showed a strong correlation between positive life satisfaction scores in the populace during election campaigns (as measured by the Eurobarometer), and the success of a governing party running for re-election. On the flip side, an unhappy electorate is much more likely to vote for populist, anti-elite, anti-establishment, authoritarian leaders and parties (as seen in support for Donald Trump, Marine Le Pen, and Brexit) [30].

Examples of Policy Issues That Can Benefit from Happiness Studies

Table 12.1 lists a somewhat random suite of policy issues faced by governments at the federal, state, or municipal level, that can presumably benefit from data and analyses carried out by the social indicators movement on communal happiness, wellbeing, life satisfaction, and quality of life [31].

Politicians have to consider both the cost of a given policy choice and its potential impact. Obviously, they will favor policies with low cost and high impact. Data and analyses from the social indicators movement provide considerable information on the impact, less so on the cost. Those who favor the use of social indicators in policy-making often bridle when high-impact policies are scuttled by presumptive high costs. John Helliwell and his co-editors of the World Happiness Report argue that the impact of a policy on communal happiness and life satisfaction is a far better criterion for good policy than the apparent willingness-to-pay among the electorate, especially for social measures in such areas as health care, environment, child welfare, and income support [32].

Most of the listings on Table 12.1 are self-explanatory, but a few require additional comment. Starting at the top of the table, for example, with the question of unemployment, it seems that government policy-makers are well aware of the costs to the economy of unemployment, and the need for financial support to those who are involuntarily out of work, but they often underestimate the social costs to those caught in the underemployment trap in the form of stress and depression, low-self esteem, family conflict, and the temptations of the criminal life. These social costs need to be included in the cost-benefit analyses that accompany policy-making decisions.

With respect to the redistributional aspects of a government's taxation structure, the social indicator literature is very clear that in their view the gain in wellbeing by the poor from such policies is much greater than the loss in wellbeing by the rich. In their eyes, the only real question is how far governments should go toward a policy of universal basic income.

On the health front, there are two takeaways. The first is that greater emphasis on preventive care almost always saves money relative to reactive care, and generally leads to higher levels of communal life satisfaction. The second is that greater emphasis on mental health relative to physical health is needed to address the fallout from mental illnesses in the form of low productivity at work, loss of employment, homelessness, addiction, depression, and misery. Richard Layard recommends programs that train therapists and improve access to preventive psychotherapy on the grounds that such measures would increase overall societal wellbeing, and would pay for themselves in reduced caseloads and reduced taxes [33]. In a more general context, it is held that any policy that is directed toward improving communal happiness, whether directly or indirectly, will lead to a healthier citizenry, less call on health-care services, and reduced health-care costs.

Table 12.1 Federal, state, and municipal policy-making that can benefit from data and analyses on communal happiness, wellbeing, life satisfaction, and quality of life

Economy	• Policies on unemployment: financial support, social support, availability and affordability of retraining programs.
	• Policies related to statutory retirement, pension plans, registered retirement plan payout schedules, taxation of retirement income.
	• Policies that address redistributional aspects of taxation structure.
	• Policies that address housing issues for homeless and elderly.
Health	• Policies that recognize the available tradeoffs between preventive and reactive health care.
	• Policies related to accessibility of mental health therapy.
	• Policies related to end-of-life treatment options.
	• Policies that relate to optimization of mix between local community-based health support and primary care system.
	• Policies that assess relative merits of publicly-available universal health care vis-a-vis private delivery.
Education	• Policies that address availability and affordability of early childhood education.
	• Policies that support well-rounded elementary and high school curricula that provide training for all aspects of life, not just careers.
	• Policies that address availability and affordability of post-secondary education.
Security and safety	• Policies that address tradeoffs between security and safety on the one hand, and freedom and privacy on the other.
	• Policies that address actual and perceived crime levels.
	• Policies that address negative youth temptations: street life, gangs, alcohol and drug addiction.
Social relationships	• Policies that support flourishing family life.
	• Policies that encourage strong neighborhood networks.
	• Policies that ensure access to leisure and sports facilities, thriving cultural amenities.
	• Policies that support a corporate culture that recognizes personal and family needs of employees.
	• Policies that promote tolerance of diversity.
Environment	• Policies that address issues of sustainable development.
	• Policy considerations that include such big-picture issues as climate change, biodiversity, and the responsibility owed to future generations.
	• Policies that address urban quality of life: efficient and affordable public transit, bikeability, parks and open spaces, air pollution.
Governance	• Policies that encourage involvement of citizenry in planning and development decisions.
	• Policy development that is democratic, inclusive, and transparent.
Infrastructure and technology	• Policies that support a healthy environment for technological innovation.

Turning to the Education box on Table 12.1, those in the social indicators movement feel that it is well-documented that the attainment of higher levels of education in the citizenry tends to raise the overall level of communal wellbeing, and that policies that support educational goals, both academic and vocational, ought to have high government priority. They also favor well-rounded curricula that train students for life, providing them not only with the three Rs, but also with a path toward self-esteem, compassion for others, social awareness, emotional resilience, recognition of the value of teamwork, sensitivity to the need for environmental stewardship, and a sense of responsibility to future generations.

There are two issues that appear on the bottom half of Table 12.1 that have led to considerable controversy in the social indicators movement. The first is the question of ethnic diversity. The second is the call for sustainable development. The World Wellbeing Panel (WWP), a collection of world leaders from the economic, psychological, and environmental wings of the wellbeing movement have wrestled with both.

The first of these issues appears as the final item in the Social Relationships box on Table 12.1. A call is made there for policies that promote a tolerance for diversity. In this form, there is probably little controversy, but the larger question as to whether government policy should promote diversity itself, through immigration policy or other means, is a political time bomb. The WWB concludes that the promotion of diversity is certainly "morally good, but sadly it often leads to divisiveness and lower subjective wellbeing" in the populace. Comparative data from social polling shows that in first-world countries, those that are smaller and more socially cohesive have happier populations [34]. On the other hand, if a country's social cohesiveness comes from coercion, as is the case in authoritarian regimes, it is unlikely to lead to happiness. The role of diversity in engendering or discouraging happiness is a thorny one.

On sustainable development, which appears as the lead item in the Environmental box on Table 12.1, the WWB notes that sustainable thinking requires a strong bequest motive, prudence and sacrifice. "Ultimately," they conclude, "things like biodiversity, climate change, and the living standards of future generations do not carry enough weight in the welfare functions of enough individuals to insure that well-intended policies will raise overall population wellbeing."

These latter issues, and perhaps some of the others on Table 12.1, raise the question as to how far governments should go in using the subjective wellbeing of the populace as a guide to policy, or whether there are issues that should be guided by expertise, even at the expense of a decline in perceived wellbeing.

In *The Politics of Happiness*, Derek Bok puts a somewhat different spin on the types of policy decisions that could benefit from social indicator data. His analysis includes many of the items listed on Table 12.1 but he organizes them under an umbrella that is worthy of our attention. He highlights government legislation from the point of view of its societal purpose: (1) to relieve suffering, (2) to reduce risk, (3) to strengthen families, (4) to provide equality of opportunity, and (5) to improve government performance. Legislation to address mental health issues would fall under the first heading. Legislation to reduce risk would include improvements to social security programs and unemployment support. Families might be strengthened by policies that address childcare support, pre-marital and pre-natal counselling, drug education programs, and the relaxation of incarceration for minor offenses. Equality of opportunity is needed in education, health care, and political access. Government performance can be improved by improving and simplifying procedures, and by discouraging pork-barrel politics, gerrymandering of election districts, and the influence of lobbyists for special interests [35].

The Effectiveness of Multi-dimensional Indexes of Wellbeing in the Policy Domain

In Chap. 9 a number of multi-dimensional indexes of wellbeing were introduced that have applicability at the national scale, and in Chap. 10 a second group was presented with applicability at regional or municipal scale. It is the dream of the social indicators movement that governments make use of these indexes in the policy domain. As is probably clear from much earlier discussion, they see two possible applications of such indexes, first as a direct competitor with the GDP as a measure of overall citizen wellbeing, and second as a guide to the design and assessment of policy initiatives.

The requirements for these two applications are somewhat different. In the first case, the index must produce a carefully-structured and well-defined single-valued measure of wellbeing that can be publically monitored and easily compared with the GDP. In the second case, a single-valued index is less suitable because the details of how a given policy initiative affects the citizenry is often lost in the aggregation process within the multi-dimensional calculations. Most policies are directed at issues that arise within a single dimension of wellbeing, so it is much more likely that individual indicators from that dimension will reveal the impact of a policy more clearly than can be gleaned from an aggregated score. Indexes that produce a dashboard of results that allow legislators to see the impact of their policies in a more nuanced fashion probably have greater value in assessing citizen response to policy change. If an index is to be used on both policy fronts, it ought to include both single-valued output and a dashboard of results at the scale of individual dimensions.

Some of the indexes introduced in the earlier chapters, like the one reported in the World Happiness Report, rely solely on subjective input gleaned from polls of the citizenry. Others, like the UN Human Development Index, depend only on objective data mined from government-sponsored, publically-available databases. Still others integrate data from both sources. In the policy domain, a strong argument can be made for using an index that includes both aspects, so that the impact of a given policy can be judged both in terms of the perceptive judgement of the citizenry and the monitoring of objective outcomes.

Perhaps the biggest perceived drawback to single-valued indexes of happiness in the policy context is their apparent temporal insensitivity. Happiness scales generally

Table 12.2 Suitability of multi-dimensional indexes of wellbeing as a measure of the effectiveness of policy

	Data		Output		
Index	Subj.	Obj.	Single no	Dashboard	Capped
UN Human Development Index (HDI)	No	Yes	Yes	No	Yes [0–1]
UN Inequality-Adjusted Human Development Index (IHDI)	No	Yes	Yes	No	Yes [0–1]
World Happiness Report (WHR)	Yes	No	Yes	Yes	Yes [0–10]
Happy Life Years (HLY)	Yes	Yes	Yes	No	Yes [0–100]
Inequality-Adjusted Happiness of Nations (IAH)	Yes	Yes	Yes	No	Yes [0–100]
Genuine Progress Indicator (GPI)	No	Yes	Yes	No	No
Canadian Index of Wellbeing (CIW)	Yes	Yes	Yes	Yes	No
Weighted Index of Social Progress (WISP)	No	Yes	Yes	No	No
Bhutan Gross National Happiness Index (GNH-B)	Yes	No	Yes	Yes	Yes [0–1]
OECD Better Life Index (BLI)	Yes	Yes	Yes	No	Yes [0–1]
Legatum Prosperity Index (LPI)	Yes	Yes	Yes	No	Yes [0–100]
Global Livability Index (GLI)	Yes	Yes	Yes	No	Yes [0–100]

do not show much short-term sensitivity to societal changes that ought to impact them. They do exhibit long-term trends, but not the day-to-day volatility that would make them more interesting to journalists and the general public. One of the reasons for this bland response is that many of these composite indexes are capped. If indexes are designed to produce a single-valued result within some specified range, then the upper limit of this range becomes a pre-determined cap. Take the Prosperity Index as an example. Its single-valued measure for a given jurisdiction must lie in the range 0–100. If happiness levels are already in the higher end of this range, they have nowhere further to go. Any curve of improvement is bound to flatten out, and annual percentage increases are bound to become muted. Indexes that do not have an upper cap are much more likely to show clear and measurable responses to government policy and legislation. Uncapped indexes are more likely to be directly comparable to the GDP and the Dow-Jones, both of which are themselves uncapped.

Table 12.2 summarizes the suitability of 12 multi-dimensional indexes of wellbeing from the points of view presented above. The first 11 are from Chap. 9, at national scale. The Global Livability index is the only representative from Chap. 10, at urban scale. The only index to display Yeses in the first four columns (indicating the use of both subjective and objective data, and the production of both single-valued and dashboard output), and a No in the fifth column (indicating that the single-valued output is not capped), is the Canadian Index of Wellbeing. If this analysis is valid, then those in the social indicators movement should look to the CIW as a model index for use in the policy domain. Neither the UN Human Development Index nor the Genuine Progress Indicator, which are the two indexes most highly touted in social indicator circles, have the optimum set of properties for use in the policy domain.

A study of the suitability of composite indexes in the policy domain was carried out in 2001 by a committee of the leading lights in the social indicators movement including Alex Michalos and Joseph Sirgy (previously referenced in Chap. 9). They had hoped to reach agreement on a set of evaluation criteria and a selection of the most-promising index to assess overall quality of life. However they were not able to reach agreement on either count. They found shortcomings in all of the 22 national-scale quality-of-life indexes that they examined. From a policy perspective, they noted that none of the indexes distinguish between the concepts of "input, through-put and output" that are used by public policy analysts, nor do they clearly show how the quality-of-life outputs of such indexes can be used as public policy inputs [36].

Where, What, How, and Why Not?

So, one is left with several questions. Where have wellbeing indexes been used to inform policy? What has been the nature of that use? How well has it worked? And to the degree that the answers to these first three questions are positive, why hasn't the usage been wider and more influential?

If one starts at the national level, it is clear that indexes of wellbeing have not found their way into the heart and soul of the policy-making cycle in very many countries. In fact, the only national government that has embraced happiness as the driver of legislation is Bhutan, where the concept of gross national happiness was born. The governments of many other countries have set up advisory boards to look into the matter, like the Sarkozy Commission in France, and the Commission on Key National Indicators in the United States, both of which were discussed in an earlier chapter, but neither of which have led to important structural changes in the machinery of national policy-making.

However it is not true that nothing has been done. Almost all countries have statistical archives like those at the US Bureau of the Census, Statistics Canada, and the UK Office of National Statistics, where datasets that often prove of interest to legislators are housed. Among those specific to the wellbeing community are Italy's Equitable and Sustainable Well-Being Measures, Israel's Sustainability and National Resilience Indicators, the Welsh Sustainable Indicator Set, the How's Austria program, and Finland's Findicator. Many countries have also created agencies or programs like the Buen Vivir Secretariat in Ecuador, the What Works Centre for Wellbeing in the UK, New Zealand's Living Standards Framework, Scotland's National Performance Framework, and the Happiness Policy Directorate of the

United Arab Emirates, and the results of studies carried out by such agencies are available to legislators in their policy deliberations. In other countries, non-governmental agencies have set up national indexes like the Canada Wellbeing Index, the Australian Unity Wellbeing Index, and the German National Welfare Index. Governments are aware of these efforts and make reference to their findings where it is seen to be to their advantage [37].

One might well ask why national governments have been so slow to incorporate the findings of more-broadly-based indexes into their legislative deliberations, especially in view of the prodding from the United Nations and other international agencies. Part of the answer, at least for developed countries, may come in the very fact that the prodding tends to come from internationalists, and that its purpose seems to be largely to point out the needs in the underdeveloped parts of the world. National governments are elected by their citizenry, and the concerns of the citizenry of most developed countries run strongly to domestic matters over international ones. It is politics, pure and simple. Governments want to be re-elected, and they recognize the primacy of domestic issues.

As a second reason, one can look to the social indicators movement itself. Proponents of more-broadly-based indexes have always assumed that the quantitative information they provide would automatically lead people to demand action. Data were expected to mobilize public opinion without further advocacy, and lead to appropriate reforms. The failure on the part of quality-of-life advocates to link knowledge to action has been partially responsible for the muted response from national governments.

Thirdly, there is the apparent necessity to raise taxes to fund the social welfare programs indicated by happiness studies. There is probably no idea more difficult to sell to the voters than the necessity to raise taxes. Few governments are willing to make the hard decisions and risk the backlash. As for the electorate, their desires are clear, if somewhat irrational; they want more services and lower taxes.

In 2014, the London-based New Economics Foundation sponsored the BRAINPOOL project (the acronym standing rather awkwardly for "Bringing Alternative Indicators into Policy"). They identified several "barriers" to the "Beyond GDP" movement, including a failure to connect with public priorities, the lack of a clear political imperative for change, the ongoing belief among the public that economic growth is the path toward shared prosperity, institutional resistance, confusion on the part of potential supporters over the merits of the many competing indexes and indicator sets, and the inability of the movement to come up with a single metric that has comparable salience to the GDP [38].

If one turns from the national to the municipal level, one finds that the use of social indicator data in policy-making has been much more widespread. The issue-by-issue, neighborhood-by-neighborhood collection and presentation of data described in Chap. 10 as part of the community indicators movement has proved ideal as a bridge between citizens and elected city legislators, and has played an important role in the design, implementation, and assessment of civic policy. Laura Musikanski, the Executive Director of the Seattle-based Happiness Alliance, is the lead author of *The Happiness Policy Handbook* which includes a Happy Community Toolkit to help municipal councils navigate the political shoals [39].

Welfare Spending and Happiness

Clearly, the findings of happiness and wellbeing studies point toward greater government activity on many fronts (mental health, environmental protection, and civic infrastructure, to name just a few), and this added activity implies increased public spending on these social welfare issues. Most of the developed nations of the world have indeed increased their levels of social expenditures over the past few decades. It seems almost axiomatic that these increases in welfare spending must have increased the levels of life satisfaction in the populace. The results of two studies carried out in the early years of the new millennium must therefore give pause to proponents of the social indicators movement. Both of them fail to find a significant correlation between welfare spending and life satisfaction.

The first one, published by the Danish economist, Christian Bjornskov, could possibly be viewed as coming from a hostile source. Bjornskov is a proponent of an economic philosophy known as public choice theory which is popular in conservative circles. It holds that governments often overstep their bounds with excessive regulations that have a detrimental effect on the quality of life of individual citizens. In the issue at hand, he was the lead author of a 2007 study that examined the correlation between the size of government and the level of life satisfaction in 74 countries. The study concluded that government social spending in a country, taken as the percent share of its GDP, has no impact on average life satisfaction, as determined by country-wide aggregation of data from the World Values Survey [40].

The second study came from Ruut Veenhoven, a decidedly non-hostile source at the very core of the social indicators movement. His 2000 study also failed to find any positive correlation between the level of welfare spending in a country and the overall happiness of its citizenry [41]. He is left to ponder: "Can these findings be true?"

A more recent study by two Norwegian economists in 2019 may offer some solace. They carried out a similar search for correlations between spending and wellbeing using data from OECD countries over the period 1980–2012. However, they looked at the data in more detail than Bjornskov or Veenhoven, teasing out the relationships, not just in an overall sense, but on an issue-by-issue basis. They confirmed the lack of correlation on the overall data, but found significant positive correlations for spending in some areas such as health care and poverty, and significant negative correlations in other areas such as labor policy [42]. Their findings add further encouragement to policy-makers to use wellbeing indexes that can provide a dashboard-style analysis rather than just a single-value result.

Of course, greater welfare spending usually comes with a higher tax burden, so another way to look at the issue at hand is to look for correlations between tax burden and subjective wellbeing (SWB) on a country by country basis. This exercise appears to give clearer results, at least for the developed countries. Using the USA, Canada, and Finland as representative, one finds the tax burden as a percentage of GDP at 25.5%, 33.5%, and 44.2% respectively. The average SWB scores reported for these three countries in the World Happiness Report are 6.88, 7.18, and 7.86 (out of 10). The difference of one full unit between the USA and Finland is very significant. Part of the difference can certainly be ascribed to the percentage of people living in poverty in the three countries: 17.3% in the USA, 10.3% in Canada, and 6.4% in Finland [43]. By this metric, citizens of countries that are more highly taxed, with correspondingly greater levels of social services, are happier than those who live in countries with lower tax burdens. Furthermore, the more progressive the tax system (that is, the greater the difference between tax rates for upper-income earners relative to those for lower-income earners) the more pronounced are the conclusions presented here [44].

The Future

No one can predict the future, but that doesn't stop people from trying, and that includes the psychologists, economists, environmentalists, and health scientists that make up the happiness and wellbeing movement. Like all soothsayers, some of their predictions are positive, some are negative, and some of them speak to the tradeoffs that characterize life on a finite planet.

On the positive side, futurists see the trends continuing toward longer life expectancy, increased literacy and numeracy, greater gender equality, more plentiful food supplies, lower incidence of childhood diseases, less smoking, more holidays, and earlier retirement [45].

On the negative side, fears of future wars and terrorism remain unabated, as do continued concerns over extreme versions of populism, the rise of authoritarian governments, and civil unrest [46]. The issues of poverty and inequality never seem to be laid to rest. On the environmental front, action seems woefully muted on global warming, ecosystem loss, and air and water pollution. Future trends seem to indicate increasing climate change and continued environmental degradation [47]. One negative prediction commonly touted in health circles is a fear of the spread of infectious diseases and this has already come to pass with the arrival of the worldwide Covid-19 health pandemic.

Some predictions are a two edged sword. There is likely to be increasing diversity in most communities with respect to race, religion, ethnicity, and sexual orientation, but it is still unclear whether this will lead to greater communal happiness, as liberals hope, or to greater community intolerance and violence. Most futurists predict increasing urbanization, but it is still not clear whether the pleasures of the "happy city" will outweigh the problems of urban poverty and congestion. The cyber revolution brings rapid access to information and more-or-less instant global communication, but also concerns over cyber dependency, cyber attack, and loss of privacy.

In the eyes of the quality-of-life movement, all the advantage that can be captured from the positive trends, and all the steps that can be taken to lessen the impact of the negative trends, would be enhanced by the increased use of social indicators and multi-dimensional indexes of wellbeing. In their view, it is imperative that legislators and decision-makers go "beyond GDP" to harvest the wealth of social data that is available, and use it to maximize the happiness, wellbeing, and quality-of-life of us all.

Given the strengths and weaknesses of both economic and social indicators, most researchers into happiness and wellbeing recommend that policy decisions be informed by both types of indicators. Social indicators are not meant to replace economic ones, but rather to complement them. If existing economic measures of prosperity are complemented with wellbeing metrics that better capture the changes in quality of life of the citizenry, decision makers will be better informed to assess and design policy. Almost all the multi-dimensional indexes presented in Chaps. 9 and 10 for use by national, state, or municipal governments, have both economic and social components.

There is also the question of "needs" and "wants." In less-developed countries where the fulfillment of basic needs is the main issue, economic indicators may be more important than social indicators. As societies grow wealthier, differences in wellbeing are less often influenced by income, and more frequently by factors such as social relationships, satisfaction at work, and environmental stewardship.

In the past decade there have been many international conferences on wellbeing and public policy sponsored by many different agencies including the UN, OECD, the International Society for Quality of Life Studies, and the International Journal of Wellbeing. The latest thinking is presented in the proceedings of these conferences which are usually available as open-access documents on the Internet. The desire for change is there, the time is ripe, and the future awaits.

References

1. Clark, A.E. et. al., The key determinants of happiness and misery, *World Happiness Report*, Chapter 5, 2017.
2. Diener, E. and M.E.P Seligman, Beyond money: Toward an economy of well-being, *Psychological Science in the Public Interest*, 5(1), 3-31, 2004; Adler, A. and M.E.P. Seligman, Using wellbeing for public policy: Theory, measurements, and recommendations, *International Journal of Wellbeing*, 6(1), 1-35, 2016.
3. Layard, R., *Happiness: Lessons from a New Science*, Penguin, 2005.
4. Marks, N., *The Happiness Manifesto: How Nations and People Can Nurture Wellbeing*, TED Books, 2011.
5. Adler, A. and M.E.P. Seligman, 2016, op.cit.
6. Forgeard, M.J.C. et.al., Doing the right thing: Measuring wellbeing for public policy, *International Journal of Wellbeing*, 1(1), 79-106, 2011.
7. Weijers, D. and A. Jarden, The science of happiness for policymakers: An overview, *Journal of Social Research and Policy*, 4(2), 21-40, 2013.

8. The quote is ascribed to Gus O'Donnell, a British economist and former Cabinet Secretary in the UK government, by Stone, A.A. and C. Mackie, eds, *Subjective Well-Being: Measuring Happiness, Suffering, and Other Dimensions of Experience*, National Research Council Panel on Measuring Subjective Well-Being in a Policy Relevant Framework, National Academies Press, 2013.
9. This chapter was informed by many books and articles on happiness and policy, including the following: Diener, E. et. al., *Wellbeing for Public Policy*, Oxford University Press, 2009; Bok, D., *The Politics of Happiness: What Government Can Learn from the New Research in WellBeing*, Princeton University Press, 2010; Boniwell, I. et. al., eds, *Oxford Handbook of Happiness*, 2013; Adler and Seligman, 2016, op. cit.; Angner, E., The politics of happiness: Subjective vs economic measures as measures of social well-being, in Bortolotti, L., ed., *Philosophy and Happiness*, 149-166, Palgrave Macmillan, 2009; De Prycker, V., Happiness on the political agenda: Pros and cons, *Jour. Happiness Studies*, 11(5), 585-603, 2010; Diener and Seligman, 2004, op. cit.; Forgeard, et. al., 2011, op. cit.; Noll, H-H., ed, Subjective social indicators: Benefits and limitations for policy-making, *Social Indicators Research*, Special Issue, 114(1), 2013; Stone and Mackie, 2013, op. cit.
10. Johns, H. and P. Ormerod, *Happiness, Economics and Public Policy*, Institute of Economic Affairs, Research Monograph 62, 60 pp., 2007. See also: Jenkins, M., Reasons to be cautious about well-being in economic development, *Intl. Jour. of Happiness and Development*, 3(2), 108-124, 2016.
11. Diego-Rosell, P., R.Tortora and J.Bird, International determinants of subjective well-being: Living in a subjectively material world, *Journal Happiness Studies*, 19, 123-143, 2018.
12. Ott, J.C., Government and happiness in 130 nations: Good governance fosters higher level and more equality of happiness, *Social Indicators Research*, 102(1), 3-22, 2011.
13. Bacon, N. et. al., *The State of Happiness: Can Public Policy Shape People's Well-Being and Resilience?*, Young Foundation, 2010.
14. Veenhoven, R., Greater happiness for a greater number: Is that possible or desirable? *Journal of Happiness Studies*, 11, 605-629, 2010; Veenhoven, R., What we have learnt about happiness, Classic qualms in the light of recent research, in *A Life Dedicated to Quality of Life*, Social Indicators Research Book Series, vol. 60, 151-170, 2015.
15. Cobb, C.W., *Measurement Tools and the Quality of Life*, Redefining Progress, 2000.
16. Radcliff, B., *The Political Economy of Human Happiness: How Voters Choices Determine the Quality of Life,* Cambridge University Press, 2013
17. Johns and Ormerod, 2007, op. cit.
18. Adler and Seligman, 2016, op. cit.; De Prycker, 2010, op. cit.; Diener et al, 2009, op.cit.
19. Diener and Seligman, 2004, op. cit.
20. Thurow, L., *The Zero-Sum Society: Distribution and the Possibilities for Economic Change*, Basic Books, 1980.
21. Angner, 2009, op. cit.: Duncan, G., Should happiness maximization be the goal of government?, *Journal Happiness Studies*, 11(2), 163-178, 2010
22. Boelhouwer, J. and C. van Campen, Steering toward happiness in the Netherlands, *Social Indicators Research*, 114 (1), 59-72, 2013.
23. Piketty, T., *Capital in the Twenty-first Century*, Harvard University Press, 2013; Keeley, B., *Income Inequality: The Gap Between Rich and Poor*, OECD, 2015; Graham, C., *Happiness for All: Unequal Hopes and Lives in Pursuit of the American Dream*, Princeton University Press, 2017; Graafland, J. and B. Louis,, Economic freedom, income inequality, and life satisfaction in OECD countries, *Journal Happiness Studies*, 19, 2071-2093, 2018.
24. Josa, I. and A. Aguado, Measuring unidimensional equality: Practical framework for the choice of an appropriate measure, *Social Indicators Research*, 149, 541-570, 2020.
25. Bok, D., 2010, op. cit.
26. Layard, R. and G. O'Donnell, How to make policy when happiness is the goal, Chapter 4, *World Happiness Report*, 2015.

27. Durand, M., Countries' experiences with well-being and happiness metrics, Chapter 8, *Global Happiness Policy Report*, 2018; Durand, M. and C. Exton, Adopting a well-being approach in central government: Policy mechanisms and practical tools, Chapter 8, *Global Happiness and Well-being Policy Report*, 2019. See also Noll, 2013, op.cit.
28. Ward, G., Happiness and voting behavior, Chapter 3, *World Happiness Report*, 2019. See also: Seaford, C., The multiple uses of subjective well-being indicators, *Social Indicators Research*, 114(1), 29-43, 2013.
29. Cobb, 2000, op. cit.
30. Ward, 2019, op. cit.
31. This section was informed by discussions in: Diener et al, 2009, op.cit.; Bacon et al, 2010, op cit; Stone and Mackie, 2013, op cit.; Clarke et al, op cit; Helliwell, J. et al, Some policy implications, Chapter 4, *World Happiness Report*, 2012; O'Donnell, G., Using well-being as a guide to policy, Chapter 6, *World Happiness Report*, 2013; Layard, R., Big ideas: Wellbeing and public policy, *Centrepiece: The Magazine for Economic Performance*, London School of Economics, Winter, 2011.
32. Helliwell et al, 2012, op.cit.
33. Layard, 2011, op. cit.
34. [barcelonagse.eu/research/world-wellbeing-panel]
35. Bok, D. , 2010, op. cit.
36. Hagerty, M.R., et. al., Quality-of-Life indexes for national policy: Review and agenda for research, *Social Indicators Research*, 55(1), 1-96, 2001; See also: Bleys, B., Beyond GDP: Classifying alternative measures for progress, *Social Indicators Research*, 109(3), 355-376, 2012.
37. Durand, 2018, op. cit.
38. [neweconomics.org/2014/04/the-brainpool-project]
39. Musikanski, L., R. Phillips and J. Crowder, *The Happiness Policy Handbook*, New Society Publ., 2019.
40. Bjornskov, C., et. al., The bigger the better? Evidence of the effect of government size on life satisfaction around the world, *Public Choice*, 130, 267-292, 2007.
41. Veenhoven, R., Well-being in the welfare state: Level not higher, distribution not more equitable, *Journal of Comparative Policy Analysis*, 2, 91-125, 2000.
42. Nordheim, O. and P.E. Martinussen, Happiness and the role of social protection: How types of social spending affected individual's life satisfaction in OECD countries, 1980-2012, *Journal of International and Comparative Social Policy*, available online, 2019.
43. [ourworldindata.org/happiness-and-life-satisfaction]
44. Oishi, S., U. Schimmack and E. Diener, Progressive taxation and the subjective wellbeing of nations, *Psychological Science*, 23(1), 86-92, 2012.
45. Moore, S. and J.L. Simon, *Its Getting Better All the Time: 100 Greatest Trends of the Last 100 Years*, Cato Institute, 2000.
46. See for example: Norris, P. and R. Inglehart, *Cultural Backlash: Trump, Brexit, and Authoritarian Populism*, Cambridge University Press, 2019; Dean, J. and R. Altemeyer, *Authoritarian Nightmare: Trump and his Followers*, Melville House, 2020.
47. [www.weforum.org/global-risks-report-2020]

